Functional and Molecular Imaging in Oncology

Editor

ANTONIO LUNA

MAGNETIC RESONANCE IMAGING CLINICS OF NORTH AMERICA

www.mri.theclinics.com

Consulting Editors
SURESH K. MUKHERJI
LYNNE S. STEINBACH

February 2016 • Volume 24 • Number 1

ELSEVIER

1600 John F. Kennedy Boulevard • Suite 1800 • Philadelphia, Pennsylvania, 19103-2899

http://www.mri.theclinics.com

MRI CLINICS OF NORTH AMERICA Volume 24, Number 1
February 2016 ISSN 1064-9689, ISBN 13: 978-0-323-41698-6

Editor: John Vassallo (j.vassallo@elsevier.com)
Developmental Editor: Meredith Clinton

Magnetic Resonance Imaging Clinics of North America (ISSN 1064-9689) is published quarterly by Elsevier Inc., 360 Park Avenue South, New York, NY 10010-1710. Months of issue are February, May, August, and November. Business and Editorial Offices: 1600 John F. Kennedy Blvd., Ste. 1800, Philadelphia, PA 19103-2899. Customer Service Office: 3251 Riverport Lane, Maryland Heights, MO 63043. Periodicals postage paid at New York, NY and additional mailing offices. Subscription prices are $380.00 per year (domestic individuals), $636.00 per year (domestic institutions), $100.00 per year (domestic students/residents), $420.00 per year (Canadian individuals), $828.00 per year (Canadian institutions), $545.00 per year (international individuals), $828.00 per year (international institutions), and $275.00 per year (international and Canadian students/residents). International air speed delivery is included in all *Clinics* subscription prices. All prices are subject to change without notice. **POSTMASTER:** Send address changes to *Magnetic Resonance Imaging Clinics*, Elsevier Health Sciences Division, Subscription Customer Service, 3251 Riverport Lane, Maryland Heights, MO 63043. Customer Service (orders, claims, online, change of address): Elsevier Health Sciences Division, Subscription **Customer Service, 3251 Riverport Lane, Maryland Heights, MO 63043. Tel:1-800-654-2452 (U.S. and Canada); 314-447-8871 (outside U.S. and Canada). Fax: 314-447-8029. E-mail: journalscustomer service-usa@elsevier.com (for print support); journalsonlinesupport-usa@elsevier.com (for online support).**

Reprints. For copies of 100 or more of articles in this publication, please contact the Commercial Reprints Department, Elsevier Inc., 360 Park Avenue South, New York, NY 10010-1710. Tel.: 212-633-3874; Fax: 212-633-3820; E-mail: reprints@elsevier.com.

Magnetic Resonance Imaging Clinics of North America is covered in the *RSNA Index of Imaging Literature*, *MEDLINE/PubMed (Index Medicus)*, and *EMBASE/Excerpta Medica*.

Contributors

CONSULTING EDITORS

SURESH K. MUKHERJI, MD, MBA, FACR
Professor and Chairman; W.F. Patenge
Endowed Chair, Department of Radiology,
Michigan State University, East Lansing,
Michigan

LYNNE S. STEINBACH, MD, FACR
Professor of Radiology and Orthopaedic
Surgery, Department of Radiology and
Biomedical Imaging, University of California
San Francisco, San Francisco, California

EDITOR

ANTONIO LUNA, MD
Chairman of Radiology, Health Time, Clinica
Las Nieves, Jaén, Spain; Assistant Professor of
Radiology, University Hospitals of Cleveland,
Case Western Reserve University, Cleveland,
Ohio

AUTHORS

RICHARD G. ABRAMSON, MD
Department of Radiology and Radiological
Sciences, Institute of Imaging Science,
Vanderbilt University, Nashville, Tennessee

LIDIA ALCALÁ-MATA, MD
Chief of Abdominal Imaging, Health Time,
Jaen, Spain

ANTONIO ALVAREZ-KINDELAN, MD, PhD
Thoracic Surgery Department, Hospital
Universitario Reina Sofía, Córdoba, Spain

LORI R. ARLINGHAUS, PhD
Department of Radiology and Radiological
Sciences, Vanderbilt University, Nashville,
Tennessee

SANDRA BALEATO-GONZÁLEZ, MD, PhD
Department of Radiology, Complexo
Hospitalario de Santiago de Compostela
(CHUS), Santiago de Compostela, Spain

MATTHIAS R. BENZ, MD
Department of Radiology, Memorial Sloan
Kettering Cancer Center, New York,
New York; Clinic of Radiology and Nuclear
Medicine, University of Basel Hospital, Basel,
Switzerland

SANJEEV BHALLA, MD
Mallinckrodt Institute of Radiology,
Washington University School of Medicine,
St Louis, Missouri

LEONARDO KAYAT BITTENCOURT, PhD
Associate Professor of Radiology,
Universidade Federal Fluminense, Niterói;
CDPI and Multi-Imagem Clinics, Rio de
Janeiro, Brazil

MATTHEW BLACKLEDGE, PhD
NIHR Post-doctorate Fellow, Institute of
Cancer Research, Sutton, United Kingdom

CLAUDIO BONINI, MD
Oroño Medical Diagnostic Center, Rosario,
Argentina

JORDI BRONCANO, MD
Cardiothoracic Department, Hospital de la
Cruz Roja, RESSALTA, Health-Time Group,
Córdoba, Spain

JAVIER CARRASCOSO-ARRANZ, MD
Department of Diagnostic Imaging,
Hospital Universitario Quirón, Madrid,
Spain

EDUARD Y. CHEKMENEV, PhD
Departments of Radiology and Radiological Sciences, Biomedical Engineering and Biochemistry, Institute of Imaging Science, Vanderbilt University, Nashville, Tennessee

DAVID J. COLLINS, BA (Hons), CPhys, MinstP
Principal Clinical Scientist, Institute of Cancer Research, Sutton, United Kingdom

DANIEL COSTA, MD
Assistant Professor of Radiology, University of Texas Southwestern Medical Center, Dallas, Texas

NANDITA M. DESOUZA, MD, FRCR, FRCP
Professor of Translational Imaging, The Institute of Cancer Research, Honorary Consultant, The Royal Marsden Hospital, London, United Kingdom

ALBERTO DIAZ DE LEON, MD
Fellow, Department of Radiology, University of Texas Southwestern Medical Center, Dallas, Texas

ADRIENNE N. DULA, PhD
Department of Radiology and Radiological Sciences, Institute of Imaging Science, Vanderbilt University, Nashville, Tennessee

SUSAN FREEMAN, FRCR
Department of Radiology, Consultant Radiologist, Cambridge University Hospitals NHS Foundation Trust, Cambridge, United Kingdom

ROBERTO GARCÍA-FIGUEIRAS, MD, PhD
Department of Radiology, Hospital Clínico Universitario de Santiago de Compostela, Santiago de Compostela, Spain

VIKAS GULANI, MD, PhD
Departments of Radiology, Urology and Biomedical Engineering, Case Comprehensive Cancer Center, University Hospitals of Cleveland, Case Western Reserve University, Cleveland, Ohio

L. CELSO HYGINO DA CRUZ Jr, MD, PhD
Magnetic Resonance Department of Clínica de Diagnóstico por Imagem (CDPI), IRM Ressonância Magnética, Rio de Janeiro, Brazil

JACOBUS F.A. JANSEN, PhD
Assistant Professor, Department of Radiology, Maastricht University Medical Center, Maastricht, The Netherlands

MARGARETH KIMURA, MD
Avenida Raymundo Magalhaes Junior, Magnetic Resonance Department of Clínica de Diagnóstico por Imagem (CDPI), Centro Médico Barrashopping, Rio de Janeiro, Brazil

DOW-MU KOH, MD, MRCP, FRCR
Professor of Functional Imaging in Cancer, Department of Radiology, Royal Marsden Hospital, Sutton, United Kingdom

JEONG-MIN LEE, MD
Sectional Chief of Abdominal Radiology and Non-vascular Intervention, Department of Radiology, Seoul National University Hospital, Sutton, United Kingdom

YONGGANG LU, PhD
Department of Radiation Oncology, University of Washington, St Louis, Missouri

ANTONIO LUNA, MD
Chairman of Radiology, Health Time Group, Clinica Las Nieves, Jaén, Spain; Assistant Professor of Radiology, University Hospitals of Cleveland, Case Western Reserve University, Cleveland, Ohio

TEODORO MARTÍN NOGUEROL, MD
Neuroradiology Section, Health – Time Group, Jaén, Spain

JOSÉ PABLO MARTÍNEZ BARBERO, MD
Neuroradiology Section, Health – Time Group, Jaén, Spain

JAMES P.B. O'CONNOR, PhD, FRCR
Cancer Research UK and EPSRC Cancer Imaging Centre, University of Manchester, Manchester, United Kingdom

ANWAR R. PADHANI, MBBS, FRCP, FRCR
Paul Strickland Scanner Centre, Mount Vernon Cancer Centre, Middlesex, United Kingdom

SHIVANI PAHWA, MD
Department of Radiology, University Hospitals of Cleveland, Case Western Reserve University, Cleveland, Ohio

CARLOS PARRA, PhD
Department of Medical Physics, Memorial Sloan Kettering Cancer Center, New York, New York

SAVANNAH C. PARTRIDGE, PhD
Research Associate Professor, Breast Imaging Section, Department of Radiology, Seattle Cancer Care Alliance, University of Washington, Seattle, Washington

IVAN PEDROSA, MD
Chief of MRI; Holder of the Jack Reynolds MD. Chair in Radiology; Associate Professor of Radiology and Advanced Imaging Research Center, Department of Radiology, University of Texas Southwestern Medical Center, Dallas, Texas

C. CHAD QUARLES, PhD
Departments of Radiology and Radiological Sciences, Biomedical Engineering and Cancer Biology, Institute of Imaging Science, Vanderbilt University, Nashville, Tennessee

HABIB RAHBAR, MD
Assistant Professor, Breast Imaging Section, Department of Radiology, Seattle Cancer Care Alliance, University of Washington, Seattle, Washington

ANDREA ROCKALL, MRCP, FRCR
Department of Radiology, Hammersmith Hospital, Consultant Radiologist, Imperial College Healthcare NHS Trust; Visiting Professor, Imperial College, London, United Kingdom

MARIA JOSÉ ROMERO, MD
Musculoskeletal Imaging, DADISA, Health Time, Zona Franca, Avenida Consejo de Europa, Cadiz, Spain

JAVIER SÁNCHEZ-GONZÁLEZ, PhD
Clinical Scientist, Philips Healthcare Iberia, Madrid, Spain

EVIS SALA, MD, PhD
Department of Radiology, Memorial Sloan Kettering Cancer Center, New York, New York

AHMED SALEM, MB ChB, FRCR
Cancer Research UK and EPSRC Cancer Imaging Centre, University of Manchester, Manchester, United Kingdom

AMITA SHUKLA-DAVE, PhD
Director Quantitative Imaging; Associate Attending Physicist, Departments of Medical Physics and Radiology, Memorial Sloan Kettering Cancer Center, New York, New York

ASHLEY M. STOKES, PhD
Department of Radiology and Radiological Sciences, Institute of Imaging Science, Vanderbilt University, Nashville, Tennessee

HEBERT ALBERTO VARGAS, MD
Department of Radiology, Memorial Sloan Kettering Cancer Center, New York, New York

JOAN C. VILANOVA, MD, PhD
Chief, Department of Radiology, Clínica Girona, IDI, Catalan Health Institute, University of Girona, Girona, Spain

JARED A. WEIS, PhD
Department of Biomedical Engineering, Vanderbilt University, Nashville, Tennessee

JENNIFER G. WHISENANT, PhD
Department of Radiology and Radiological Sciences, Institute of Imaging Science, Vanderbilt University, Nashville, Tennessee

JASON M. WILLIAMS, PhD
Institute of Imaging Science, Vanderbilt University, Nashville, Tennessee

KATHERINE L. WRIGHT, PhD
Department of Radiology, University Hospitals of Cleveland, Case Western Reserve University, Cleveland, Ohio

THOMAS E. YANKEELOV, PhD
Departments of Radiology and Radiological Sciences, Biomedical Engineering, Cancer Biology and Physics, Institute of Imaging Science, Vanderbilt University, Nashville, Tennessee

IGOR ZHUKOV, PhD
National Research Nuclear University MEPhI, Moscow, Russia

Contents

DCE-MR imaging applications are largely centered on lesion detection, characterization, and localization. In research, DCE-MR imaging helps inform decision making in early-phase clinical trials by showing efficacy and by selecting dose and schedule. However, the role of these techniques in patient selection is uncertain. Future research is required to optimize existing DCE-MR imaging methods and to fully validate these biomarkers for wider use in patient care and in drug development.

Magnetic resonance spectroscopy (MRS) is a noninvasive functional technique to evaluate the biochemical behavior of human tissues. This property has been widely used in assessment and therapy monitoring of brain tumors. MRS studies can be implemented outside the brain with successful and promising results in the evaluation of prostate and breast cancer, but still with limited reproducibility. As a result of technical improvements, malignancies of the musculoskeletal system and abdominopelvic organs can benefit from the molecular information that MRS provides. The technical challenges and main applications in oncology of ^{1}H MRS in a clinical setting are the focus of this review.

Functional MR imaging methods make possible the quantification of dynamic physiologic processes that occur in the brain. Moreover, the use of these advanced imaging techniques in the setting of oncologic treatment of the brain is widely accepted and has found worldwide routine clinical use.

Head and neck cancer is one of the most common cancers worldwide. MR imaging–based diffusion and perfusion techniques enable the noninvasive assessment of tumor biology and physiology, which supplement information obtained from standard structural scans. Diffusion and perfusion MR imaging techniques provide novel biomarkers that can aid monitoring in pretreatment, during treatment, and posttreatment stages to improve patient selection for therapeutic strategies, provide evidence for change of therapy regime, and evaluate treatment response. This review discusses pertinent aspects of the role of diffusion and perfusion MR imaging, and computational analysis methods in studying head and neck cancer.

With recent advances in MR imaging, its application in the thorax has been feasible. The performance of both morphologic and functional techniques in the evaluation of thoracic malignances has improved not only differentiation from benign etiologies, but also treatment monitoring based on a multiparametric approach. Several MR imaging–derived parameters have been described as potential biomarkers linked with prognosis and survival. Therefore, an integral approach with a nonradiating and noninvasive technique could be an optimal alternative for evaluating those patients.

Multiparametric MR Imaging in Abdominal Malignancies

Antonio Luna, Shivani Pahwa, Claudio Bonini, Lidia Alcalá-Mata, Katherine L. Wright, and Vikas Gulani

Modern MR imaging protocols can yield both anatomic and functional information for the assessment of hepatobiliary and pancreatic malignancies. Diffusion-weighted imaging is fully integrated into state-of-the-art protocols for tumor detection, characterization, and therapy monitoring. Hepatobiliary contrast agents have gained ground in the evaluation of focal liver lesions during the last years. Perfusion MR imaging is expected to have a central role for monitoring therapy in body tumors treated with antivascular drugs. Approaches such as magnetic resonance (MR) elastography and ^{1}H-MR spectroscopy are still confined to research centers, but with the potential to grow in a short time frame.

Role of Multiparametric MR Imaging in Malignancies of the Urogenital Tract

Alberto Diaz de Leon, Daniel Costa, and Ivan Pedrosa

Multiparametric MR imaging (mpMRI) combine different sequences that, when properly tailored, can provide qualitative and quantitative information about the tumor microenvironment beyond traditional tumor size measures and/or morphologic assessments. This article focuses on mpMRI in the evaluation of urogenital tract malignancies by first reviewing technical aspects and then discussing its potential clinical role. This includes insight into histologic subtyping and grading of renal cell carcinoma and assessment of tumor response to targeted therapies. The clinical utility of mpMRI in the staging and grading of ureteral and bladder tumors is presented. Finally, the evolving role of mpMRI in prostate cancer is discussed.

Functional MR Imaging in Gynecologic Cancer

Nandita M. deSouza, Andrea Rockall, and Susan Freeman

Dynamic-contrast enhanced (DCE) and diffusion-weighted (DW) MR imaging are invaluable in the detection, staging, and characterization of uterine and ovarian malignancies, for monitoring treatment response, and for identifying disease recurrence. When used as adjuncts to morphologic T2-weighted (T2-W) MR imaging, these techniques improve accuracy of disease detection and staging. DW-MR imaging is preferred because of its ease of implementation and lack of need for an extrinsic contrast agent. MR spectroscopy is difficult to implement in the clinical workflow and lacks both sensitivity and specificity. If used quantitatively in multi-center clinical trials, standardization of DCE- and DW-MR imaging techniques and rigorous quality assurance is mandatory.

Multiparametric MR Imaging of Breast Cancer

Habib Rahbar and Savannah C. Partridge

Breast MR imaging has increased in popularity over the past 2 decades due to evidence of its high sensitivity for cancer detection. Current clinical MR imaging approaches rely on the use of a dynamic contrast-enhanced acquisition that facilitates morphologic and semiquantitative kinetic assessments of breast lesions. The use of more functional and quantitative parameters holds promise to broaden the utility of MR imaging and improve its specificity. Because of wide variations in approaches for measuring these parameters and the considerable technical challenges, robust multicenter data supporting their routine use are not yet available, limiting current applications of many of these tools to research purposes.

Functional MR imaging is the technique of choice to evaluate and manage malignant musculoskeletal masses. Advanced MR imaging sequences include chemical shift MR imaging, diffusion-weighted imaging with apparent diffusion coefficient mapping, MR spectroscopy imaging, and dynamic contrast-enhanced perfusion imaging. Functional MR imaging adds value to morphologic sequences in the detection, characterization, staging, and post therapy assessment of malignant musculoskeletal malignancies. This article reviews the technical role of each functional sequence and their clinical applications to allow more confident decisions to be made. Multiparametric analysis of functional and anatomic MR sequences allows musculoskeletal tumors analysis to be improved.

Cancer therapy is mainly based on different combinations of surgery, radiotherapy, and chemotherapy. Additionally, targeted therapies (designed to disrupt specific tumor hallmarks, such as angiogenesis, metabolism, proliferation, invasiveness, and immune evasion), hormonotherapy, immunotherapy, and interventional techniques have emerged as alternative oncologic treatments. Conventional imaging techniques and current response criteria do not always provide the necessary information regarding therapy success particularly to targeted therapies. In this setting, MR imaging offers an attractive combination of anatomic, physiologic, and molecular information, which may surpass these limitations, and is being increasingly used for therapy response assessment.

MAGNETIC RESONANCE IMAGING CLINICS OF NORTH AMERICA

RELATED INTEREST

Radiologic Clinics of North America, May 2015 (Vol. 53, No. 3)
Advanced MR Imaging in Clinical Practice
Hersh Chandarana, *Editor*
Available at: www.radiologic.theclinics.com

VISIT THE CLINICS ONLINE!
Access your subscription at:
www.theclinics.com

PROGRAM OBJECTIVE
The goal of *Magnetic Resonance Imaging Clinics of North America* is to keep practicing physicians up to date with current clinical practice by providing timely articles reviewing the state of the art in patient care.

TARGET AUDIENCE
All practicing physicians and healthcare professionals who provide patient care utilizing findings from Magnetic Resonance Imaging.

LEARNING OBJECTIVES
Upon completion of this activity, participants will be able to:
1. Review imaging techniques in brain, head, and neck tumors.
2. Discuss use of multiparametric imaging in breast cancers and cancers of the abdomen and urogenital track.
3. Recognize fMRI techniques in oncology in the era of personalized medicine.

ACCREDITATION
The Elsevier Office of Continuing Medical Education (EOCME) is accredited by the Accreditation Council for Continuing Medical Education (ACCME) to provide continuing medical education for physicians.

The EOCME designates this enduring material for a maximum of 15 *AMA PRA Category 1 Credit*(s)™. Physicians should claim only the credit commensurate with the extent of their participation in the activity.

All other health care professionals requesting continuing education credit for this enduring material will be issued a certificate of participation.

DISCLOSURE OF CONFLICTS OF INTEREST
The EOCME assesses conflict of interest with its instructors, faculty, planners, and other individuals who are in a position to control the content of CME activities. All relevant conflicts of interest that are identified are thoroughly vetted by EOCME for fair balance, scientific objectivity, and patient care recommendations. EOCME is committed to providing its learners with CME activities that promote improvements or quality in healthcare and not a specific proprietary business or a commercial interest.

The planning committee, staff, authors and editors listed below have identified no financial relationships or relationships to products or devices they or their spouse/life partner have with commercial interest related to the content of this CME activity:
Richard G. Abramson, MD; Hebert Alberto Vargas, MD; Lidia Alcal-a-Mata, MD; Antonio Alvarez-Kindelan, MD, PhD; Lori R. Arlinghaus, PhD; Sandra Baleato-González, MD, PhD; Matthias R. Benz, MD; Sanjeev Bhalla, MD; Matthew Blackledge, PhD; Claudio Bonini, MD; Jordi Broncano, MD; Javier Carrascoso-Arranz, MD; Eduard Y. Chekmenev, PhD; David J. Collins, BA (Hons), CPhys, MinstP; Daniel Costa, MD; L. Celso Hygino da Cruz Jr, MD, PhD; Alberto Diaz de Leon, MD; Nandita M. deSouza, MD, FRCR, FRCP; Adrienne N. Dula, PhD; Anjali Fortna; Susan Freeman, FRCR; Roberto García-Figueiras, MD, PhD; Jacobus F.A. Jansen, PhD; Leonardo Kayat Bittencourt, PhD; Margareth Kimura, MD; Dow-Mu Koh, MD, MRCP, FRCR; Jeong-Min Lee, MD; Yonggang Lu, PhD; Antonio Luna, MD; Teodoro Martín Noguerol, MD; Jose Pablo Martínez Barbero, MD; Suresh K. Mukherji, MD, MBA, FACR; James P.B. O'Connor, PhD, FRCR; Carlos Parra, PhD; Savannah C. Partridge, PhD; Ivan Pedrosa, MD; C. Chad Quarles, PhD; Habib Rahbar, MD; Andrea Rockall, MRCP, FRCR; Maria José Romero, MD; Evis Sala, MD, PhD; Ahmed Salem, MB ChB, FRCR; Erin Scheckenbach; Amita Shukla-Dave, PhD; Ashley Stokes, PhD; Karthik Subramaniam; John Vassallo; Joan C. Vilanova, MD, PhD; Jared Weis, PhD; Jennifer Whisenant, PhD; Jason Williams, PhD; Katherine L. Wright, PhD; Thomas Yankeelov, PhD; Igor Zhukov, PhD.

The planning committee, staff, authors and editors listed below have identified financial relationships or relationships to products or devices they or their spouse/life partner have with commercial interest related to the content of this CME activity:
Vikas Gulani, MD, PhD and his spouse have research support from Siemens AG.
Anwar R. Padhani, MBBS, FRCP, FRCR is on the speakers' bureau for, and a consultant/advisor for, Siemens AG.
Shivani Pahwa, MD has research support from Siemens AG.
Javier Sánchez – González, MD has an emplyoment affiliation with Koninklijke Phillips N.V.

UNAPPROVED/OFF-LABEL USE DISCLOSURE
The EOCME requires CME faculty to disclose to the participants:
1. When products or procedures being discussed are off-label, unlabelled, experimental, and/or investigational (not US Food and Drug Administration [FDA] approved); and
2. Any limitations on the information presented, such as data that are preliminary or that represent ongoing research, interim analyses, and/or unsupported opinions. Faculty may discuss information about pharmaceutical agents that is outside of FDA-approved labelling. This information is intended solely for CME and is not intended to promote off-label use of these medications. If you have any questions, contact the medical affairs department of the manufacturer for the most recent prescribing information.

TO ENROLL

To enroll in the *Magnetic Resonance Imaging Clinics of North America* Continuing Medical Education program, call customer service at 1-800-654-2452 or sign up online at http://www.theclinics.com/home/cme. The CME program is available to subscribers for an additional annual fee of USD 250.

METHOD OF PARTICIPATION

In order to claim credit, participants must complete the following:

1. Complete enrolment as indicated above.
2. Read the activity.
3. Complete the CME Test and Evaluation. Participants must achieve a score of 70% on the test. All CME Tests and Evaluations must be completed online.

CME INQUIRIES/SPECIAL NEEDS

For all CME inquiries or special needs, please contact elsevierCME@elsevier.com.

Foreword
Functional MR Imaging in Oncology

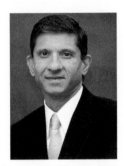

Suresh K. Mukherji, MD, MBA, FACR
Consulting Editor

We are currently in the era of personalized therapy, which has a direct impact on oncologic therapies. The emphasis on precision medicine is driving the field of molecular diagnostics and creating the burgeoning arena of imaging proteomics and genomics. This issue of *Magnetic Resonance Imaging Clinics of North America* is incredibly timed with the recent announcement of the Precision Medicine Initiative by the National Institutes of Health. The role of imaging in modern oncology will clearly be impactful as oncologic diagnostics and therapeutics become more targeted and personalized. This issue provides state-of-the-art reviews of numerous current techniques, such as diffusion-weighted imaging, dynamic contrast-enhanced MR imaging, blood-oxygen–dependent level, and MR spectroscopy. This issue also has articles covering evolving techniques, such as chemical exchange saturation transfer, hyperpolarized MR imaging, MR elastography, and various nanoparticles.

I wish to thank Dr Antonio Luna for his wonderful contribution and all of the authors for their superb efforts. The timing of this issue could not have been better, and it creates an excellent roadmap of the potential role of MR imaging in the era of Precision Medicine.

Suresh K. Mukherji, MD, MBA, FACR
Department of Radiology
Michigan State University
846 Service Road
160 Radiology Building
East Lansing, MI 48824, USA

E-mail address:
mukherji@rad.msu.edu

Magn Reson Imaging Clin N Am 24 (2016) xv
http://dx.doi.org/10.1016/j.mric.2015.10.002
1064-9689/16/$ – see front matter © 2016 Published by Elsevier Inc.

Preface
MR Imaging Pushes Radiologists to Move Forward in Oncologic Imaging

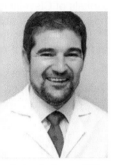

Antonio Luna, MD
Editor

Treatment of oncologic patients has recently changed to personalized therapy, driven by both the development of new-targeted drugs and an increasing use of genetic and molecular diagnostics. Now, cancer is considered a heterogeneous and multifocal disease with different cell clones involved, and unique and specific features in each patient. Furthermore, cancer changes constantly due to random mutations and genetic interactions with the microenvironment. Additionally, cancer reacts to the specific therapies, demonstrating secondary changes, which determine variable response patterns with time.

Imaging is used for the "in vivo" phenotyping of this diversity of cancer. In this setting, functional and molecular information from imaging techniques, classically provided by nuclear medicine, and specifically PET, has been considered essential to understand the insights of cancer and its microenvironment, and the changes induced with therapy. MR imaging has emerged with the potential to represent different tumor characteristics using a multiparametric protocol. Combining morphologic and functional sequences, MR imaging is able to inform different tumor hallmarks,

such as cellularity, microstructure, metabolism, angiogenesis, and hypoxia. All of this quantitative information helps to perform precision diagnostics, which can create impact as tailored treatment to the individual patient. Now, the radiologist must integrate these numeric biomarkers in our classical descriptive reports and learn how to transmit them to clinicians, and to become a central part of multidisciplinary oncologic teams. In addition, research in collaboration with informatics, biotechnologists, and engineers is needed to expand its clinical role. Hence, all of these steps are necessary for radiologists to advance in the goal of improving the personalized care of oncologic patients in this new molecular era as functional imaging information, specifically MR imaging, can create a paradigm shift in the diagnosis and therapy of different tumors.

Thanks to an enthusiastic group of researchers, this issue resumes the role of MR imaging in modern oncology, revealing its potential role in personalized medicine and clinical trials of oncologic drugs. A succinct technical overview of the most "popular" functional sequences, such as diffusion-weighted imaging (DWI) and dynamic contrast-enhanced

Magn Reson Imaging Clin N Am 24 (2016) xvii–xviii
http://dx.doi.org/10.1016/j.mric.2015.10.001
1064-9689/16/$ – see front matter © 2016 Published by Elsevier Inc.

(DCE) MR imaging, and molecular one (meaning sequence), such as MR spectroscopy, are also performed. In addition, novel MR imaging probes, such as chemical exchange saturation transfer MR imaging, hyperpolarized MR imaging, blood-oxygen–dependent level, MR elastography, specific contrast, such as hepatobiliary contrast agents, superparamagnetic particles of iron oxide, or activatable nanoparticles, are also reviewed. A deeper understanding of the clinical use of all of these techniques can be obtained in the specific articles that deal with the applications of functional and molecular MR imaging in the detection, characterization, and therapy monitoring of malignancies in the brain and the body.

Antonio Luna, MD
Department of Radiology
Health Time
Clinica Las Nieves
Carmelo Torres 2
Jaén 23007, Spain

Department of Radiology
University Hospitals of Cleveland
Case Western Reserve University
11100 Euclid Avenue
Cleveland, OH 44106, USA

E-mail address:
aluna70@htime.org

Functional MR Imaging Techniques in Oncology in the Era of Personalized Medicine

Matthias R. Benz, MD[a,b,*], Hebert Alberto Vargas, MD[a],
Evis Sala, MD, PhD[a]

KEYWORDS

• DWI • DCE • Hepatobiliary contrast agent • SPIO • MRS • DNP

KEY POINTS

• Several functional MR imaging techniques are being used to detect biological processes in vivo, for example, to evaluate tissue organization with diffusion-weighted imaging, to assess tumor vascularity with dynamic contrast-enhanced MR imaging or tumor metabolites using magnetic resonance spectroscopy or dynamic nuclear polarization.
• The most important strength of functional MR imaging is its capacity for whole-body imaging, to capture whole-tumor heterogeneity in vivo, and the noninvasive assessment of changes over time.
• Standardization of these imaging techniques needs to be addressed in the future.

INTRODUCTION

The National Cancer Institute defines personalized cancer medicine as "a form of medicine that uses [...] specific information about a person's tumor to help diagnose, plan treatment, find out how well treatment is working, or make a prognosis."[1] Functional imaging allows visual analysis and quantification of biological processes in vivo, such as tumor metabolism, chemical composition, and blood flow. Its most important strength in comparison with other laboratory-based tests of tumor biology is its capacity for whole-body imaging, to capture whole-tumor heterogeneity in vivo, and the noninvasive assessment of (treatment-related) changes over time. Genetic tumor analysis based on single/few tumor biopsy samples may not reflect intratumoral heterogeneity and phenotypic diversity. A study in primary renal carcinoma and associated metastatic sites revealed that intratumoral heterogeneity can lead to underestimation of the tumor genomic landscape represented from single tumor biopsy samples[2] and thus may contribute to treatment failure.

Multiple functional/molecular imaging technologies are available,[3,4] with PET/computed tomography (PET/CT), single-photon emission computed tomography (SPECT), and MR imaging being represented in clinical routine. Because these modalities image different biologic processes, they have the potential to be used in conjunction rather than in competition with one another. Irrespective of their field of application, the advantages of MR imaging in comparison with PET and SPECT relate

Disclosure Statement: Dr. M.R. Benz receives support from MSK Cancer Center Support Grant/Core Grant, P30 CA008748.
[a] Department of Radiology, Memorial Sloan Kettering Cancer Center, 1275 York Avenue, New York, NY 10065, USA; [b] Clinic of Radiology and Nuclear Medicine, University of Basel Hospital, Petersgraben 4, Basel 4031, Switzerland
* Corresponding author. Clinic of Radiology and Nuclear Medicine, University of Basel Hospital, Petersgraben 4, Basel 4031, Switzerland.
E-mail address: matthias.benz@usb.ch

Magn Reson Imaging Clin N Am 24 (2016) 1–10
http://dx.doi.org/10.1016/j.mric.2015.08.001
1064-9689/16/$ – see front matter © 2016 Elsevier Inc. All rights reserved.

to its high spatial and temporal resolution, the superior soft tissue contrast, the capacity of multiparametric imaging, and the lack of ionizing radiation, which is relevant in vulnerable populations, such as children and women of childbearing age,[5] but might be less relevant in adult patients with cancer who undergo chemotherapy and/or radiation therapy.

Several functional MR imaging techniques are being used to, for example, evaluate tissue organization with diffusion-weighted imaging (DWI), to assess tumor vascularity with dynamic contrast-enhanced (DCE) MR imaging, and to detect tumor metabolites using magnetic resonance spectroscopy (MRS)/spectroscopic imaging (MRSI) or dynamic nuclear polarization (DNP). In addition, several specific and nonspecific MR contrast agents are clinically applicable or under investigation.[3,4] On T2*-weighted imaging, hypoxia can be detected based on an increase in the transverse relaxation rate of water caused by the paramagnetic effect of endogenous deoxyhemoglobin using blood oxygen level–dependent (BOLD) MR. This technique has been used for imaging tumor hypoxia and treatment response.[6–8]

Radiogenomics is another exiting field that aims to correlate cancer-imaging features and genetic data for the evaluation of imaging biomarkers. For example, imaging features extracted from MR imaging have been shown to be correlated with gene expression in breast cancer[9] and glioblastoma.[10] Texture analysis describes mathematical parameters computed from the distribution of pixels and is a noninvasive method of assessing heterogeneity within the tumor. Features derived by texture analysis have, for example, been shown to act as a potential imaging biomarker of tumoral response to neoadjuvant chemotherapy/radiation therapy in rectal cancer.[11]

DIFFUSION-WEIGHTED IMAGING

DWI uses the incoherent 3-dimensional motion of water molecules in vivo (Brownian motion) to generate contrast. The degree of water diffusion within intracellular and extracellular fluid and between intracellular and extracellular compartments is impeded by tissue cellularity, intracellular elements, membranes, and macromolecules.[12] The motion of water molecules, for example, in tumor tissue, cytotoxic edema, abscess, and fibrosis is more restricted and displays higher DWI signal intensity. The apparent diffusion coefficient (ADC) is a measure of the magnitude of diffusion and is lower in tissue with restricted diffusion compared with normal parenchyma (Fig. 1). ADC is expressed in units of mm²/s.

Diffusion-based contrast primarily depends on the selection of b-values (the degree of diffusion weighting that is applied during image acquisition), with improved contrast-to-noise ratio at higher b-values, at the expense of lower signal-to-noise ratios.

In general, malignant tumors exhibit higher DWI signal and lower ADC values compared with normal/reactive tissue or benign tumors. DWI has been shown to improve detection and diagnostic accuracy in several primary malignancies; for example, in prostate[13] or endometrial[14] cancer. DWI in conjunction with morphologic MR imaging sequences improves detection of metastatic spread to the peritoneal cavity,[15] in particular in gynecologic malignancies with a reported sensitivity and specificity for the detection of peritoneal implants of 90.0% and 95.5%, respectively.[16]

In several studies, lower ADC values have been associated with a more aggressive tumor.[17–20] However, DWI signal intensity and ADC values are dependent on histologic characteristics, such as tumor type, tumor grade/differentiation, and extent of necrosis.[12] False negatives may occur particularly in well-differentiated tumors, in cystic or necrotic lesions. Abscess and infection might cause false-positive findings.

Low pretreatment tumor ADC has been found to predict a favorable treatment response; for example, in colorectal and gastric carcinomas.[21,22] This observation might be explained by the relationship between tumor necrosis and unfavorable patient outcomes.

Successful treatment is generally reflected by decreases in signal intensity on high *b* value images and corresponding increases in ADC values due to treatment-induced necrosis, edema, or cellular lysis; all of them induce an increase in water diffusion in the extracellular space. However, transient early decreases in ADC values can be seen after treatment.[23]

The development of echoplanar imaging, high gradient amplitudes, multichannel coils, and parallel imaging facilitated DWI to be extended to whole-body imaging[23] (Fig. 2). Whole-body DW MR imaging is an exciting field to image systemic disease, such as multiple myeloma, lymphoma, and leukemia, but also solid tumors with associated metastatic spread, particularly those involving the skeleton. Whole-body DWI can provide complementary information to CT, PET/CT, and SPECT or might be able to replace tests using ionizing radiation. However, published data on staging/restaging accuracy and treatment response assessment are limited. Whole-body DWI for tumor staging has some limitations, especially with regard to the limited anatomic coverage

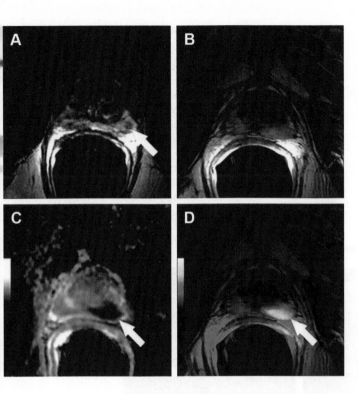

Fig. 1. Pretreatment transverse T2-weighted image (A) showed a tumor focus in the left peripheral zone (arrow). The patient was treated with radiation therapy. MR imaging was performed 2 years later due to rising prostate-specific antigen (PSA). A discrete abnormality was difficult to appreciate on the transverse T2-weighted images at this time (B); however, the ADC map (b-values of b = 0, 1000 s/mm²) (C) and the fused T2-weighted and DW MR images (D) clearly depict the presence of recurrent tumor (arrows).

for intravenous contrast-enhanced sequences. Some solutions have been proposed. For example, Klenk and colleagues[24] used ferumoxytol (AMAG Pharmaceuticals, Inc, Waltham, MA) enhanced whole-body DWI for staging of children and young adults with malignant lymphoma and sarcoma in comparison with ^{18}F-fluorodeoxyglucose (FDG) PET/CT. Ferumoxytol increases the signal intensity on T1-weighted images and decreases the signal intensity on T2-weighted images (hereby improving the contrast between tumor and the reticuloendothelial system). The fusion of ferumoxytol-enhanced whole-body DWI scans with ferumoxytol-enhanced anatomic T1-weighted scans provided diagnostic images very similar to an ^{18}F-FDG PET/CT scan with equivalent sensitivities, specificities, and staging results of both imaging modalities.[24]

Short-term and midterm test-retest variability of repeated ADC measurements in a healthy population has been reported to be not significant with a mean coefficient of variation of 14%.[25] However, the investigators suggest that treatment effects of less than approximately 27% (1.96 × coefficient of variation) will not be meaningfully detectable.[25] Interestingly, this definition of tumor response is very similar to what was reported in several studies investigating metabolic tumor response by ^{18}F-FDG PET and which was suggested as a cutoff in the recently introduced

PET Response Criteria In Solid Tumors (PERCIST) criteria.[26]

The lack of standardization and the limited published data on interscanner variability hinder the comparison of DWI results between studies. A recent prospective study[27] evaluated the variability of ADC values in various anatomic regions in the upper abdomen measured with systems from different vendors and with different field strengths. The investigators found no significant differences between ADC values measured at 1.5 T and at 3.0 T in any anatomic region. However, in 2 of 7 regions at 1.5 T (left and right liver lobes) and in 4 of 7 regions at 3.0 T (left liver lobe, pancreas, and renal cortex and medulla), intervendor differences were significant.

DYNAMIC CONTRAST-ENHANCED MR IMAGING AND MR CONTRAST AGENTS
Perfusion Imaging

Extracellular paramagnetic gadolinium-based contrast agents (EGBCA) distribute nonspecifically in the blood plasma and interstitial space and are administered to reduce the T1 relaxation time of nearby protons, and therewith increase the signal intensity on T1-weighted images. In oncologic imaging, DCE MR imaging uses a bolus injection of EGBCA to acquire multiple serial images as the contrast agent passes through

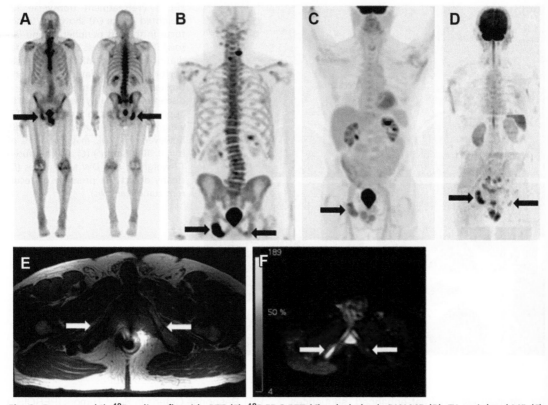

Fig. 2. Bone scan (*A*), ^{18}F-sodium fluoride PET (*B*), ^{18}F-FDG PET (*C*), whole-body DW MR (*D*), T1-weighted MR (*E*), and b50/900 fused MR (*F*) of a patient with metastasized prostate cancer. All scans readily depicted a bone metastasis in the right pubic bone (*right arrows* on all images). ^{18}F-sodium fluoride PET (*B*) and whole-body DW MR (*D/F*) detected an additional T1 low signal lesion in the left pubic bone suspicious for metastatic disease (*left arrows* on *B*, *D–F*). Degenerative ^{18}F-sodium fluoride avidity of the spine (*B*).

tissue to obtain information on altered blood flow and vascularization of tumors. The perfusion data extracted from DCE MR imaging can be investigated qualitatively (visual), in a semiquantitative or quantitative manner to obtain data on enhancement fraction and permeability, respectively. Most of the pharmacologic models used for the quantitative approach are based on determining the rate of contrast exchange between blood plasma and extracellular space using transfer rate constants, such as K^{trans} (forward volume transfer constant) and k_{ep} (reverse reflux rate constant between extracellular space and plasma).

The absence of enhancement is a strong predictor of benignity in several tumors, for example, in breast cancer,[28] whereas the semiquantitative enhancement criterion that suggests malignancy is a rapid initial enhancement (**Fig. 3**). Quantitative DCE MR imaging also allows differentiation of malignant from benign tumors, as has been shown for example, in adnexal masses.[29] On the other hand, qualitative DCE MR imaging time curve

type analysis was found to perform poorly for the differentiation of prostate cancer from healthy prostatic tissue.[30] DCE is currently considered to add relatively little incremental value to the combination of T2-weighted and DWI for the detection of prostate cancer, as reflected in the recently updated Prostate Imaging and Reporting and Data Systems: Version 2 (PIRADS v2.0), which ascribed DCE a minor role in determining the PIRADS Assessment Category when T2-weighted and DWI are of diagnostic quality.[31] The addition of DCE MR imaging to T2-weighted and DWI also did not contribute significant incremental value in the detection of locally recurrent prostate cancer after radiation therapy.[32]

Anatomic tumor size measurements using standard World Health Organization, Response Evaluation Criteria In Solid Tumors (RECIST), and RECIST 1.1 criteria[33] have limitations, particularly in assessing early treatment response and in assessing the effects of molecularly targeted therapies and antiangiogenic strategies that stabilize disease rather than induce fast tumor shrinkage.

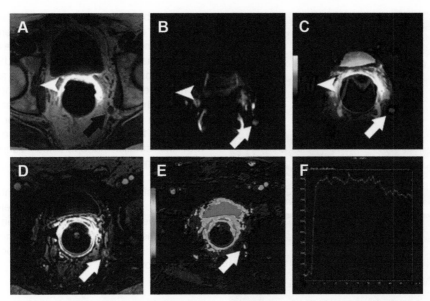

Fig. 3. Patient with rising PSA after radical prostatectomy. Hypointense lesion in the right acetabulum (*arrowhead*) and enlarged left internal iliac lymph node (*arrow*) are suspicious for metastatic disease on T1-weighted MR imaging (*A*). DWI (*B*) and fused T2-weighted and DWI data (*C*) show hyperintense signal in the right acetabulum (*arrowhead*) as well as in the left internal iliac lymph node (*arrow*). DCE MR imaging (*D*) shows early contrast media uptake of both lesions (*arrowhead* and *arrow*). The parametric map (*E*) and the time-signal intensity curve (*F*) confirm the early contrast media uptake (*arrow* in *E*).

DCE MR imaging parameters can serve as predictive biomarkers and enable early treatment response assessment in patients who undergo treatment with antiangiogenic drugs and other therapies.[34–38] However, the clinical application of the potentially powerful biomarkers derived from DCE MR imaging has been limited by the lack of standardization to permit interscanner/interinstitutional comparison of DCE MR imaging studies. Initiatives such as the Quantitative Imaging Biomarker Alliance[39] will help to address these issues in the future.

Hepatobiliary Contrast Agents

Three hepatobiliary contrast agents (HBCAs) have been developed for liver MR imaging: gadoxetic acid (Gd-EOB-DTPA; Eovist [Bayer, USA], Primovist [Bayer, Germany]), gadobenate dimeglumine (Gd-BOPTA; MultiHance [Bracco, Italy]), and mangafodipir trisodium (Mn-DPDP; Teslascan [GE Healthcare, USA]; marketing status: discontinued). Gd-BOPTA and Gd-EOB-DTPA are taken up to varying degrees by functioning hepatocytes via organic anion transporters and are subsequently excreted in the bile (**Fig. 4**). The relatively stronger hepatic signal intensity and biliary tree enhancement of Gd-EOB-DTPA in comparison with Gd-BOPTA results due to approximately 50% and 3% to 5% of excretion via the bile route, respectively.[40]

T1 shortening of the liver and biliary tree results in an increased difference in signal intensity for nonhepatocellular lesions compared with normal liver background. Therefore, HBCAs allow dynamic imaging in the arterial phase (20 s post injection [p.i.]), portal venous phase (60–70 s p.i.) and late venous phase (2–3 min p.i.), as well as liver-specific imaging with regard to a lesion's hepatocyte function and hepatocyte content during the hepatobiliary phase (20 min p.i.).[41] The results of several studies have shown that MR imaging with HBCA depicts more metastatic lesions in the liver than contrast-enhanced MR imaging with EGBCA and adds diagnostic information and confidence.[42,43] Gd-BOPTA and Gd-EOB-DTPA have been shown to be equivalent to EGBCA dynamic imaging for lesion characterization.[44,45] However, the relatively short bolus transit time due to the lower approved dose of Gd-EOB-DTPA (0.025 mmol/kg) in comparison with conventional EGBCA (1.0 mmol/kg) may result in weaker arterial enhancement of liver lesions and impaired lesion characterization. Therefore, the acquisition of the arterial phase needs specific attention and might benefit from modified injection strategies.[46,47] In addition, acute self-limiting dyspnea was observed significantly more often using gadoxetate disodium compared with gadobenate dimeglumine and might affect arterial-phase MR image quality.[48]

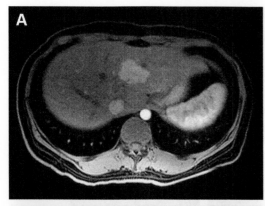

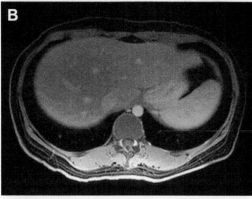

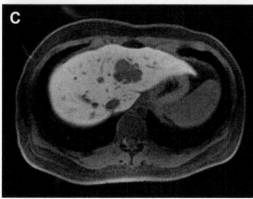

Fig. 4. Hypervascular hepatic tumor (*A*), no washout of extracellular contrast agent (*B*) but hypointense on delayed hepatobiliary phase with Eovist (*C*). The biopsy was consistent with adrenocortical metastasis. (*Courtesy of* Dr Richard Kinh Gian Do, Memorial Sloan Kettering Cancer Center, New York, NY.)

Superparamagnetic Particles of Iron Oxide

Superparamagnetic particles of iron oxide (SPIOs) are composed of a crystalline iron oxide core (ferri [Fe^{3+}] magnetic and ferro [Fe^{2+}] magnetic material in the form of maghemite [γFe_2O_3] and magnetite [Fe_3O_4]) and a stabilizing coating material, usually made of low molecular weight dextran. SPIOs are divided into different classes according to their global size: standard SPIOs (SSPIOs) have a diameter of greater than 50 nm, whereas SPIOs with a diameter of less than 50 nm are referred to as ultra small particles of iron oxide (USPIO). Due to their shortening of T2/T2* they are also known as negative, that is, signal eliminating, contrast agents with darkening of the contrast-enhanced tissue at a given echo time. However, enhancement on T1-weighted images also can be seen with the smaller nanoparticles. Various SPIOs have been tested in clinical and preclinical settings.[49]

The passive uptake of SPIOs in the mononuclear phagocyte system or reticuloendothelial system after intravenous application has been shown to increase the sensitivity of detecting metastasis in the liver,[50] the spleen,[51] lymph nodes,[52] and bone marrow.[53]

Other MR Imaging Agents

Nanoparticles also can be targeted toward specific receptors or molecules by conjugating specific ligands to their surface, such as antibodies, peptides, or small molecules.[3]

Activatable MR contrast agents are able to induce an imaging signal only when a particular disease state is present.[54,55]

Due to the 100% natural abundance and relatively high sensitivity of ^{19}F for MR imaging (83% to that of protons), ^{19}F MR imaging has been used in preclinical and clinical studies to track drug biodistribution,[56] and to assess regional tumor hypoxia among others.[57]

Another example is chemical exchange saturation transfer (CEST) agents, in which contrast enhancement is based on selectively reducing the magnetization of the water signal, with only minimal effect on its longitudinal relaxation rate.[58]

Multimodality probes aim to combine MR imaging with nuclear or optical imaging to obtain high spatial resolution and high sensitivity or enable preoperative staging and intraoperative molecular imaging.[3]

IMAGING OF TUMOR METABOLITES USING "TRADITIONAL" MAGNETIC RESONANCE SPECTROSCOPY/SPECTROSCOPIC IMAGING AND DYNAMIC NUCLEAR POLARIZATION

"Traditional" Magnetic Resonance Spectroscopy

MRS/MRSI permits noninvasive acquisition of signals from cancer metabolites. Accessible nuclei are, for example, ^{1}H, ^{31}P, [23]Na, ^{19}F, ^{13}C,[59] with differences in detectability and signal intensity related to variations in signal susceptibility, percentage isotope concentration, and tissue concentration. Clinical MRS/MRSI studies use signals from ^{1}H nuclei of compounds in tissue because ^{1}H nuclei provide the largest signal, and do not require hardware modification to the scanner.[60] The major metabolites evaluated in ^{1}H MRS include choline (cell membrane marker), creatine (energy marker), lipids (tissue breakdown and cell death), lactate (metabolic acidosis), and in the brain N-acetyl aspartate (normal neuronal marker).[61]

The metabolic fingerprints of several malignancies have been studied; however, the main field of investigation is the brain (Fig. 5), followed by prostate and breast imaging. Most brain tumors manifest with relative reduction of N-acetyl aspartate and elevation of choline. MRS in brain tumors has been shown to be a useful tool in the initial diagnosis, tumor grading, imaging-guided biopsy, and treatment response assessment.[62,63] Elevated choline signal, however, also can be observed in other tumors, such as prostate cancer[64] and breast cancer.[65] Early studies in prostate cancer reported an ability of MRS to help differentiate cancer from benign/necrotic tissue[66–68]; however, a prospective multicenter study, conducted by the American College of Radiology Imaging Network (ACRIN), reported that the addition of MR spectroscopic imaging to anatomic MR imaging did not improve the accuracy for localization of peripheral zone prostate cancer.[69] In breast cancer, a prospective single-center study reported that MRS in addition to DCE MR imaging and DWI improves the accuracy of breast cancer diagnosis.[70] The evaluation of MRS using newer platforms with improved spatial and temporal resolution and comparisons to current standard of care functional techniques, such as DWI, is warranted.

Dynamic Nuclear Polarization (Hyperpolarization)

MR imaging signal intensity is proportional to the spin polarization (the difference in the fraction of nuclei aligned with or against an applied magnetic field). Because polarization is typically very small on the order of 0.0001% to 0.0005% depending on the nucleus and field, nuclei other than protons (with its high concentration in water and fat, which overcomes poor polarization) are difficult to image using standard techniques.[71] Hyperpolarization refers to a procedure that drives nuclei (such as ^{15}N or ^{13}C), temporarily, into a significant redistribution of the ordinary population of energy levels to gain signals 10,000-fold or more.[71]

After the administration of a hyperpolarized agent (such as [1-^{13}C] pyruvate) the agent's delivery as well as its metabolic substrates can be monitored using MR imaging.

Measurements of hyperpolarized ^{13}C label flux between pyruvate and lactate in lymphoma-bearing[72] and glioblastoma-bearing[73] mice has been shown to be able to detect response to chemotherapy. In addition, the amount of hyperpolarized lactate measured after injection of hyperpolarized [1- ^{13}C] pyruvate showed great potential as a new biomarker capable of noninvasively grading prostate cancer in mice.[74]

The first in-man imaging study of MR imaging with hyperpolarized [1- ^{13}C] pyruvate in 31 patients with untreated biopsy-proven prostate cancer[75] confirmed the safety of the agent (no dose-limiting toxicities were observed) and showed elevated [1- ^{13}C] lactate/[1- ^{13}C] pyruvate ratio in regions of biopsy-proven prostate cancer.[75]

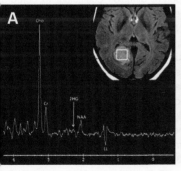 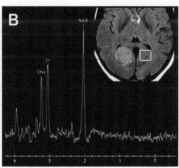

Fig. 5. Single-voxel spectroscopy in a fluid-attenuated inversion recovery hyperintense isocitrate dehydrogenase (IDH) mutant low-grade astrocytoma. The tumor (A) shows high choline (Cho, a cell membrane marker) at 3.2 ppm, low creatine (Cr, an energy marker) at 3.0 ppm, low N-acetylaspartate (NAA, a neuronal marker) at 2.0 ppm, and inverted lipid/lactate (LL, an anaerobic glycolysis marker) at 1.3 ppm. The high Cho and LL are consistent with malignancy. Using a variable TE1/TE2, a small 2HG (2-hydroxyglutarate, an oncometabolite formed exclusively by IDH mutant tumors) peak is also present at 2.25 ppm. Compare with normal spectrum seen in contralateral brain (B) with absent 2HG peak. (Courtesy of Dr Robert J. Young, Memorial Sloan Kettering Cancer Center, New York, NY.)

SUMMARY: FUNCTIONAL MR IMAGING TODAY AND TOMORROW

DW and DCE MR imaging already contribute significantly to several aspects of personalized cancer medicine, namely diagnosis, treatment planning, response assessment, and prognosis. Nevertheless, the need for further standardization of these imaging techniques is beyond question, and needs to be addressed. Whole-body DWI is an exciting field; however, future studies need to investigate in more depth the biologic significance of the findings depicted, their prognostic relevance, and cost-effectiveness in comparison with MDCT and PET/CT. New MR imaging probes, such as targeted or activatable contrast agents and dynamic nuclear hyperpolarization, show great promise to further improve the care of patients with cancer in the near future.

REFERENCES

1. Available at: http://www.cancer.gov/dictionary?cdrid=561717.
2. Gerlinger M, Rowan AJ, Horswell S, et al. Intratumor heterogeneity and branched evolution revealed by multiregion sequencing. N Engl J Med 2012; 366(10):883–92.
3. Kircher MF, Willmann JK. Molecular body imaging: MR imaging, CT, and US. Part I. Principles. Radiology 2012;263(3):633–43.
4. Kircher MF, Willmann JK. Molecular body imaging: MR imaging, CT, and US. Part II. Applications. Radiology 2012;264(2):349–68.
5. Pearce MS, Salotti JA, Little MP, et al. Radiation exposure from CT scans in childhood and subsequent risk of leukaemia and brain tumours: a retrospective cohort study. Lancet 2012;380(9840): 499–505.
6. Gross S, Gilead A, Scherz A, et al. Monitoring photodynamic therapy of solid tumors online by BOLD-contrast MRI. Nat Med 2003;9(10):1327–31.
7. Jiang L, Weatherall PT, McColl RW, et al. Blood oxygenation level-dependent (BOLD) contrast magnetic resonance imaging (MRI) for prediction of breast cancer chemotherapy response: a pilot study. J Magn Reson Imaging 2013;37(5):1083–92.
8. Lin YC, Wang JJ, Hong JH, et al. Noninvasive monitoring of microvascular changes with partial irradiation using dynamic contrast-enhanced and blood oxygen level-dependent magnetic resonance imaging. Int J Radiat Oncol Biol Phys 2013;85(5):1367–74.
9. Grimm LJ, Zhang J, Mazurowski MA. Computational approach to radiogenomics of breast cancer: luminal A and luminal B molecular subtypes are associated with imaging features on routine breast MRI extracted using computer vision algorithms. J Magn Reson Imaging 2015. [Epub ahead of print].
10. Zinn PO, Mahajan B, Sathyan P, et al. Radiogenomic mapping of edema/cellular invasion MRI-phenotypes in glioblastoma multiforme. PLoS One 2011;6(10):e25451.
11. De Cecco CN, Ganeshan B, Ciolina M, et al. Texture analysis as imaging biomarker of tumoral response to neoadjuvant chemoradiotherapy in rectal cancer patients studied with 3-T magnetic resonance. Invest Radiol 2015;50(4):239–45.
12. Padhani AR, Liu G, Koh DM, et al. Diffusion-weighted magnetic resonance imaging as a cancer biomarker: consensus and recommendations. Neoplasia 2009;11(2):102–25.
13. Jung SI, Donati OF, Vargas HA, et al. Transition zone prostate cancer: incremental value of diffusion-weighted endorectal MR imaging in tumor detection and assessment of aggressiveness. Radiology 2013;269(2):493–503.
14. Beddy P, Moyle P, Kataoka M, et al. Evaluation of depth of myometrial invasion and overall staging in endometrial cancer: comparison of diffusion-weighted and dynamic contrast-enhanced MR imaging. Radiology 2012;262(2):530–7.
15. Low RN, Sebrechts CP, Barone RM, et al. Diffusion-weighted MRI of peritoneal tumors: comparison with conventional MRI and surgical and histopathologic findings–a feasibility study. AJR Am J Roentgenol 2009;193(2):461–70.
16. Fujii S, Matsusue E, Kanasaki Y, et al. Detection of peritoneal dissemination in gynecological malignancy: evaluation by diffusion-weighted MR imaging. Eur Radiol 2008;18(1):18–23.
17. Woodfield CA, Tung GA, Grand DJ, et al. Diffusion-weighted MRI of peripheral zone prostate cancer: comparison of tumor apparent diffusion coefficient with Gleason score and percentage of tumor on core biopsy. AJR Am J Roentgenol 2010;194(4):W316–22.
18. Hilario A, Ramos A, Perez-Nunez A, et al. The added value of apparent diffusion coefficient to cerebral blood volume in the preoperative grading of diffuse gliomas. AJNR Am J Neuroradiol 2012;33(4):701–7.
19. Nakanishi M, Chuma M, Hige S, et al. Relationship between diffusion-weighted magnetic resonance imaging and histological tumor grading of hepatocellular carcinoma. Ann Surg Oncol 2012;19(4):1302–9.
20. Curvo-Semedo L, Lambregts DM, Maas M, et al. Diffusion-weighted MRI in rectal cancer: apparent diffusion coefficient as a potential noninvasive marker of tumor aggressiveness. J Magn Reson Imaging 2012;35(6):1365–71.
21. Cui Y, Zhang XP, Sun YS, et al. Apparent diffusion coefficient: potential imaging biomarker for prediction and early detection of response to chemotherapy in hepatic metastases. Radiology 2008; 248(3):894–900.

22. Heijmen L, Ter Voert EE, Oyen WJ, et al. Multimodality imaging to predict response to systemic treatment in patients with advanced colorectal cancer. PLoS One 2015;10(4):e0120823.

23. Koh DM, Collins DJ. Diffusion-weighted MRI in the body: applications and challenges in oncology. AJR Am J Roentgenol 2007;188(6):1622–35.

24. Klenk C, Gawande R, Uslu L, et al. Ionising radiation-free whole-body MRI versus (18)F-fluorodeoxyglucose PET/CT scans for children and young adults with cancer: a prospective, non-randomised, single-centre study. Lancet Oncol 2014;15(3):275–85.

25. Braithwaite AC, Dale BM, Boll DT, et al. Short- and midterm reproducibility of apparent diffusion coefficient measurements at 3.0-T diffusion-weighted imaging of the abdomen. Radiology 2009;250(2): 459–65.

26. Wahl RL, Jacene H, Kasamon Y, et al. From RECIST to PERCIST: evolving considerations for PET response criteria in solid tumors. J Nucl Med 2009; 50(Suppl 1):122S–50S.

27. Donati OF, Chong D, Nanz D, et al. Diffusion-weighted MR imaging of upper abdominal organs: field strength and intervendor variability of apparent diffusion coefficients. Radiology 2014;270(2):454–63.

28. Schnall MD, Blume J, Bluemke DA, et al. Diagnostic architectural and dynamic features at breast MR imaging: multicenter study. Radiology 2006;238(1):42–53.

29. Thomassin-Naggara I, Balvay D, Aubert E, et al. Quantitative dynamic contrast-enhanced MR imaging analysis of complex adnexal masses: a preliminary study. Eur Radiol 2012;22(4):738–45.

30. Hansford BG, Peng Y, Jiang Y, et al. Dynamic contrast-enhanced MR imaging curve-type analysis: is it helpful in the differentiation of prostate cancer from healthy peripheral zone? Radiology 2015; 275(2):448–57.

31. Available at: http://www.acr.org/Quality-Safety/Resources/PIRADS.

32. Donati OF, Jung SI, Vargas HA, et al. Multiparametric prostate MR imaging with T2-weighted, diffusion-weighted, and dynamic contrast-enhanced sequences: are all pulse sequences necessary to detect locally recurrent prostate cancer after radiation therapy? Radiology 2013;268(2):440–50.

33. Tirkes T, Hollar MA, Tann M, et al. Response criteria in oncologic imaging: review of traditional and new criteria. Radiographics 2013;33(5):1323–41.

34. Barrett T, Gill AB, Kataoka MY, et al. DCE and DW MRI in monitoring response to androgen deprivation therapy in patients with prostate cancer: a feasibility study. Magn Reson Med 2012;67(3):778–85.

35. Gollub MJ, Gultekin DH, Akin O, et al. Dynamic contrast enhanced-MRI for the detection of pathological complete response to neoadjuvant chemotherapy for locally advanced rectal cancer. Eur Radiol 2012;22(4):821–31.

36. Jensen LR, Garzon B, Heldahl MG, et al. Diffusion-weighted and dynamic contrast-enhanced MRI in evaluation of early treatment effects during neoadjuvant chemotherapy in breast cancer patients. J Magn Reson Imaging 2011;34(5): 1099–109.

37. Kim JH, Kim CK, Park BK, et al. Dynamic contrast-enhanced 3-T MR imaging in cervical cancer before and after concurrent chemoradiotherapy. Eur Radiol 2012;22(11):2533–9.

38. Padhani AR, Leach MO. Antivascular cancer treatments: functional assessments by dynamic contrast-enhanced magnetic resonance imaging. Abdom Imaging 2005;30(3):324–41.

39. Available at: https://www.rsna.org/QIBA.aspx.

40. Reimer P, Schneider G, Schima W. Hepatobiliary contrast agents for contrast-enhanced MRI of the liver: properties, clinical development and applications. Eur Radiol 2004;14(4):559–78.

41. Jhaveri K, Cleary S, Audet P, et al. Consensus statements from a multidisciplinary expert panel on the utilization and application of a liver-specific MRI contrast agent (gadoxetic acid). AJR Am J Roentgenol 2015;204(3):498–509.

42. Hammerstingl R, Huppertz A, Breuer J, et al. Diagnostic efficacy of gadoxetic acid (Primovist)-enhanced MRI and spiral CT for a therapeutic strategy: comparison with intraoperative and histopathologic findings in focal liver lesions. Eur Radiol 2008;18(3):457–67.

43. Zech CJ, Herrmann KA, Reiser MF, et al. MR imaging in patients with suspected liver metastases: value of liver-specific contrast agent Gd-EOB-DTPA. Magn Reson Med Sci 2007;6(1):43–52.

44. Huppertz A, Haraida S, Kraus A, et al. Enhancement of focal liver lesions at gadoxetic acid-enhanced MR imaging: correlation with histopathologic findings and spiral CT–initial observations. Radiology 2005; 234(2):468–78.

45. Kuwatsuru R, Kadoya M, Ohtomo K, et al. Comparison of gadobenate dimeglumine with gadopentetate dimeglumine for magnetic resonance imaging of liver tumors. Invest Radiol 2001;36(11):632–41.

46. Motosugi U, Ichikawa T, Sou H, et al. Dilution method of gadolinium ethoxybenzyl diethylenetriaminepentaacetic acid (Gd-EOB-DTPA)-enhanced magnetic resonance imaging (MRI). J Magn Reson Imaging 2009;30(4):849–54.

47. Schmid-Tannwald C, Herrmann K, Oto A, et al. Optimization of the dynamic, Gd-EOB-DTPA-enhanced MRI of the liver: the effect of the injection rate. Acta Radiol 2012;53(9):961–5.

48. Davenport MS, Viglianti BL, Al-Hawary MM, et al. Comparison of acute transient dyspnea after intravenous administration of gadoxetate disodium and gadobenate dimeglumine: effect on arterial phase image quality. Radiology 2013;266(2):452–61.

49. Ittrich H, Peldschus K, Raabe N, et al. Superparamagnetic iron oxide nanoparticles in biomedicine: applications and developments in diagnostics and therapy. Rofo 2013;185(12):1149–66.

50. Fretz CJ, Stark DD, Metz CE, et al. Detection of hepatic metastases: comparison of contrast-enhanced CT, unenhanced MR imaging, and iron oxide-enhanced MR imaging. AJR Am J Roentgenol 1990;155(4):763–70.

51. Ferrucci JT, Stark DD. Iron oxide-enhanced MR imaging of the liver and spleen: review of the first 5 years. AJR Am J Roentgenol 1990;155(5):943–50.

52. Weissleder R, Elizondo G, Wittenberg J, et al. Ultrasmall superparamagnetic iron oxide: an intravenous contrast agent for assessing lymph nodes with MR imaging. Radiology 1990;175(2):494–8.

53. Kotoura N, Sakamoto K, Fukuda Y, et al. Evaluation of magnetic resonance signal intensity in bone marrow after administration of super paramagnetic iron oxide (SPIO). Nihon Hoshasen Gijutsu Gakkai Zasshi 2011;67(3):212–20 [in Japanese].

54. Querol M, Bogdanov A Jr. Environment-sensitive and enzyme-sensitive MR contrast agents. Handb Exp Pharmacol 2008;185(Pt 2):37–57.

55. Chauvin T, Durand P, Bernier M, et al. Detection of enzymatic activity by PARACEST MRI: a general approach to target a large variety of enzymes. Angew Chem Int Ed Engl 2008;47(23):4370–2.

56. Wolters M, Mohades SG, Hackeng TM, et al. Clinical perspectives of hybrid proton-fluorine magnetic resonance imaging and spectroscopy. Invest Radiol 2013;48(5):341–50.

57. Chen JJ, Lanza GM, Wickline SA. Quantitative magnetic resonance fluorine imaging: today and tomorrow. Wiley Interdiscip Rev Nanomed Nanobiotechnol 2010;2(4):431–40.

58. Hancu I, Dixon WT, Woods M, et al. CEST and PARACEST MR contrast agents. Acta Radiol 2010;51(8):910–23.

59. Negendank W. Studies of human tumors by MRS: a review. NMR Biomed 1992;5(5):303–24.

60. Winfield JM, Payne GS, deSouza NM. Functional MRI and CT biomarkers in oncology. Eur J Nucl Med Mol Imaging 2015;42(4):562–78.

61. Wang LL, Leach JL, Breneman JC, et al. Critical role of imaging in the neurosurgical and radiotherapeutic management of brain tumors. Radiographics 2014;34(3):702–21.

62. Brandao LA, Shiroishi MS, Law M. Brain tumors: a multimodality approach with diffusion-weighted imaging, diffusion tensor imaging, magnetic resonance spectroscopy, dynamic susceptibility contrast and dynamic contrast-enhanced magnetic resonance imaging. Magn Reson Imaging Clin N Am 2013;21(2):199–239.

63. Hollingworth W, Medina LS, Lenkinski RE, et al. A systematic literature review of magnetic resonance spectroscopy for the characterization of brain tumors. AJNR Am J Neuroradiol 2006;27(7):1404–11.

64. Kurhanewicz J, Vigneron D, Carroll P, et al. Multiparametric magnetic resonance imaging in prostate cancer: present and future. Curr Opin Urol 2008;18(1):71–7.

65. Begley JK, Redpath TW, Bolan PJ, et al. In vivo proton magnetic resonance spectroscopy of breast cancer: a review of the literature. Breast Cancer Res 2012;14(2):207.

66. Mueller-Lisse UG, Vigneron DB, Hricak H, et al. Localized prostate cancer: effect of hormone deprivation therapy measured by using combined three-dimensional 1H MR spectroscopy and MR imaging: clinicopathologic case-controlled study. Radiology 2001;221(2):380–90.

67. Parivar F, Hricak H, Shinohara K, et al. Detection of locally recurrent prostate cancer after cryosurgery: evaluation by transrectal ultrasound, magnetic resonance imaging, and three-dimensional proton magnetic resonance spectroscopy. Urology 1996;48(4):594–9.

68. Pickett B, Kurhanewicz J, Coakley F, et al. Use of MRI and spectroscopy in evaluation of external beam radiotherapy for prostate cancer. Int J Radiat Oncol Biol Phys 2004;60(4):1047–55.

69. Weinreb JC, Blume JD, Coakley FV, et al. Prostate cancer: sextant localization at MR imaging and MR spectroscopic imaging before prostatectomy–results of ACRIN prospective multi-institutional clinicopathologic study. Radiology 2009;251(1):122–33.

70. Pinker K, Bogner W, Baltzer P, et al. Improved diagnostic accuracy with multiparametric magnetic resonance imaging of the breast using dynamic contrast-enhanced magnetic resonance imaging, diffusion-weighted imaging, and 3-dimensional proton magnetic resonance spectroscopic imaging. Invest Radiol 2014;49(6):421–30.

71. Kurhanewicz J, Vigneron DB, Brindle K, et al. Analysis of cancer metabolism by imaging hyperpolarized nuclei: prospects for translation to clinical research. Neoplasia 2011;13(2):81–97.

72. Day SE, Kettunen MI, Gallagher FA, et al. Detecting tumor response to treatment using hyperpolarized C-13 magnetic resonance imaging and spectroscopy. Nat Med 2007;13(11):1382–7.

73. Park I, Larson PEZ, Zierhut ML, et al. Hyperpolarized C-13 magnetic resonance metabolic imaging: application to brain tumors. Neuro Oncol 2010;12(2):133–44.

74. Albers MJ, Bok R, Chen AP, et al. Hyperpolarized C-13 lactate, pyruvate, and alanine: noninvasive biomarkers for prostate cancer detection and grading. Cancer Res 2008;68(20):8607–15.

75. Nelson SJ, Kurhanewicz J, Vigneron DB, et al. Metabolic imaging of patients with prostate cancer using hyperpolarized [1-(1)(3)C]pyruvate. Sci Transl Med 2013;5(198):198ra08.

MR Imaging Biomarkers in Oncology Clinical Trials

Richard G. Abramson, MD[a], Lori R. Arlinghaus, PhD[b], Adrienne N. Dula, PhD[a],
C. Chad Quarles, PhD[a,c,d], Ashley M. Stokes, PhD[a], Jared A. Weis, PhD[e],
Jennifer G. Whisenant, PhD[a], Eduard Y. Chekmenev, PhD[a,c,f], Igor Zhukov, PhD[g],
Jason M. Williams, PhD[h], Thomas E. Yankeelov, PhD[a,c,d,i],*

KEYWORDS

- DCE-MR imaging • DSC-MR imaging • Diffusion • CEST • Elastography • Hyperpolarized
- Multiparametric

KEY POINTS

- The fundamental limitations of RECIST (Response Evaluation Criteria in Solid Tumors) must be addressed by more quantitative imaging methods; MR imaging offers many existing and emerging methods to fill this need.
- DCE-MR imaging, DSC-MR imaging, and diffusion MR imaging have advanced to the point where they can offer quantitative insights into tumor characteristics, and these techniques are now frequently used in clinical trials either alone or in concert.
- Magnetic resonance (MR) elastography, CEST (chemical exchange saturation transfer), and hyperpolarized MR imaging are 3 emerging techniques that can offer insights complementary to those provided by the diffusion and perfusion MR imaging methods.
- The ability to acquire multiple data types in a single MR imaging session provides the opportunity to combine these methods in a multiparametric approach, which has been shown to have increased clinical value over single parameter methods.

INCORPORATING QUANTITATIVE MR IMAGING IN CLINICAL TRIALS

The last decade has seen tremendous interest and research effort devoted to the use of quantitative imaging within oncology.[1,2] Quantitative imaging techniques can measure various properties within medical images that might serve as reliable surrogates for various pathophysiological processes with which to personalize cancer therapy and

Disclosure Statement: The authors have nothing to disclose.
[a] Department of Radiology and Radiological Sciences, Institute of Imaging Science, Vanderbilt University, VUIIS 1161 21st Avenue South, AA 1105 MCN, Nashville, TN 37232-2310, USA; [b] Department of Radiology and Radiological Sciences, Vanderbilt University, 1161 21st Avenue South, AA 1105 MCN, Nashville, TN 37232-2310, USA; [c] Department of Biomedical Engineering, Institute of Imaging Science, Vanderbilt University, VUIIS 1161 21st Avenue South, AA 1105 MCN, Nashville, TN 37232-2310, USA; [d] Department of Cancer Biology, Institute of Imaging Science, Vanderbilt University, 1161 21st Avenue South, AA 1105 MCN, Nashville, TN 37232-2310, USA; [e] Department of Biomedical Engineering, Vanderbilt University, VUIIS 1161 21st Avenue South, AA 1105 MCN, Nashville, TN 37232-2310, USA; [f] Department of Biochemistry, Institute of Imaging Science, Vanderbilt University, 1161 21st Avenue South, AA 1105 MCN, Nashville, TN 37232-2310, USA; [g] National Research Nuclear University MEPhI, Kashirskoye highway, 31, Moscow 115409, Russia; [h] Department of Radiology and Radiological Sciences, Institute of Imaging Science, Vanderbilt University, 1161 21st Avenue South, AA 1105 MCN, Nashville, TN 37232-2310, USA; [i] Department of Physics, Institute of Imaging Science, Vanderbilt University, VUIIS 1161 21st Avenue South, AA 1105 MCN, Nashville, TN 37232-2310, USA
* Corresponding author. 1161 21st Avenue South, AA 1105 MCN, Nashville, TN.
E-mail address: thomas.yankeelov@vanderbilt.edu

Magn Reson Imaging Clin N Am 24 (2016) 11–29
http://dx.doi.org/10.1016/j.mric.2015.08.002
1064-9689/16/$ – see front matter © 2016 Elsevier Inc. All rights reserved.

accelerate drug development.[3] Furthermore, the prospect of combining several quantitative imaging measures for establishing radiologic phenotypes predictive of clinical trajectories is particularly appealing, and MR imaging has emerged as a promising modality for this purpose.[4] MR imaging continues to be a mainstay for conventional size-based tumor assessments (ie, the Response Evaluation Criteria in Solid Tumors, RECIST; see next section) that are standard efficacy endpoints within clinical trials and increasingly common in routine, standard-of-care settings. Moreover, MR imaging applications that can quantitatively report on various aspects of tumor biology, including perfusion, cellularity, metabolism, and protein deposition, offer the potential to supplement and enhance conventional anatomic information, which when used alone provides an incomplete assessment of solid tumors.[5] This review spotlights some of the leading technological developments in MR imaging that are laying the groundwork for quantitative MR imaging to transition from being viewed as an advanced research paradigm to becoming a widely established clinical reality for the cancer community. This transition presents a number of unique challenges as well as exciting opportunities for imaging science.

There are several key steps for the development and evaluation of a particular quantitative imaging measure before it can be considered a true biomarker and safely incorporated into clinical practice[6] (Box 1). Perhaps one of the most essential tools for the evaluation of biomarkers is the multicenter clinical trial. Over the last several years, the National Cancer Institute (NCI) has spearheaded efforts to coordinate multicenter biomarker studies for imaging. The NCI's Quantitative Imaging Network currently includes 17 Centers of Imaging Excellence in the United States, several of which are actively engaged in validation of imaging based biomarkers.[7] Other groups, including the Radiological Society of North America Quantitative Imaging Biomarker Alliance[1] and

the American College of Radiology Imaging Network, recently merged with the Eastern Cooperative Oncology Group to form ECOG-ACRIN,[8] have also been rigorously pursuing multicenter quantitative imaging clinical trials. These groups have developed their own clinical trial designs and workflows, image acquisition and analysis procedures, and regulatory processes. There are also efforts to harmonize procedures and practices across these groups in order to arrive at a comprehensive set of standards for the clinical validation and implementation of quantitative imaging biomarkers. The authors draw from collective insights to emphasize a few key commonalities with their own experiences and discuss some administrative, regulatory, and logistical considerations facing trials of a putative MR imaging biomarker.

One of the most crucial aspects of successful integration of MR imaging biomarker research with an oncology clinical trial will be the level of engagement and collaboration the imaging scientists and radiologists have with the medical oncologists and clinical trial sponsors. Investigator-initiated trials offer certain advantages in this regard relative to industry-sponsored trials, because the latter often requires a higher level of engagement and a greater emphasis on allocating resources for data management and regulatory compliance. Furthermore, because these studies are frequently designed at the industrial sponsor months—or years—before academic investigators become aware of it, integrating an advanced imaging technique can be difficult. Regardless of the type of trial, there are several characteristics pertaining to the design and execution of an MR-based imaging biomarker study that need to be considered within the context of a therapeutic oncology trial. Ideally, the biomarker study design would be rationally tailored to address a clearly defined clinical problem (eg, predicting which patients will benefit from neoadjuvant therapy) and would test the ability of a candidate MR imaging

---

Box 1
Key steps for the development and evaluation of quantitative imaging measures

1. Validation tests the accuracy, precision, repeatability, and reproducibility of the biomarker measurement.

2. Qualification establishes the biomarker as a surrogate for tumor pathophysiology, response to therapy, or other clinical endpoint of interest.

3. Utilization examines the performance and implementation of the biomarker within the specific context of its proposed use, especially across multiple institutions and clinical settings.

Adapted from Refs.[2,9,10]

technique, or group of techniques, to predict or correlate with a desired clinical outcome (eg, pathologic complete response). The predictive value of a particular imaging measure will likely vary depending on the choice of clinical endpoint. When progression-free or overall survival (OS) is a primary endpoint, incorporation of multiple strategically chosen imaging time points during follow-up is recommended (**Box 2**).

The first scientific body to review, advise, and ultimately approve an imaging-based biomarker study is the institutions' Scientific Review Committee (SRC), which consists of clinicians, basic scientists, biostatisticians, nurses, pharmacists, and other medical professionals whose primary mission is to scrutinize the scientific merit and clinical prioritization of a new study in the context of an institution's existing menu of studies. For most institutions, a new clinical trial protocol will undergo review by the SRC before it is reviewed by the local Institutional Review Board (IRB). A critical aspect of the SRC review entails thorough scrutiny of the statistical methodology proposed in the study. Before protocol submission, it is highly worthwhile, and at some institutions required, to meet with a qualified biostatistician, particularly one well versed in the analysis of imaging data, to ensure that the aims and study design are in keeping with a sound statistical framework appropriate for the development of imaging biomarkers.[11] Studies must be demonstrated as having accrual goals capable of satisfying a predefined level of statistical power (typically, 80%) to determine the predictive association between the MR biomarker or biomarkers in question and the primary clinical endpoint. Sample sizes must also be justified on the basis of historical accrual data within identical or very similar patient populations and clinical settings. Feedback from the SRC is one of the primary opportunities for constructive criticism so that the aims, design, and future conduct of a study are consistent with institutional standards for statistical rigor, clinical relevance, and scientific quality.

Once SRC approval is obtained, the next step in opening a new imaging study is protocol review and approval by the local IRB. Although scientific rigor and clinical relevance are the primary concerns in SRC review, the IRB is typically most focused on ensuring that the study meets all federal, state, and local policies pertaining to patient safety and confidentiality. For MR imaging studies, one of the most important aspects of IRB review will be centered on the patient screening process to ensure compatibility with the large magnetic field the patient will encounter as part of the imaging procedure. The IRB will verify that prospective patients will be given every means necessary to disclose the presence of ferromagnetic materials and will also allow designated key study personnel to access the prospective patient's medical record to verify MR compatibility of implants; this is especially important in patients with cancer receiving chemotherapy or other procedures (biopsy, surgery), because vascular access ports, biopsy marker clips, and stents are constructed of materials whose MR compatibility can vary widely. The IRB will heavily scrutinize methods for verifying the manufacturer and model number for an implant or device in question. Rigorous rating standards from the American Society for Testing and Materials (ASTM) International exist for virtually all implantable biomaterials and have been approved by the US Food and Drug Administration. The IRB will mandate that only implanted materials having an ASTM rating of "MR Safe" at the particular field strength in question are included within the study. Implants having a rating of "MR Conditional" are often excluded, but there are instances where a particular MR imaging environment with specific conditions may be acceptable. For example, at 3.0 T, the only implants or devices currently accepted on study are those classified as MR Conditional 6 (ASTM Standard F2503).[12]

While the IRB is reviewing the imaging protocol, there are several steps that can be taken to help ensure no delays are experienced in opening to accrual. Like therapeutic trials, studies devoted to validating a perspective imaging biomarker should be nationally registered at ClinicalTrials.gov and/or the NCI. At many institutions, national study registration is required of all clinical studies as a matter of local policy, and recent changes

---

Box 2
Helpful factors when determining the timing of follow-up scans

1. The expected mechanism, onset, and duration of action of the therapeutic agent or intervention under investigation in the clinical trial.

2. The schedule of events (ie, timing of biomarker scan should coincide whenever possible with the patient's clinical appointments) within the trial.

3. Potential interference from use of contrast media in other clinical trial radiological procedures.

4. Interscan interval in relation to reimbursement policies of the sponsor, patient's insurance provider, or Centers for Medicate and Medicaid Services.

to the registration rules put forward by the International Committee of Medical Journal Editors now necessitate registration even for noninterventional imaging studies. Another critical logistical step before opening to accrual is to ensure that all imaging-related study materials have been distributed to the appropriate study personnel. The most convenient venue for such interactions is the Site Initiation Visit, where imaging scientists, clinicians, research nurses, and others can meet to review key aspects of the study to establish an adequate recruitment plan and clinical workflow. This Site Initiation Visit is particularly important in situations whereby the acquisition of imaging data is to occur on dedicated research scanners in facilities that are separated from the cancer clinics where recruitment will take place, because the processes and procedures involved in advanced imaging studies are often unfamiliar to clinical staff.

CURRENT USE OF MR IMAGING FOR CLINICAL TRIALS

In modern clinical oncology practice, MR imaging is widely used as a tool for cancer screening, lesion detection, lesion characterization, and therapy monitoring. Within cancer clinical trials, MR imaging is used for assessing response to treatment, although its role varies depending on the anatomic site of disease. For many clinical trials in solid malignancies, MR imaging may play a secondary role to computed tomography (CT) and may be used only when there is a contraindication to iodinated intravenous contrast media. For certain tumor types (eg, brain and head/neck cancers), MR imaging may be the preferred modality for response assessment due to its excellent soft tissue contrast resolution.

When MR imaging is used for treatment response assessment, most current cancer clinical trials use one of several standardized response assessment guidelines based on changes in gross lesion size. These guidelines specify how to identify and measure target lesions at baseline imaging before therapy, how to evaluate disease burden at follow-up time points following initiation of treatment, and how to place patients into response categories at successive time points over the course of the clinical trial.[13] The most widely used response assessment guideline, incorporated into most modern solid tumor clinical trials, is RECIST.[14] Because its emphasis is on changes in tumor size measurement over time, RECIST necessitates high-spatial resolution MR imaging techniques optimized for capturing anatomic detail.

Measuring changes in tumor size on anatomic imaging has been the mainstay of imaging-based response assessment for decades[15] and is supported by research linking tumor shrinkage in early-stage trials with subsequent survival benefits.[16–19] However, an exclusive focus on anatomic imaging has recently been called into question with the emergence of functional imaging techniques that provide information on tumor status beyond lesion size. These techniques, many of which are MR-based and are described later, offer the promise of reporting on response at an earlier time point than traditional tumor size-based approaches, which may lag weeks to months behind a physiologic tumor response. Functional imaging techniques may also succeed in better capturing and measuring the antitumor efficacy of newer targeted agents, the cytostatic effects of which may be underestimated by traditional size-based approaches.

QUANTITATIVE MR IMAGING TECHNIQUES CURRENTLY AVAILABLE FOR CLINICAL TRIALS

Three techniques are focused on that have advanced to the point where they are frequently used in clinical trials to report on therapeutic response. In the section entitled "Emerging MR Imaging Methods for Cancer," 4 emerging techniques are described.

Dynamic Susceptibility Contrast MR Imaging

Abnormal angiogenesis is a common characteristic of malignant brain tumors, and dynamic susceptibility contrast MR imaging (DSC-MR imaging) is frequently used to noninvasively interrogate the hemodynamic features of the expanding vascular network. In DSC-MR imaging, dynamic MR images are acquired before and after an intravenous bolus injection of a contrast agent (CA), which is typically one of several clinically approved gadolinium chelates. As the CA passes through tissue, it decreases the relaxation times (T_1, T_2, and T_2^*) of tissue water and the associated MR imaging signal intensity. The magnitude of the change in the relaxation rate is determined by the concentration of the CA and the geometry of the tissue structures containing the CA. Pharmacokinetic models can be applied to DSC-MR imaging data to estimate blood volume, blood flow, and mean transit time.[20–22]

Given the known association between brain tumor pathologic abnormality and angiogenesis, early DSC-MR imaging studies demonstrated the clinical utility of this technique by verifying a positive correlation between tumor blood volume and brain tumor grade.[21,23–27] As an example, Boxerman and colleagues[25] found relative blood volume values (ie, relative to normal appearing white matter) of 1.52, 2.84, and 3.96 in a cohort of patients with World Health Organization grades II (n = 11), II (n = 9), and IV (n = 23), respectively. Furthermore, the correlation between blood volume and tumor grade was significant (r = 0.60; P<.0001). It was noted that designating tumor grade based on blood volume maps alone, however, may be confounded by intragrade variability, particularly between grades III and IV.

Although such diagnostic studies served to support the consideration of DSC-MR imaging in brain tumor patient management, its clinical potential was more fully realized when studies emerged demonstrating its prognostic capabilities. Law and colleagues[28] investigated the ability of pretreatment blood volume maps to predict clinical response (complete response, stable disease, progressive disease [PD], and death) in patients with low-grade gliomas undergoing standard-of-care treatments. The patients with lesions exhibiting blood volume values less than 1.75 (relative to normal appearing white matter) had a median time to progression of 4620 days, whereas those with values higher than 1.75 had a median time to progression of 245 days. An important conclusion in this study is that while DSC-MR imaging may have low specificity for diagnosing low-grade gliomas, it has a much higher specificity for predicting clinical endpoints in patients receiving standard treatment regimens.

In the context of routine therapy and clinical trials, standard MR imaging techniques are unable to reliably differentiate between PD and pseudoprogression (PsP). Because of the heightened angiogenic response in recurring gliomas, DSC-MR imaging–derived cerebral blood volume (CBV) maps have been explored as a means to overcome this limitation.[29–31] In a phase II clinical trial of temozolomide, paclitaxel poliglumex, and concurrent radiation, the mean CBV measured at initial progressive enhancement and the change in CBV after therapy were used to distinguish PD and PsP.[29] The single time point CBV values acquired after therapy were similar between patients exhibiting PsP and PD (2.35 vs 2.17, P = .67). However, changes in CBV between follow-up examinations were significantly different between PsS and PD (−0.84 and 0.84, P = .001) as were the trends in CBV (negative vs positive slope; P = .04). It was concluded that longitudinal changes in posttherapy CBV values may be more useful for tracking treatment response than static values (Fig. 1).

The identification of early predictors of clinical endpoints (eg, OS) could reduce the duration and cost of clinical trials. Toward this end, the predictive potential of DSC-MR imaging in glioblastoma multiforme (GBM) patients was recently evaluated in ACRIN 6677/RTOG 0625, a multicenter, randomized, phase II trial of bevacizumab with irinotecan or temozolomide.[32] Changes in tumor CBV before and at 2, 8 and 16 weeks after treatment initiation were correlated with OS. Significant

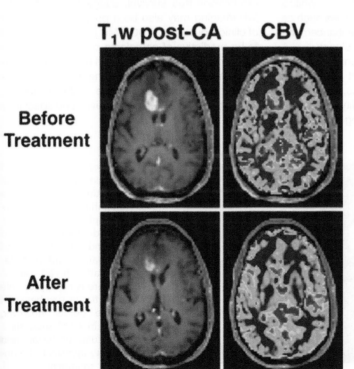

T₁w post-CA   **CBV**

Before Treatment

After Treatment

Fig. 1. Example of DSC-MR imaging–based assessment of bevacizumab-induced CBV changes in recurrent high-grade glioma. Two weeks of bevacizumab treatment reduced CA extravasation and the enhancing tumor volume (*left column*). Treatment also decreased CBV throughout most of the enhancing tumor, with a mean tumor decrease of 22% (*right column*).

decreases in CBV at 2 weeks were observed in patients with an OS greater than 1 year, whereas patients with increases in tumor CBV were found to have significantly shorter OS. This trial highlights the potential of CBV as a prognostic biomarker of treatment response in recurrent GBM patients, particularly in the context of therapeutic agents targeting angiogenic pathways.

With the increasing use of DSC-MR imaging in clinical trials and routine practice, there is growing interest in the field to standardize image acquisition and postprocessing strategies.[33] Although there is a general consensus on the most robust acquisition strategies (eg, pulse sequence type and parameters, CBV quantification, correction techniques for CA leakage effects), current efforts aim to address the challenges of harmonizing these techniques across MR imaging vendors and data analysis packages.

Dynamic Contrast-Enhanced MR Imaging

DCE-MR imaging acquires heavily T_1-weighted images before, during, and after injection of a CA leading to an increase in signal intensity on T_1-weighted images yielding a time-intensity curve reflecting the delivery and retention of CA within the tissue of interest. DCE-MR imaging is a class of techniques characterized by whether a qualitative, semiquantitative, or quantitative approach is used for data analysis. A qualitative analysis examines the shape (eg, plateau or persistent) of the time-intensity curve,[34,35] while a semi-quantitative analysis provides values such as the area under the curve (AUC), enhancement, time to peak, and wash-in/wash-out slopes.[34,36] A quantitative analysis fits the time-intensity curve to pharmacokinetic models to extract parameters that reflect physiologic characteristics, such as tumor vessel perfusion and permeability and tissue volume fractions.[36] Although applying quantitative models to the DCE-MR imaging data is more complex than qualitative or semiquantitative approaches, the extracted parameters provide (in principle) a more direct measure of vascular characteristics. The Tofts-Kety model is most frequently used and considers the CA distributed between 2 compartments, the blood/plasma space (C_p) and the tissue space (C_t).[37] In 1999, Tofts and colleagues[38] standardized quantitative DCE-MR imaging notation where K^{trans} is the volume transfer constant between C_p and C_t, k_{ep} is the redistribution rate constant between C_t and C_p, and the plasma and tissue volume fractions are denoted as v_p and v_e, respectively.

DCE-MR imaging has played a role in the assessment of anticancer therapies as well as in the prediction of eventual response in a variety of cancers[39–43] (**Fig. 2**). An early report using DCE-MR imaging as a study endpoint in a phase I clinical trial was in 2002 when 5,6-dimethylxanthenone-4-acetic acid was used to treat patients with advanced solid tumors.[44] Despite the small sample size, significant reductions in the AUC were reported in 9 of the 16 patients at 24 hours after the first dose.[44] More recently, DCE-MR imaging was investigated in a phase I trial of patients with prostate cancer treated with cediranib. In most of the patients, Dahut and colleagues[45] observed rapid and sustained reductions in AUC and K^{trans} from baseline up to 2 or more cycles of therapy. In addition, K^{trans} at baseline was associated with progression-free survival, suggesting that DCE-MR imaging may also be a predictive biomarker of clinical outcome.[45] DCE-MR imaging was found to be predictive of pathologic complete response (pCR) in patients with stage II/III breast cancer undergoing neoadjuvant chemotherapy. Li and colleagues[46] found that after one cycle of therapy, k_{ep} predicted pCR with a sensitivity and specificity of 0.83 and 0.65, respectively.

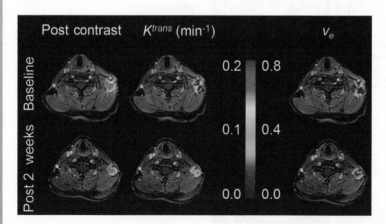

Fig. 2. Representative example of DCE-MR imaging used in a clinical trial investigating the efficacy of a novel PI3K inhibitor in combination with cisplatin. Quantitative MR imaging data were collected at baseline and after 2 weeks of therapy in a patient with metastatic triple-negative breast cancer. Note that there is no appreciable difference in tumor size between imaging time points; however, the decrease in K^{trans} suggests a decrease vascular perfusion and permeability. v_e appears to be unchanged after treatment.

Even with these successes, several limitations of DCE-MR imaging have been identified[41,47,48] emphasizing the need for its systematic evaluation in assessing treatment response and predicting clinical outcomes. Accuracy and precision of the estimated quantitative parameters can be affected by the estimation of the arterial input function, spatial and temporal resolutions, pharmacokinetic models, and curve fitting strategies. On the subject of model fitting, Huang and colleagues[49] were the first to compare 12 DCE-MR imaging software tools in a multicenter data analysis challenge. K^{trans}, k_{ep}, v_e, and v_p from 10 patients before and after the first cycle of neoadjuvant chemotherapy (BAC) were analyzed using site-specific models and algorithms. Although considerable parameter variations were observed, agreement in parameter percentage change was better than that in absolute parameters. Further systematic evaluations assessing reproducibility, evaluating efficacy in a specific patient population and therapy, and finally, expanding into a multicenter study are required. Reproducibility studies are important in order to establish the range outside of which any observed changes would be due to therapy and not measurement error.[50,51] The reproducibility of several semiquantitative and quantitative parameters has been investigated in patients with solid tumors.[51,52] Although there have been some excellent efforts at evaluating semiquantitative DCE-MR imaging in a large multicenter trial (see Ref.[53]), more studies are needed before DCE-MR imaging can be fully used in routine clinical care.

Diffusion-Weighted Imaging

In diffusion-weighted imaging (DWI), the image contrast reflects the distance water molecules can migrate or diffuse from their original spatial position over a short time interval due to random, thermally induced motion (ie, Brownian motion). By acquiring 2 or more images with different degrees of diffusion weighting (obtained by applying the diffusion sensitizing gradients with different amplitudes on successive image acquisitions), an estimate of the amount of molecular water diffusion, termed the apparent diffusion coefficient (ADC), can be calculated at each voxel using the equation

$$S = S_0 \cdot \exp(-b \cdot ADC) \qquad [1]$$

where S is the signal intensity measured with application of a diffusion-sensitizing gradient, S_0 is the signal intensity with no diffusion-sensitizing gradient, and b is a composite variable reflecting various acquisition parameters (including the strength of the gradient pulse, duration of the pulse, and interval between pulses).[54] For a more extensive review of the physics of DWI, the reader is referred to Ref.[55]

Cancers often exhibit significantly reduced ADC values when compared with healthy tissues, a finding typically attributed to the increased cell density of many malignancies.[56] With treatment, intratumoral ADC values typically increase, presumably because of decreases in cell density consequent to apoptosis and cell death, with concomitant disruption of cell membranes, allowing water molecules to diffuse more freely. This basic paradigm—low tumor ADC values before treatment followed by rising tumor ADC values with effective treatment—provides the basic model for DWI as a technique for response assessment (**Fig. 3** for an illustrative example).

One of the potential advantages of DWI for evaluating treatment response over standard response criteria, such as RECIST, is that it is sensitive to changes occurring at the cellular level before changes in gross tumor size. Recent studies have demonstrated changes in ADC after a single cycle of neoadjuvant treatment for breast cancer, and these changes correlate with pathologic outcome.[46,57] Changes in ADC 1 month after transcatheter arterial chemoembolization were predictive of progression-free survival in hepatocellular carcinoma.[58] DWI also provides a means of evaluating the response of antiangiogenic drugs. For example, studies of patients receiving bevacizumab for newly diagnosed[59] and for recurrent glioblastoma[60] both demonstrated that characteristics of the tumor ADC histograms at early time points in treatment may be useful for determining patient outcome.

Even with these promising results, there still remain several challenges that must be overcome before DWI is routinely used in the clinical setting. The standard image acquisition techniques used to acquire DWIs are susceptible to image artifacts.[55] In the ACRIN 6677/RTOG 0625 trial,[61] only 47% of the 123 patients had high-quality diffusion data free of image distortion, and only 68% were considered usable. The complex physiologic factors that affect ADC measurements are also a limitation. It is generally assumed that the measured ADC primarily reflects tumor cellularity; however, there are several biological processes (eg, edema and perfusion) that can affect ADC values. Ellingson and colleagues[61] hypothesized that the increase in ADC they measured in patients who showed early disease progression was an indicator that the drug was not effectively reducing vascular edema rather than a change in tumor cellularity. Data analysis methods must be validated as well. Analyses using mean tumor ADC alone may not be able to predict patient response

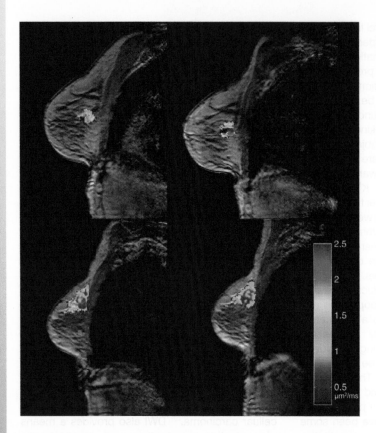

Fig. 3. Changes in ADC in response to neoadjuvant therapy in breast cancer can be measured early in the course of therapy. Shown here are examples of ADC maps acquired before the start of therapy (*left column*) and after one cycle of therapy (*right column*) for a patient who went on to have a pCR (*top row*) and a patient who did not respond (*bottom row*). ADC values are shown in units of μm²/ms.

as well as more advanced analysis methods, such as functional diffusion mapping[57] or multiparametric analyses[46] (see section entitled Multiparameter MR Imaging Methods).

In summary, DWI is a valuable tool for quantitative imaging and treatment assessment, relying only on endogenous contrast mechanisms. It can be applied in a variety of applications and disease sites. Future work includes standardizing protocols, improving image quality, and performing additional multicenter trials.

EMERGING MR IMAGING METHODS FOR CANCER
Chemical Exchange Saturation Transfer MR Imaging

Chemical exchange saturation transfer (CEST) is a technique enabling indirect detection of tissue metabolites via exchangeable protons. The exchangeable protons that resonate at a frequency distinct from bulk water protons are selectively saturated via many off-resonance (with respect to water protons) pulses before imaging.[62] The saturated species are thought to interact with the magnetization of the bulk water through direct chemical exchange, which reduces the observed water signal. Of particular interest for cancer

imaging is the amide proton transfer (APT) metric (**Fig. 4**), reflective of the concentration of amide protons and their exchange rate with the free proton pool.[63] This APT metric has been used to assess physical and physiologic characteristics of the tissue microenvironment, such as temperature, pH, and metabolite concentration.[64–66]

A z-spectrum, which is the measured water signal, $S(\Delta\omega)$, normalized by the signal without saturation (S_0) plotted as a function the offset frequency ($\Delta\omega$) of the saturating irradiation, is used to assess the CEST effects present in a tissue.[67] The z-spectrum is characterized by a symmetric direct saturation around the water frequency ($\Delta\omega = 0$ ppm) and aberrations from this symmetry at the resonances of the exchangeable protons, particularly that due to APT ($\Delta\omega = 3.5$ ppm). These asymmetries are quantified via magnetization transfer ratio (MTR) asymmetry analysis[68] calculated by subtracting the right ($-\Delta\omega$) and left ($\Delta\omega$) signal intensity ratios:

$$MTR_{asym}(\Delta\omega) = MTR(\Delta\omega) - MTR(-\Delta\omega)$$
$$= S_{sat}(-\Delta\omega)/S_0 - S_{sat}(\Delta\omega)/S_0$$
[2]

which can be used to examine the z-spectra asymmetry caused by the APT ($\Delta\omega = 3.5$ ppm), termed APT_{asym}:

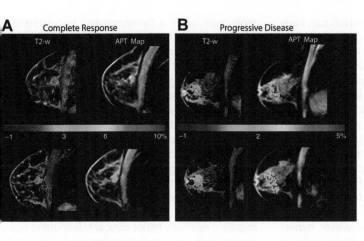

A Complete Response
T2-w APT Map

B Progressive Disease
T2-w APT Map

Fig. 4. The figure displays APT maps in patients with breast cancer who underwent MR imaging examination at 3 T before (*top row*) and after a single cycle (*bottom row*) of neoadjuvant therapy. (*A*) T_2-weighted images on the left and APT maps on the right for a patient who achieved a pCR at the end of therapy. (*B*) Similar results for a patient that had residual disease at the conclusion of neoadjuvant therapy. The mean APT values decreased by 27% for the responder (*A*), whereas this metric increased by 78% for the nonresponder (*B*).

$$APT_{asym} = S_{sat}(-3.5 \text{ ppm})/S_0$$
$$- S_{sat}(3.5 \text{ ppm})/S_0 \qquad [3]$$

The APT_{asym} was initially applied in humans to assess amide proton content (thought to be proportional to mobile protein or peptides[64]) and their exchange rate (thought to be reflective of tissue pH)[64,66,69] in brain tumors at 3 T.[70] This study, as well as those following[71] including migration to 7 T,[72,73] demonstrate that APT_{asym} is increased in glioma relative to surrounding tissue. This increase in APT contrast is hypothesized to be a result of tumor cells accumulating defective proteins at a higher rate than normal while also experiencing alterations in pH due to hypoxia.[74] Contrary to MR spectroscopy (MRS), CEST MR imaging has sufficient sensitivity to allow imaging due to the signal enhancement, which facilitates clinical translation. Preclinical[75] and clinical[70,71] studies indicate the ability to distinguish tumor from edema as well as perform tumor grading.[71,76]

APT_{asym} is a unique contrast offering complementary information to that provided by standard clinical MR imaging measures; however, it is not without limitations. For example, CEST imaging in vivo is a complex technique because of interferences with direct water saturation (spillover effect[77]), the involvement of other exchanging pools,[78] in particular, macromolecular systems (magnetization transfer[79]), and nuclear Overhauser effects.[80] Moreover, there is a strong dependence of the measured effects on the sequence parameters of radiofrequency irradiation for selective saturation, which makes the comparison of results obtained at different laboratories difficult.[81]

Hyperpolarized MR Imaging

MR hyperpolarization technology allows increasing nuclear spin polarization to the order unity (or

100%) significantly above the equilibrium P level; thus, the process of hyperpolarization enables unprecedented MR imaging sensitivity gains by more than 10,000-fold, which is achieved through transient manipulation with the agent molecule. The hyperpolarized substrate molecule can be administered via intravenous injection or inhalation (typically as a bolus) into a living organism.[82] There are multiple biomedical hyperpolarization technologies that have already demonstrated their potential in humans[82,83]: dissolution Dynamic Nuclear Polarization (d-DNP),[84] Parahydrogen Induced Polarization,[85,86] Signal Amplification by Reversible Exchange (SABRE),[87] and Spin Exchange Optical Pumping.[88] The main goal of the hyperpolarization process is to produce a sufficiently large batch of hyperpolarized contrast agent (HCA) with a sufficiently long lifetime (ie, long T_1) for its administration and in vivo distribution and subsequent metabolism. As a result, most HCA include a low-γ heteronucleus (129Xe, 13C, 15N, 3He, etc.) used for hyperpolarization storage and detection,[82] because protons typically have low T_1 values on the order of a few seconds, although there are exceptions when long-lived states of protons are used, such as those in hyperpolarized propane gas.[89,90] HCAs are nonradioactive, and they can report on both uptake and metabolism, because it is possible to discern multiple metabolites and report on their distribution[91] using the difference in chemical shifts[92] or in J-couplings of multiple metabolites.[93] Moreover, HCAs' T_1 and lifetimes are typically within minutes, and therefore, HCAs signals are quickly cleared, and multiple administrations of HCAs can be conducted within the same imaging session. Furthermore, a hyperpolarized MR imaging scan requires only a few seconds.[94,95] In addition, the detection sensitivity of hyperpolarized MR imaging does not depend on B_0 of the main scanner,[96] and high-quality images can be potentially obtained with low-field MR imaging (ie, ≤ 0.3 T), which can have significantly lower costs and greater patient throughput than high-field MR imaging. High-resolution human images were reported at magnetic field strengths of 0.2 T with hyperpolarized 129Xe[97] and 0.007 T with hyperpolarized 3He.[98]

HCAs can be successfully used for quantitative imaging (Box 3). For example, the ratio of injected hyperpolarized 13C-pyruvate to produced 13C-lactate in tumors is correlated with the aggressiveness of prostate cancer,[99] and the hyperpolarized 13C-lactate intensity is correlated with response to treatment.[100] The ratio of injected hyperpolarized bicarbonate and produced hyperpolarized CO_2 can directly report on pH.[101] However, hyperpolarized MR imaging has a major shortcoming in that the actual produced signal is proportional to the product of P and metabolite concentration, and the exact knowledge of the concentration is hindered by the differential T_1 relaxation processes of multiple metabolites (eg, 13C-pyruvate and 13C-lactate pair) in multiple compartments (eg, relaxation in blood and in tumor). These challenges can be potentially overcome with the use of a single metabolite: for example, the use of hyperpolarized 15N-heterocycles produced by d-DNP[102] and SABRE[103] technologies can be used for pH sensing, whereby the chemical shift itself of the molecular probe is highly sensitive to the pH environment,[102] with potential application to cancer imaging, because acidic pH is frequently a property of cancer.[104,105]

Despite the above advantages of hyperpolarized MR imaging, there are 2 major translational barriers. First, the preparation of HCAs requires (frequently expensive) isotopic labeling, and expensive hyperpolarization equipment with relatively low throughput. Second, most HCA

molecules have a heteronuclear hyperpolarized site (eg, 13C or 129Xe) requiring multinuclear MR imaging scanner capability, a feature not widely available on MR imaging scanners. These fundamental challenges can be potentially solved through the use of less expensive hyperpolarization techniques (eg, SABRE vs d-DNP), or through innovation in hyperpolarization hardware,[95] or through the invention of HCAs with long-lived proton sites versus heteronuclear-based HCAs (eg, hyperpolarized 1H-propane vs hyperpolarized 129Xe). Moreover, heteronuclear-based HCAs can also potentially be detected via indirect proton detection[34]; the latter would require a relatively minor clinical MR imaging scanner upgrade and would therefore enable this technology on most clinical MR imaging scanners.

Magnetic Resonance Elastography

The fundamental link between tissue mechanics and disease has led to the development of technologies for quantitative assessment of mechanical stiffness in tissue through noninvasive imaging, termed elastography.[120–127] A primary motivation for the use of elastography in cancer response assessment and prediction is based on direct evidence linking the progression of cancerous tissue to the disruption and concurrent stiffening of the stromal extracellular matrix structural architecture.[128–131] Elevated interstitial fluid pressure within tumors also contributes to observations of elevated stiffness and correlates with cancer progression and therapeutic resistance.[132] Many new cancer therapeutics seek to directly target the abnormal cancer niche,[133] including drugs with specific anti-fibrotic activity.[134] Thus, it is of great import to develop imaging-based methods to provide a noninvasive measure of the mechanical stiffness of the tissue extracellular matrix.

As a general method, elastography involves applying mechanical excitation, imaging the displacement response, and computing spatial estimates of tissue mechanical elasticity. Although first demonstrated using ultrasound,[120] elastography has been applied in many imaging modalities, including MR, CT, and optical imaging. MR elastography (MRE), in particular, allows for quantitative evaluation of tissue mechanical stiffness over a large field of view and deep within the body.[135] Mechanical excitation, either dynamic or quasi-static, is typically applied externally by coupling to an acoustic, piezoelectric, or pneumatic deformation source. In the dynamic case, tissue response to mechanical excitation is typically visualized using phase-contrast imaging and motion-sensitive pulse sequences synchronized to the

---

Box 3
Hyperpolarized contrast agents for quantitative imaging

In less than 20 years,[106] hyperpolarization technologies enabled validation of many HCAs in animal models of human diseases, including the use of 13C-pyruvate,[92,100,107] 13C-lactate,[108] 13C-glucose,[109] 13C-fructose,[110] 13C-succinate,[111] 13C-fumarate,[101] 13C-glutamine[112] in cancer imaging, 13C-bicarbonate[113] for pH imaging, 13C-tetrafluoropropionate[114] for plaque imaging, 129Xe and 3He for lung imaging,[115] 129Xe for brown fat imaging[116] among others.[82,117] Moreover, hyperpolarized 129Xe, 3He, and 13C-pyruvate have already been successfully tested in clinical trials.[94,118,119]

requency of applied excitation.[135] In the quasi-static case, image volumes are acquired before and after the application of mechanical deformation.[136,137] Quantitative estimates of tissue stiffness are then calculated based on the observed tissue displacement and an assumed material constitutive relationship (typically linear elasticity), through direct inversion or biomechanical model-based methods. An example of quasi-static MRE with biomechanical model-based reconstruction of tissue stiffness as applied to breast cancer assessment is shown in **Fig. 5**.

Preliminary applications of MRE in the clinic have been made for assessing hepatic fibrosis and are rapidly emerging as a successful noninvasive image-based alternative to percutaneous tissue biopsy.[126] Although the number of MRE studies in cancer is limited, recent investigations have begun to show promise for the use of MRE in characterization of this disease. For example, Venkatesh and colleagues[138] used MRE to show that mechanical stiffness could differentiate malignant focal liver lesions from benign lesions, normal liver tissue, and fibrotic liver tissue. In this preliminary study, malignant liver lesions were found to be significantly stiffer than benign lesions (10.1 kPa vs 2.7 kPa, $P<.001$) with 100% accuracy. MRE for lesion characterization has

also shown promise in breast[139–141] and prostate[142] cancers. Challenging the simplifying assumptions of linear biomechanical constitutive relationships, Garteiser and colleagues[143] used a viscoelastic mechanical model and extracted estimates of the storage modulus (elasticity component) and the loss modulus (viscous component) and found a significant elevation in the viscous component of the viscoelastic MRE signal in malignant breast tumors as compared with benign breast tumors.

Although MRE has recently shown promise for response assessment in several preclinical cancer studies,[144–146] significantly more work needs to be performed in order to advance MRE for use in clinical therapy response assessment and prediction. Many more patients in this setting must be examined with MRE in order to evaluate the predictive performance. In addition, methodological advancements will be necessary to address the limited spatial resolution and signal quality of traditional MRE examinations. These technical challenges must be overcome for robust longitudinal response assessment for small lesions and within-lesion heterogeneity. Finally, correlations of MRE with histopathology will be important for further understanding of the biological basis of these examinations.

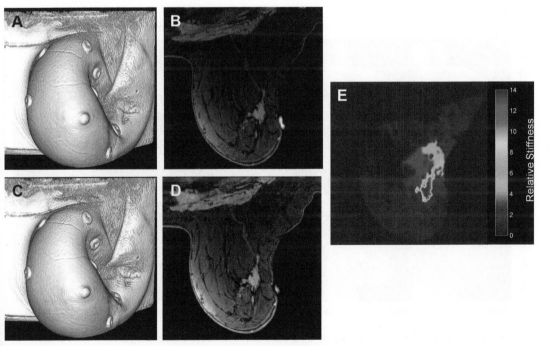

Fig. 5. An example of quasi-static MR elastography in breast cancer. Image volumes and central slice images before (A, B) and after (C, D) the application of an external mechanical deformation are used, along with a biomechanical model, to estimate the tissue mechanical stiffness (E). Cancer is typically revealed to be significantly stiffer than surrounding healthy tissue.

Multiparameter MR Imaging Methods

As indicated above, quantitative MR imaging techniques are playing an increasingly important role in oncology for detecting lesions, monitoring therapy, or predicting treatment response. A relatively new approach to increase the accuracy of tumor identification or prediction of therapy response is to integrate the data available from multiparametric MR imaging. The general hypothesis is that combining the (potentially) complementary information on tumor properties available from multiple MR imaging measures will increase the ability to detect, monitor, and predict outcome. For example, there have been many studies showing that multiparameter MR imaging can achieve this goal in prostate cancer.[147–151] In the study by Turkbey and colleagues,[147] 70 patients with biopsy-proved prostate cancer with a median Gleason score of 7 were imaged by T_2-weighted MR imaging, DCE-MR imaging, and MRS. On T_2-weighted images, the criterion to detect prostate cancer was a well-circumscribed, round-ellipsoid low-intensity lesion. On MRS, the criterion for identifying tumor tissue was a choline-citrate ratio of 3 or greater standard deviations above the mean value of healthy tissue. On DCE-MR imaging, tumor location was evaluated by visual interpretation as well as K^{trans} and k_{ep} parametric maps. The results showed

that the combination of T_2, DCE-MR imaging, and MRS increased the probability of tumor detection from approximately 0.38 (DCE-MR imaging alone) to 0.78 (combining all measures).

There have also been efforts investigating multiparameter MR imaging methods for assessing or predicting the response of breast tumors to neoadjuvant chemotherapy, and several recent publications have demonstrated that combining multiple parameters improves predictive ability.[46,53,152–156] Fig. 6 demonstrates an illustrative example. In the study by Hylton and colleagues,[56] 216 patients with invasive breast cancer of 3 cm or greater were imaged by MR at 4 time points: before NAC, after one cycle of anthracyline-based treatment, between the anthracycline-based regimen and taxane, and after all cycles of NAC. The longest diameter of the primary tumor, tumor volume, signal enhancement ratio at MR imaging, and clinical tumor size was assessed, and changes in each parameter from baseline to each time point were fit to a univariate random-effects logistic regression model to predict pCR and residual cancer burden. A multivariate model was also performed and adjusted for race and age. Higher area under the receiver operating characteristic curve (AUCs) were found for longest diameter and tumor volume than for clinical size at all the time points in the univariate analysis. When all 4 variables were

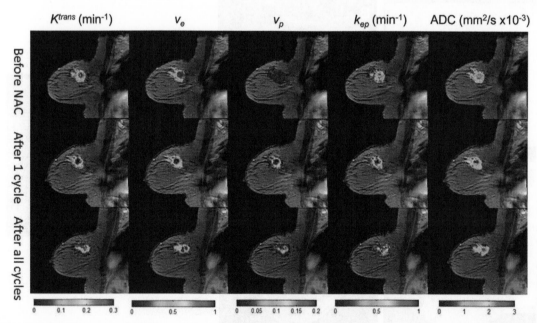

Fig. 6. Parametric maps of K^{trans}, v_e, v_p, k_{ep}, and ADC are displayed before (*top row*), after 1 cycle (*middle row*), and after all cycles (*bottom row*) of neoadjuvant chemotherapy for a patient that had residual tumor burden. It is clear that each one of these maps displays their own spatial variations and report on different aspects of tumor status. Thus, combining them to increase (for example) the predictive value of quantitative MR imaging is a natural line of investigation.

considered in the multivariate analysis, the AUCs for predicting pCR increased to 0.75 and 0.84, at the early time point and before surgery, respectively. Similarly, the AUCs for predicting residual cancer burden also increased to 0.71 and 0.81.

Two relatively new areas of multiparametric imaging include using such data to initialize and constrain predictive mechanistic models of tumor growth and treatment response (see, eg, Ref.[157] and references cited therein), and to relate tumor phenotype to genomic signatures.[158] Both of these approaches have seen much interest in recent years, although with many technical improvements and initial applications in patients. However, much work is required to bring these methods to routine application in clinical trials. More broadly, although multiparametric methods are gaining more attention in oncology, consensus on the optimal practice in image acquisition, data processing, and interpretation has yet to be determined and is an active area of investigation. Indeed, for each of the above MR imaging methods described, the authors have tried to list current shortcomings of the techniques, and these issues are only compounded when 2 (or more) methods are combined.

SUMMARY

Quantitative MR imaging in oncology had undergone enormous advances in the last decade with many techniques now routinely used in clinical trials. Furthermore, there are many methods that are rapidly evolving and have shown early promise in preliminary clinical studies. Going forward, it is imperative that consensus among data acquisition and analysis methods is achieved, and repeatability and reproducibility are established so that quantitative MR imaging can be intelligently applied for particular disease types and therapeutic regimens.

ACKNOWLEDGMENTS

The authors thank the National Institutes of Health, the National Science Foundation, and the Department of Defense for funding through NCI U01CA142565, NCI R25CA092043, NCI U01CA174706, NCI R01CA158079, NCATS KL2 RR024977, NIBIB 1R21EB020323, NSF CHE-1416268, NIH 1R21EB018014, and the DOD CDMRP breast cancer award W81XWH-12-1-0159/BC112431. RGA was funded in part by the Association of University Radiologist's GE Radiology Research Academic Fellowship.

REFERENCES

1. Buckler AJ, Bresolin L, Dunnick NR, et al. A collaborative enterprise for multi-stakeholder participation in the advancement of quantitative imaging. Radiology 2011;258(3):906–14.
2. Rosenkrantz AB, Mendiratta-Lala M, Bartholmai BJ, et al. Clinical utility of quantitative imaging. Acad Radiol 2015;22(1):33–49.
3. Yankeelov TE, Abramson RG, Quarles CC. Quantitative multimodality imaging in cancer research and therapy. Nat Rev Clin Oncol 2014;11(11):670–80.
4. Gore JC, Manning HC, Quarles CC, et al. Magnetic resonance in the era of molecular imaging of cancer. Magn Reson Imaging 2011;29(5):587–600.
5. Wahl RL, Jacene H, Kasamon Y, et al. From RECIST to PERCIST: evolving considerations for pet response criteria in solid tumors. J Nucl Med 2009;50(Suppl 1):122S–50S.
6. Kurland BF, Gerstner ER, Mountz JM, et al. Promise and pitfalls of quantitative imaging in oncology clinical trials. Magn Reson Imaging 2012;30(9):1301–12.
7. Clarke LP, Nordstrom RJ, Zhang H, et al. The quantitative imaging network: NCI's historical perspective and planned goals. Transl Oncol 2014;7(1):1–4.
8. Comis RL, Schnall MD. Opportunities for the ECOG-ACRIN cancer research group within the new National Clinical Trials network. Semin Oncol 2015;42(1):1–3.
9. Micheel C, Ball J, Institute of Medicine (U.S.). Committee on qualification of biomarkers and surrogate endpoints in chronic disease. Evaluation of biomarkers and surrogate endpoints in chronic disease. Washington, DC: National Academies Press; 2010. p. 97–116.
10. Abramson RG, Burton KR, Yu JP, et al. Methods and challenges in quantitative imaging biomarker development. Acad Radiol 2015;22(1):25–32.
11. Raunig DL, McShane LM, Pennello G, et al. Quantitative imaging biomarkers: a review of statistical methods for technical performance assessment. Stat Methods Med Res 2015;24(1):27–67.
12. Shellock FG, Spinazzi A. MRI safety update 2008: part 2, screening patients for MRI. AJR Am J Roentgenol 2008;191(4):1140–9.
13. Abramson RG, McGhee CR, Lakomkin N, et al. Pitfalls in RECIST data extraction for clinical trials: beyond the basics. Acad Radiol 2015;22(6):779–86.
14. Eisenhauer EA, Therasse P, Bogaerts J, et al. New response evaluation criteria in solid tumours: revised RECIST guideline (version 1.1). Eur J Cancer 2009;45(2):228–47.
15. Miller AB, Hoogstraten B, Staquet M, et al. Reporting results of cancer treatment. Cancer 1981;47(1):207–14.
16. Jain RK, Lee JJ, Ng C, et al. Change in tumor size by RECIST correlates linearly with overall survival in phase I oncology studies. J Clin Oncol 2012;30(21):2684–90.
17. Buyse M, Thirion P, Carlson RW, et al. Relation between tumour response to first-line chemotherapy

and survival in advanced colorectal cancer: a meta-analysis. Meta-analysis group in cancer. Lancet 2000;356(9227):373–8.

18. Pazdur R. Response rates, survival, and chemotherapy trials. J Natl Cancer Inst 2000;92(19): 1552–3.

19. Paesmans M, Sculier JP, Libert P, et al. Response to chemotherapy has predictive value for further survival of patients with advanced non-small cell lung cancer: 10 years experience of the European lung cancer working party. Eur J Cancer 1997; 33(14):2326–32.

20. Aronen HJ, Cohen MS, Belliveau JW, et al. Ultrafast imaging of brain tumors. Top Magn Reson Imaging 1993;5(1):14–24.

21. Aronen HJ, Gazit IE, Louis DN, et al. Cerebral blood volume maps of gliomas: comparison with tumor grade and histologic findings. Radiology 1994;191(1):41–51.

22. Ostergaard L, Weisskoff RM, Chesler DA, et al. High resolution measurement of cerebral blood flow using intravascular tracer bolus passages. Part I: mathematical approach and statistical analysis. Magn Reson Med 1996;36(5):715–25.

23. Donahue KM, Krouwer HG, Rand SD, et al. Utility of simultaneously acquired gradient-echo and spin-echo cerebral blood volume and morphology maps in brain tumor patients. Magn Reson Med 2000;43(6):845–53.

24. Schmainda KM, Rand SD, Joseph AM, et al. Characterization of a first-pass gradient-echo spin-echo method to predict brain tumor grade and angiogenesis. AJNR Am J Neuroradiol 2004;25(9):1524–32.

25. Boxerman JL, Schmainda KM, Weisskoff RM. Relative cerebral blood volume maps corrected for contrast agent extravasation significantly correlate with glioma tumor grade, whereas uncorrected maps do not. AJNR Am J Neuroradiol 2006;27(4): 859–67.

26. Law M, Yang S, Wang H, et al. Glioma grading: sensitivity, specificity, and predictive values of perfusion MR imaging and proton MR spectroscopic imaging compared with conventional MR imaging. AJNR Am J Neuroradiol 2003;24(10): 1989–98.

27. Weber MA, Zoubaa S, Schlieter M, et al. Diagnostic performance of spectroscopic and perfusion MRI for distinction of brain tumors. Neurology 2006; 66(12):1899–906.

28. Law M, Oh S, Babb JS, et al. Low-grade gliomas: dynamic susceptibility-weighted contrast-enhanced perfusion MR imaging–prediction of patient clinical response. Radiology 2006;238(2): 658–67.

29. Boxerman JL, Ellingson BM, Jeyapalan S, et al. Longitudinal DSC-MRI for distinguishing tumor recurrence from pseudoprogression in patients with a high-grade glioma. Am J Clin Oncol 2014. [Epub ahead of print].

30. Gahramanov S, Raslan AM, Muldoon LL, et al. Potential for differentiation of pseudoprogression from true tumor progression with dynamic susceptibility-weighted contrast-enhanced magnetic resonance imaging using ferumoxytol vs. gadoteridol: a pilot study. Int J Radiat Oncol Biol Phys 2011;79(2): 514–23.

31. Tsien C, Galban CJ, Chenevert TL, et al. Parametric response map as an imaging biomarker to distinguish progression from pseudoprogression in high-grade glioma. J Clin Oncol 2010;28(13): 2293–9.

32. Schmainda KM, Zhang Z, Prah M, et al. Dynamic susceptibility contrast MRI measures of relative cerebral blood volume as a prognostic marker for overall survival in recurrent glioblastoma: results from the ACRIN 6677/RTOG 0625 multicenter trial. Neuro-oncology 2015;17(8): 1148–56.

33. Welker K, Boxerman J, Kalnin A, et al. ASFNR recommendations for clinical performance of MR dynamic susceptibility contrast perfusion imaging of the brain. AJNR Am J Neuroradiol 2015;36(6): E41–51.

34. Barnes SL, Whisenant JG, Loveless ME, et al. Practical dynamic contrast enhanced MRI in small animal models of cancer: data acquisition, data analysis, and interpretation. Pharmaceutics 2012; 4(3):442–78.

35. Kuhl CK, Mielcareck P, Klaschik S, et al. Dynamic breast MR imaging: are signal intensity time course data useful for differential diagnosis of enhancing lesions? Radiology 1999;211(1):101–10.

36. Yankeelov TE, Gore JC. Dynamic contrast enhanced magnetic resonance imaging in oncology: theory, data acquisition, analysis, and examples. Curr Med Imaging Rev 2009;3(2):91–107.

37. Kety SS. The theory and applications of the exchange of inert gas at the lungs and tissues. Pharmacol Rev 1951;3(1):1–41.

38. Tofts PS, Brix G, Buckley DL, et al. Estimating kinetic parameters from dynamic contrast-enhanced T(1)-weighted MRI of a diffusable tracer: standardized quantities and symbols. J Magn Reson Imaging 1999;10(3):223–32.

39. Padhani AR, Hayes C, Assersohn L, et al. Prediction of clinicopathologic response of breast cancer to primary chemotherapy at contrast-enhanced MR imaging: initial clinical results. Radiology 2006; 239(2):361–74.

40. Johansen R, Jensen LR, Rydland J, et al. Predicting survival and early clinical response to primary chemotherapy for patients with locally advanced breast cancer using DCE-MRI. J Magn Reson Imaging 2009;29(6):1300–7.

41. Hahn OM, Yang C, Medved M, et al. Dynamic contrast-enhanced magnetic resonance imaging pharmacodynamic biomarker study of sorafenib in metastatic renal carcinoma. J Clin Oncol 2008; 26(28):4572–8.

42. Kelly RJ, Rajan A, Force J, et al. Evaluation of KRAS mutations, angiogenic biomarkers, and DCE-MRI in patients with advanced non-small-cell lung cancer receiving sorafenib. Clin Cancer Res 2011;17(5):1190–9.

43. Meyer JM, Perlewitz KS, Hayden JB, et al. Phase I trial of preoperative chemoradiation plus sorafenib for high-risk extremity soft tissue sarcomas with dynamic contrast-enhanced MRI correlates. Clin Cancer Res 2013;19(24):6902–11.

44. Galbraith SM, Rustin GJ, Lodge MA, et al. Effects of 5,6-dimethylxanthenone-4-acetic acid on human tumor microcirculation assessed by dynamic contrast-enhanced magnetic resonance imaging. J Clin Oncol 2002;20(18):3826–40.

45. Dahut WL, Madan RA, Karakunnel JJ, et al. Phase II clinical trial of cediranib in patients with metastatic castration-resistant prostate cancer. BJU Int 2013;111(8):1269–80.

46. Li X, Abramson RG, Arlinghaus LR, et al. Multiparametric magnetic resonance imaging for predicting pathological response after the first cycle of neoadjuvant chemotherapy in breast cancer. Invest Radiol 2015;50(4):195–204.

47. Kim KA, Park MS, Ji HJ, et al. Diffusion and perfusion MRI prediction of progression-free survival in patients with hepatocellular carcinoma treated with concurrent chemoradiotherapy. J Magn Reson Imaging 2014;39(2):286–92.

48. Barnes SL, Quarles CC, Yankeelov TE. Modeling the effect of intra-voxel diffusion of contrast agent on the quantitative analysis of dynamic contrast enhanced magnetic resonance imaging. PLoS One 2014;9(9):e108726.

49. Huang W, Li X, Chen Y, et al. Variations of dynamic contrast-enhanced magnetic resonance imaging in evaluation of breast cancer therapy response: a multicenter data analysis challenge. Transl Oncol 2014;7(1):153–66.

50. Barnes SL, Whisenant JG, Loveless ME, et al. Assessing the reproducibility of dynamic contrast enhanced magnetic resonance imaging in a murine model of breast cancer. Magn Reson Med 2013;69(6):1721–34.

51. Galbraith SM, Lodge MA, Taylor NJ, et al. Reproducibility of dynamic contrast-enhanced MRI in human muscle and tumours: comparison of quantitative and semi-quantitative analysis. NMR Biomed 2002;15(2):132–42.

52. Jackson A, Jayson GC, Li KL, et al. Reproducibility of quantitative dynamic contrast-enhanced MRI in newly presenting glioma. Br J Radiol 2003;76(903):153–62.

53. Hylton NM, Blume JD, Bernreuter WK, et al. Locally advanced breast cancer: MR imaging for prediction of response to neoadjuvant chemotherapy–results from ACRIN 6657/I-SPY TRIAL. Radiology 2012;263(3):663–72.

54. Le Bihan D, Breton E, Lallemand D, et al. MR imaging of intravoxel incoherent motions: application to diffusion and perfusion in neurologic disorders. Radiology 1986;161(2):401–7.

55. Arlinghaus LR, Yankeelov TE. Diffusion-weighted MRI. In: Yankeelov T, Pickens DR, Price RR, editors. Quantitative MRI in cancer, imaging in medical diagnosis and therapy. Boca Raton (FL): CRC Press; 2012. p. 81–97.

56. Charles-Edwards EM, deSouza NM. Diffusion-weighted magnetic resonance imaging and its application to cancer. Cancer Imaging 2006;6: 135–43.

57. Galban CJ, Ma B, Malyarenko D, et al. Multi-site clinical evaluation of DW-MRI as a treatment response metric for breast cancer patients undergoing neoadjuvant chemotherapy. PLoS One 2015;10(3):e0122151.

58. Vandecaveye V, Michielsen K, De Keyzer F, et al. Chemoembolization for hepatocellular carcinoma: 1-month response determined with apparent diffusion coefficient is an independent predictor of outcome. Radiology 2014;270(3):747–57.

59. Wen Q, Jalilian L, Lupo JM, et al. Comparison of ADC metrics and their association with outcome for patients with newly diagnosed glioblastoma being treated with radiation therapy, temozolomide, erlotinib and bevacizumab. J Neurooncol 2015; 121(2):331–9.

60. Pope WB, Qiao XJ, Kim HJ, et al. Apparent diffusion coefficient histogram analysis stratifies progression-free and overall survival in patients with recurrent GBM treated with bevacizumab: a multi-center study. J Neurooncol 2012;108(3):491–8.

61. Ellingson BM, Kim E, Woodworth DC, et al. Diffusion MRI quality control and functional diffusion map results in ACRIN 6677/RTOG 0625: a multi-center, randomized, phase II trial of bevacizumab and chemotherapy in recurrent glioblastoma. Int J Oncol 2015;46(5):1883–92.

62. Wolff SD, Balaban RS. Magnetization transfer contrast (MTC) and tissue water proton relaxation in vivo. Magn Reson Med 1989;10(1):135–44.

63. van Zijl PC, Zhou J, Mori N, et al. Mechanism of magnetization transfer during on-resonance water saturation. A new approach to detect mobile proteins, peptides, and lipids. Magn Reson Med 2003;49(3):440–9.

64. Zhou J, Payen JF, Wilson DA, et al. Using the amide proton signals of intracellular proteins and peptides to detect pH effects in MRI. Nat Med 2003; 9(8):1085–90.

65. Sun PZ, Zhou J, Sun W, et al. Detection of the ischemic penumbra using pH-weighted MRI. J Cereb Blood Flow Metab 2007;27(6):1129–36.

66. Ward KM, Balaban RS. Determination of pH using water protons and chemical exchange dependent saturation transfer (CEST). Magn Reson Med 2000;44(5):799–802.

67. Bryant RG. The dynamics of water-protein interactions. Annu Rev Biophys Biomol Struct 1996;25:29–53.

68. Guivel-Scharen V, Sinnwell T, Wolff SD, et al. Detection of proton chemical exchange between metabolites and water in biological tissues. J Magn Reson 1998;133(1):36–45.

69. Sun PZ, Murata Y, Lu J, et al. Relaxation-compensated fast multislice amide proton transfer (APT) imaging of acute ischemic stroke. Magn Reson Med 2008;59(5):1175–82.

70. Jones CK, Schlosser MJ, van Zijl PC, et al. Amide proton transfer imaging of human brain tumors at 3T. Magn Reson Med 2006;56(3):585–92.

71. Zhou J, Blakeley JO, Hua J. Practical data acquisition method for human brain tumor amide proton transfer (APT) imaging. Magn Reson Med 2008; 60(4):842–9.

72. Jones CK, Polders D, Hua J, et al. In vivo three-dimensional whole-brain pulsed steady-state chemical exchange saturation transfer at 7 T. Magn Reson Med 2012;67(6):1579–89.

73. Mougin OE, Coxon RC, Pitiot A, et al. Magnetization transfer phenomenon in the human brain at 7 T. Neuroimage 2010;49(1):272–81.

74. Salhotra A, Lal B, Laterra J, et al. Amide proton transfer imaging of 9L gliosarcoma and human glioblastoma xenografts. NMR Biomed 2008; 21(5):489–97.

75. Zhou J, Lal B, Wilson DA, et al. Amide proton transfer (APT) contrast for imaging of brain tumors. Magn Reson Med 2003;50(6):1120–6.

76. Wen Z, Hu S, Huang F, et al. MR imaging of high-grade brain tumors using endogenous protein and peptide-based contrast. Neuroimage 2010; 51(2):616–22.

77. Mulkern RV, Williams ML. The general solution to the Bloch equation with constant RF and relaxation terms: application to saturation and slice selection. Med Phys 1993;20(1):5–13.

78. van Zijl PC, Jones CK, Ren J, et al. MRI detection of glycogen in vivo by using chemical exchange saturation transfer imaging (glycoCEST). Proc Natl Acad Sci U S A 2007;104(11):4359–64.

79. Desmond KL, Stanisz GJ. Understanding quantitative pulsed CEST in the presence of MT. Magn Reson Med 2012;67(4):979–90.

80. Li H, Zu Z, Zaiss M, et al. Imaging of amide proton transfer and nuclear Overhauser enhancement in ischemic stroke with corrections for competing effects. NMR Biomed 2015;28(2):200–9.

81. Sun PZ, van Zijl PC, Zhou J. Optimization of the irradiation power in chemical exchange dependent saturation transfer experiments. J Magn Reson 2005;175(2):193–200.

82. Kurhanewicz J, Vigneron DB, Brindle K, et al. Analysis of cancer metabolism by imaging hyperpolarized nuclei: prospects for translation to clinical research. Neoplasia 2011;13(2):81–97.

83. Nikolaou P, Goodson BM, Chekmenev EY. NMR hyperpolarization techniques for biomedicine. Chemistry 2015;21(8):3156–66.

84. Ardenkjaer-Larsen JH, Fridlund B, Gram A, et al. Increase in signal-to-noise ratio of > 10,000 times in liquid-state NMR. Proc Natl Acad Sci U S A 2003;100(18):10158–63.

85. Bowers CR, Weitekamp DP. Transformation of symmetrization order to nuclear-spin magnetization by chemical-reaction and nuclear-magnetic-resonance. Phys Rev Lett 1986;57(21):2645–8.

86. Eisenschmid TC, Kirss RU, Deutsch PP, et al. Para hydrogen induced polarization in hydrogenation reactions. J Am Chem Soc 1987;109(26): 8089–91.

87. Adams RW, Aguilar JA, Atkinson KD, et al. Reversible interactions with para-hydrogen enhance NMR sensitivity by polarization transfer. Science 2009; 323(5922):1708–11.

88. Walker TG, Happer W. Spin-exchange optical pumping of noble-gas nuclei. Rev Mod Phys 1997;69(2):629–42.

89. Kovtunov KV, Truong ML, Barskiy DA, et al. Long-lived spin states for low-field hyperpolarized gas MRI. Chem Eur J 2014;20(45):14629–32.

90. Kovtunov KV, Truong ML, Barskiy DL, et al. Propane-d_6 heterogeneously hyperpolarized by para-hydrogen. J Phys Chem C Nanomater Interfaces 2014;118(48):28234–43.

91. Larson PEZ, Hu S, Lustig M, et al. Fast dynamic 3D MR spectroscopic imaging with compressed sensing and multiband excitation pulses for hyperpolarized C-13 studies. Magn Reson Med 2011; 65(3):610–9.

92. Golman K, in't Zandt R, Thaning M. Real-time metabolic imaging. Proc Natl Acad Sci U S A 2006; 103(30):11270–5.

93. Kennedy BWC, Kettunen MI, Hu D-E, et al. Probing lactate dehydrogenase activity in tumors by measuring hydrogen/deuterium exchange in hyperpolarized L-[1- C-13,U-H-2]lactate. J Am Chem Soc 2012;134(10):4969–77.

94. Mugler JP, Altes TA. Hyperpolarized 129Xe MRI of the human lung. J Magn Reson Imaging 2013; 37(2):313–31.

95. Nikolaou P, Coffey AM, Walkup LL, et al. Near-unity nuclear polarization with an 'open- source' 129Xe hyperpolarizer for NMR and MRI. Proc Natl Acad Sci U S A 2013;110(35):14150–5.

96. Coffey AM, Truong ML, Chekmenev EY. Low-field MRI can be more sensitive than high- field MRI. J Magn Reson 2013;237:169–74.

97. Patz S, Muradian I, Hrovat MI, et al. Human pulmonary imaging and spectroscopy with hyperpolarized Xe-129 at 0.2T. Acad Radiol 2008;15(6): 713–27.

98. Tsai LL, Mair RW, Rosen MS, et al. An open-access, very-low-field MRI system for posture-dependent He-3 human lung imaging. J Magn Reson 2008;193(2):274–85.

99. Lupo JM, Chen AP, Zierhut ML, et al. Analysis of hyperpolarized dynamic C-13 lactate imaging in a transgenic mouse model of prostate cancer. Magn Reson Imaging 2010;28(2):153–62.

100. Day SE, Kettunen MI, Gallagher FA, et al. Detecting tumor response to treatment using hyperpolarized C-13 magnetic resonance imaging and spectroscopy. Nat Med 2007;13(11):1382–7.

101. Gallagher FA, Kettunen MI, Hu DE, et al. Production of hyperpolarized [1,4-C-13(2)]malate from [1,4-C-13(2)]fumarate is a marker of cell necrosis and treatment response in tumors. Proc Natl Acad Sci U S A 2009;106(47):19801–6.

102. Jiang W, Lumata L, Chen W, et al. Hyperpolarized 15N-pyridine derivatives as pH-sensitive MRI agents. Sci Rep 2015;5:9104.

103. Shchepin RV, Truong ML, Theis T, et al. Hyperpolarization of "Neat" liquids by NMR signal amplification by reversible exchange. J Phys Chem Lett 2015;6(10):1961–7.

104. Gatenby RA, Gillies RJ. Why do cancers have high aerobic glycolysis? Nat Rev Cancer 2004;4(11): 891–9.

105. Truong ML, Coffey AM, Shchepin RV, et al. Subsecond proton imaging of 13C hyperpolarized contrast agents in water. Contrast Media Mol Imaging 2014;9(5):333–41.

106. Golman K, Axelsson O, Johannesson H, et al. Parahydrogen-induced polarization in imaging: subsecond C-13 angiography. Magn Reson Med 2001; 46(1):1–5.

107. Park I, Bok R, Ozawa T, et al. Detection of early response to temozolomide treatment in brain tumors using hyperpolarized (13)C MR metabolic imaging. J Magn Reson Imaging 2011;33(6): 1284–90.

108. Chen AP, Kurhanewicz J, Bok R, et al. Feasibility of using hyperpolarized [1-C-13]lactate as a substrate for in vivo metabolic C-13 MRSI studies. Magn Reson Imaging 2008;26(6):721–6.

109. Rodrigues TB, Serrao EM, Kennedy BWC, et al. Magnetic resonance imaging of tumor glycolysis using hyperpolarized 13C-labeled glucose. Nat Med 2014;20(1):93–7.

110. Keshari KR, Wilson DM, Chen AP, et al. Hyperpolarized 2-C-13-fructose: a hemiketal DNP substrate for in vivo metabolic imaging. J Am Chem Soc 2009;131(48):17591–6.

111. Zacharias NM, Chan HR, Sailasuta N, et al. Real-time molecular imaging of tricarboxylic acid cycle metabolism in vivo by hyperpolarized 1-C-13 diethyl succinate. J Am Chem Soc 2012;134(2):934–43.

112. Gallagher FA, Kettunen MI, Day SE, et al. C-13 MR spectroscopy measurements of glutaminase activity in human hepatocellular carcinoma cells using hyperpolarized C-13-labeled glutamine. Magn Reson Med 2008;60(2):253–7.

113. Gallagher FA, Kettunen MI, Day SE, et al. Magnetic resonance imaging of pH in vivo using hyperpolarized C-13-labelled bicarbonate. Nature 2008; 453(7197):940–73.

114. Bhattacharya P, Chekmenev EY, Reynolds WF, et al. Parahydrogen-induced polarization (PHIP) hyperpolarized MR receptor imaging in vivo: a pilot study of 13C imaging of atheroma in mice. NMR Biomed 2011;24(8):1023–8.

115. Patz S, Hersman FW, Muradian I, et al. Hyperpolarized Xe-129 MRI: a viable functional lung imaging modality? Eur J Radiol 2007;64(3):335–44.

116. Branca RT, He T, Zhang L, et al. Detection of brown adipose tissue and thermogenic activity in mice by hyperpolarized xenon MRI. Proc Natl Acad Sci U S A 2014;111(50):18001–6.

117. Brindle KM. Imaging metabolism with hyperpolarized 13C-labeled cell substrates. J Am Chem Soc 2015;137(20):6418–27.

118. Nelson SJ, Kurhanewicz J, Vigneron DB, et al. Metabolic imaging of patients with prostate cancer using hyperpolarized 1-C-13 pyruvate. Sci Transl Med 2013;5(198):198ra108.

119. Conradi MS, Saam BT, Yablonskiy DA, et al. Hyperpolarized He-3 and perfluorocarbon gas diffusion MRI of lungs. Prog Nucl Magn Reson Spectrosc 2006;48(1):63–83.

120. Ophir J, Cespedes I, Ponnekanti H, et al. Elastography—a quantitative method for imaging the elasticity of biological tissues. Ultrason Imaging 1991; 13(2):111–34.

121. Muthupillai R, Lomas DJ, Rossman PJ, et al. Magnetic-resonance elastography by direct visualization of propagating acoustic strain waves. Science 1995;269(5232):1854–7.

122. Rose GH, Dresner MA, Rossman PJ, et al. "Palpation of the brain" using magnetic resonance elastography. Radiology 1998;209P:425.

123. Dresner MA, Rose GH, Rossman PJ, et al. Magnetic resonance elastography of the prostate. Radiology 1998;209P:181.

124. Kallel F, Price RE, Konofagou E, et al. Elastographic imaging of the normal canine prostate in vitro. Ultrason Imaging 1999;21(3):201–15.

125. Sandrin L, Fourquet B, Hasquenoph JM, et al. Transient elastography: a new noninvasive method for

assessment of hepatic fibrosis. Ultrasound Med Biol 2003;29(12):1705–13.

126. Yin M, Talwalkar JA, Glaser KJ, et al. Assessment of hepatic fibrosis with magnetic resonance elastography. Clin Gastroenterol Hepatol 2007;5(10): 1207–13.

127. Barr RG, Destounis S, Lackey LB 2nd, et al. Evaluation of breast lesions using sonographic elasticity imaging: a multicenter trial. J Ultrasound Med 2012;31(2):281–7.

128. Paszek MJ, Weaver VM. The tension mounts: mechanics meets morphogenesis and malignancy. J Mammary Gland Biol Neoplasia 2004;9(4):325–42.

129. Paszek MJ, Zahir N, Johnson KR, et al. Tensional homeostasis and the malignant phenotype. Cancer Cell 2005;8(3):241–54.

130. Paszek MJ, Zahir N, Lakins JN, et al. Mechanosignaling in mammary morphogenesis and tumorigenesis. Mol Biol Cell 2004;15:241A.

131. Huang S, Ingber DE. Cell tension, matrix mechanics, and cancer development. Cancer Cell 2005;8(3):175–6.

132. Jain RK, Martin JD, Stylianopoulos T. The role of mechanical forces in tumor growth and therapy. Annu Rev Biomed Eng 2014;16:321–46.

133. Jain RK. Normalizing tumor microenvironment to treat cancer: bench to bedside to biomarkers. J Clin Oncol 2013;31(17):2205–18.

134. Diop-Frimpong B, Chauhan VP, Krane S, et al. Losartan inhibits collagen I synthesis and improves the distribution and efficacy of nanotherapeutics in tumors. Proc Natl Acad Sci U S A 2011;108(7): 2909–14.

135. Mariappan YK, Glaser KJ, Ehman RL. Magnetic resonance elastography: a review. Clin Anat 2010;23(5):497–511.

136. Miga MI. A new approach to elastography using mutual information and finite elements. Phys Med Biol 2003;48(4):467–80.

137. Weis JA, Miga MI, Arlinghaus LR, et al. A mechanically coupled reaction-diffusion model for predicting the response of breast tumors to neoadjuvant chemotherapy. Phys Med Biol 2013; 58(17):5851–66.

138. Venkatesh SK, Yin M, Glockner JF, et al. MR elastography of liver tumors: preliminary results. AJR Am J Roentgenol 2008;190(6):1534–40.

139. McKnight AL, Kugel JL, Rossman PJ, et al. MR elastography of breast cancer: preliminary results. Am J Roentgenol 2002;178(6):1411–7.

140. Siegmann KC, Xydeas T, Sinkus R, et al. Diagnostic value of MR elastography in addition to contrast-enhanced MR imaging of the breast-initial clinical results. Eur Radiol 2010;20(2): 318–25.

141. Weis JA, Miga MI, Li X, et al. Predicting the response of breast cancer to neoadjuvant

chemotherapy using a mechanically coupled reaction-diffusion model. Cancer Res, in press.

142. Sahebjavaher RS, Nir G, Honarvar M, et al. MR elastography of prostate cancer: quantitative comparison with histopathology and repeatability of methods. NMR Biomed 2015;28(1):124–39.

143. Garteiser P, Doblas S, Daire JL, et al. MR elastography of liver tumours: value of viscoelastic properties for tumour characterisation. Eur Radiol 2012; 22(10):2169–77.

144. Pepin KM, Chen J, Glaser KJ, et al. MR elastography derived shear stiffness–a new imaging biomarker for the assessment of early tumor response to chemotherapy. Magn Reson Med 2014;71(5):1834–40.

145. Li J, Jamin Y, Boult JK, et al. Tumour biomechanical response to the vascular disrupting agent ZD6126 in vivo assessed by magnetic resonance elastography. Br J Cancer 2014;110(7):1727–32.

146. Weis JA, Flint KM, Sanchez V, et al. Assessing the accuracy and reproducibility of modality independent elastography in a murine model of breast cancer. J Med Imaging (Bellingham) 2015;2(3): 036001.

147. Turkbey B, Pinto P, Mani H, et al. Prostate cancer: value of multiparametric MRI Imaging at 3T for detection—histopathologic correlation. Radiology 2012;255:89–99.

148. Turkbey B, Mani H, Shah V, et al. Multiparametric 3T prostate magnetic resonance imaging to detect cancer: histopathological correlation using prostatectomy specimens processed in customized magnetic resonance imaging based molds. J Urol 2011;186:1818–24.

149. Delongchamps N, Rouanne M, Flam T, et al. Multiparametric magnetic resonance imaging for the detection and localization of prostate cancer: combination of T2-weighted, dynamic contrast-enhanced and diffusion-weighted imaging. BJU Int 2010;107:1411–8.

150. Fütterer JJ, Engelbrecht MR, Huisman HJ, et al. Staging prostate cancer with dynamic contrast-enhanced endorectal MR imaging prior to radical prostatectomy: experienced versus less experienced readers. Radiology 2005;237(2): 541–9.

151. Hoeks CMA, Barentsz JO, Hambrock T, et al. Prostate cancer: multiparametric MR imaging for detection, localization, and staging. Radiology 2011;261: 46–66.

152. Yankeelov TE, Lepage M, Chakravarthy A, et al. Integration of quantitative DCEMRI and ADC mapping to monitor treatment response in human breast cancer: initial results. Magn Reson Imaging 2007;25:1–13.

153. Belli P, Costantini M, Ierardi C, et al. Diffusion-weighted imaging in evaluating the response to

neoadjuvant breast cancer treatment. Breast J 2011;17:610–9.

154. Fangberget A, Nilsen LB, Hole KH, et al. Neoadjuvant chemotherapy in breast cancer-response evaluation and prediction of response to treatment using dynamic contrast-enhanced and diffusion-weighted MR imaging. Eur Radiol 2011;21:1188–99.

155. Hahn SY, Ko EY, Han BK, et al. Role of diffusion-weighted imaging as an adjunct to contrast-enhanced breast MRI in evaluating residual breast cancer following neoadjuvant chemotherapy. Eur J Radiol 2014;83:283–8.

156. Jensen LR, Garzon B, Heldahl MG, et al. Diffusion-weighted and dynamic contrast-enhanced MRI in evaluation of early treatment effects during neoadjuvant chemotherapy in breast cancer patients. J Magn Reson Imaging 2011;34:1099–109.

157. Yankeelov TE, Atuegwu N, Hormuth D, et al. Clinically relevant modeling of tumor growth and treatment response. Sci Transl Med 2013;5(187): 187ps9.

158. Colen R, Foster I, Gatenby R, et al. NCI workshop report: clinical and computational requirements for correlating imaging phenotypes with genomics signatures. Transl Oncol 2014;7(5):556–69.

Body Diffusion-weighted MR Imaging in Oncology
Imaging at 3 T

Dow-Mu Koh, MD, MRCP, FRCR[a],*, Jeong-Min Lee, MD[b],
Leonardo Kayat Bittencourt, PhD[c,d],
Matthew Blackledge, PhD[e],
David J. Collins, BA (Hons), CPhys, MinstP[e]

KEYWORDS

- Diffusion MR • Oncology • Cancer • MR Imaging

KEY POINTS

- Advances in hardware and software enable high-quality body diffusion-weighted images to be acquired for oncologic assessment.
- 3.0 T affords improved signal/noise for higher spatial resolution and smaller field-of-view diffusion-weighted imaging (DWI).
- DWI at 3.0 T can be applied as at 1.5 T to improve tumor detection, disease characterization, and the assessment of treatment response.
- DWI at 3.0 T can be acquired on a hybrid PET-MR imaging system, to allow functional MR information to be combined with molecular imaging.

INTRODUCTION

In the past few years, diffusion-weighted imaging (DWI) has become a standard imaging sequence for the evaluation of patients with cancer, especially those on 1.5-Tesla (T) magnetic resonance (MR) systems. This transformation in clinical practice has been brought about by improvements in MR hardware and software, as well as the growing clinical evidence for its use to detect disease, characterize lesions, and assess tumor response to treatment. Furthermore, because the technique is quick to perform, without the need for exogenous contrast administration, it can be routinely deployed for body MR imaging studies without significantly increasing the examination time.

In clinical practice, DWI is largely used as a qualitative tool, although it is a quantitative functional MR imaging technique. Imaging performed at higher diffusion weightings (typically at b-values of 750–1000 s/mm^2 in the body) effectively suppresses the signal from normal background tissue, thus enhancing the conspicuity of cellular disease, which remains high signal intensity. Such qualitative deployment of DWI is widely used in daily practice as a tool to improve tumor detection that may be missed on conventional or contrast-enhanced imaging sequences. However, quantitative DWI is likely to become more important in oncology because these measurements provide objective quantification of water mobility in tissues, which can be applied to aid tissue characterization and

Disclosure: The authors have nothing to disclose.
[a] Department of Radiology, Royal Marsden Hospital, Downs Road, Sutton, SM2 5PT, UK; [b] Department of Radiology, Seoul National University Hospital, Seoul, South Korea; [c] Department of Radiology, Universidade Federal Fluminense, Niterói, Rio de Janeiro, Brazil; [d] CDPI and Multi-Imagem Clinics, Rio de Janeiro, Brazil; [e] Institute of Cancer Research, Sutton, UK
* Corresponding author.
E-mail address: dow-mu.koh@icr.ac.uk

Magn Reson Imaging Clin N Am 24 (2016) 31–44
http://dx.doi.org/10.1016/j.mric.2015.08.007
1064-9689/16/$ – see front matter © 2016 Elsevier Inc. All rights reserved.

mri.theclinics.com

to evaluate tumor response to treatment. There is emerging evidence that quantitative DWI can also yield novel predictive or prognostic information.

The apparent diffusion coefficient (ADC), calculated using 2 or more b-values, remains the most widely used quantitative DWI parameter and has been shown to have good measurement repeatability within and between scanners, particularly at 1.5 T. However, there is widening recognition of the nonmonoexponential signal attenuation at increasing b-values in tissues. Consequently, there is now significant interest in applying nonmonoexponential diffusion models to derive additional quantitative parameters that inform on tissue water diffusivity. These nonmonoexponential diffusion models include intravoxel incoherent motion (IVIM), stretched exponential, and diffusion kurtosis models. To enable these models to be used with confidence, there is a need for meticulous image acquisition using more than 2 b-values, to ensure that images have good signal/noise ratio and to ascertain their measurement repeatability. For example, it has been shown that the perfusion-sensitive parameters of perfusion fraction (f) and pseudodiffusion coefficient (D*) have poor measurement repeatability, particularly in hypovascular lesions, which has limited wider translation of IVIM DWI into everyday clinical practice.

Until recently, DWI performed in the body has been significantly more robust at 1.5 T compared with 3.0 T. Initial experience of the technique in oncology has been largely gained through developments at 1.5 T. However, recent hardware and software innovations have stimulated the development of body DWI at 3.0 T. This article considers the advantages and disadvantages of performing body DWI at 3.0 T, followed by a discussion of the technical implementation of body DWI at 3.0 T in oncology, including whole-body DWI. The current evidence for clinical applications of DWI at 3.0 T for oncologic evaluation is discussed. In addition, the potential of body DWI at 3.0 T combined within a PET-MR hybrid imaging system is highlighted. Knowledge of the basics of DWI and the implementation of the technique for body imaging at 1.5 T is assumed and so this is not discussed. The reader is referred to several review articles published on the subject.[1–3]

BODY DIFFUSION-WEIGHTED IMAGING AT 3.0 TESLA: ADVANTAGES AND DISADVANTAGES

In theory, the measured MR signal is proportional to the square of the static magnetic field, suggesting that there should be a 4-fold increase in signal at 3.0 T compared with at 1.5 T. However, in practice, because of several factors, including changes in tissue relaxation rates and increased magnetic susceptibility in tissues at 3.0 T, the signal gain is usually of the order of 30% to 60%. Furthermore, image noise also scales linearly with the increase in field strength. Nonetheless, the increased image signal/noise at 3.0 T can be harnessed for reduced-field-of-view imaging over specific anatomic locations, such as the prostate, cervix, uterus, pancreas, and breast, as well as the head and neck regions; this can translate to higher spatial resolution DWI of these areas.

The main disadvantages of performing body DWI at 3.0 T are the increased sensitivity to susceptibility artifacts and the higher likelihood of chemical-shift artifacts from poor fat suppression as a consequence of B1 magnetic field inhomogeneity. However, there are now technical implementations that can help to overcome these limitations. Using the readout-segmented echo-planar imaging (EPI) technique, it is possible to reduce the degree of susceptibility artifacts and geometric distortion encountered. In addition, advances in hardware and software shimming (eg, using advanced or image-based shimming options) improves magnetic field homogeneity, leading to more uniform fat suppression across large fields of view, thus reducing the number of poor-quality DWI studies that are degraded by chemical-shift artifacts as a consequence of poor fat suppression. Dual (parallel) radiofrequency transmit systems have reduced the B1 inhomogeneity, which has improved fat suppression at 3.0 T.

Combinatorial chemical and fat-suppression techniques can also be harnessed to advantage at 3.0 T DWI because of the larger differences in the MR precessional frequencies between tissues. For example, when performing DWI in women with silicone breast implants, combining spectral fat suppression technique with a slice-selective gradient reversal scheme allows successful dual suppression of fat and silicone at 3.0 T, which is difficult to achieve at 1.5 T (Fig. 1). In this regard, DWI of the breasts in women with silicone breast implants is more likely to yield meaningful results at 3.0 T compared with at 1.5 T.

TECHNICAL IMPLEMENTATION OF BODY DIFFUSION-WEIGHTED IMAGING AT 3.0 TESLA

Modern state-of-the-art MR systems at 3.0 T have evolved considerably in the past few years with improvement in surface coil technologies, gradient performance, and advanced shimming options. This progress has led to an overall improvement in

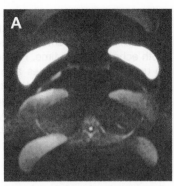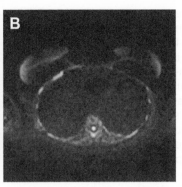

Fig. 1. A 36-year-old woman with bilateral silicone breast implants. (A) DWI at 3.0 T performed using short-tau inversion recovery (STIR) single-shot echo-planar technique. Note that although fat suppression is achieved, ghosting artifacts are seen arising from the high-signal-intensity silicone breast implants. (B) DWI at 3.0 T performed using the combination of STIR fat suppression with slice-selective gradient reversal technique. This combinatorial signal suppression scheme allows both the fat and silicone signals to be effective suppressed.

the quality of body DWI achievable at 3.0 T, including whole-body DWI (WB-DWI).

When performing body DWI at 3.0 T, the guiding principles applicable to imaging at 1.5 T remain important at 3.0 T. Sequence optimization to ensure good image signal/noise and to minimize associated artifacts are paramount in obtaining consistent high-quality images. Important considerations for the optimization of DWI acquisitions are summarized in Table 1. In addition to these general measures, there are specific technical approaches that merit further discussions.

Magnetic Resonance Shimming

Shimming refers to the process of adjusting the homogeneity of the static MR magnetic field. On modern scanners, shimming is both passive and active. Passive shimming is achieved by placing pieces of steel around the superconducting magnetic such that these produce their own magnetic fields, which work in synergy with the main field to improve field homogeneity. Active shimming is effected by adjusting electrical currents through specific shim coils to generate corrective magnetic fields, thus overcoming local field inhomogeneity.

In the past few years, active shimming technologies have become more sophisticated, with advanced higher-order shimming options becoming available on many 3.0-T MR platforms. More recently, individualized image-based shimming has been successfully implemented, which makes use of the measured individual voxel signal intensities to effect field corrections. These

Table 1
General considerations for optimization of DWI protocol

Imaging Parameter	Optimization for DWI
TE	Choose lowest possible TE to maximize signal/noise ratio
Matrix size	Use small matrix size to improve image signal/noise
Field of view	Large field of view improves image signal/noise
Section thickness	Thick image section improves image signal/noise
Fat suppression	Inversion-recovery fat-suppression technique more robust over large fields of view
Diffusion gradient application scheme	Monopolar gradient ensures lowest TE values Bipolar gradients can help to reduce geometric distortions Simultaneous gradient application schemes (eg, 3 scan trace) technique helps to minimize TE
b-Values	Choose b-values appropriate for the tissue of study Ensure sufficient signal averages for good image signal/noise at high b-values
Receiver bandwidth	Optimized receiver bandwidth helps to reduce TE, geometric distortion, and chemical shift artifacts

Abbreviation: TE, echo time.

more sophisticated shimming options are often more time consuming to perform, but can significantly improve the quality of DWI at 3.0 T. Consequently, it is now possible to obtain high-quality diffusion-weighted images, including multistation or whole-body images, using commercial 3.0-T systems (**Fig. 2**). Station-to-station spinal misalignment, which used to be an issue with multistation body DWI at 3.0 T, can largely be averted when advanced shimming techniques are applied.

Reduced-field-of-view Imaging

The increased signal/noise at 3.0 T can be harnessed to obtain high-spatial-resolution diffusion-weighted images, by using smaller fields of view. Reduced-field–of-view DWI has been implemented on all the major MR vendor systems, which use inner-volume excitation, outer-volume signal suppression, or a combination of both techniques to enhance image quality. The technique has been harnessed to advantage, especially on parallel-transmit MR systems, in which two-dimensional–selective parallel-transmit excitation can be used to prescribe a selected field of view for evaluation.

Reduced-field–of-view diffusion-weighted MR techniques have been applied for the evaluation of the breast,[4–6] pancreas, prostate,[7–10] spinal cord,[11–14] peripheral nerves,[15] head/neck

tumors,[16] and the thyroid glands.[17,18] By reducing the number of phase-encoding steps within the smaller imaged volume, it is possible to reduce both echo and scan time. Furthermore, the ability to use shorter echo times also means improved image signal/noise and reduced sensitivity to susceptibility artifacts.[10] Harnessing the dual-source parallel-transmit radiofrequency excitation technique also improves B1 field homogeneity at 3.0 T, thus improving image quality and reducing artifacts.[8,9,19]

Readout-segmented Echo-planar Imaging

Diffusion-weighted MR imaging based on readout-segmented EPI was introduced to reduce geometric distortions, image blurring, and artifacts. Using the readout-segmented technique allows reduction in the echo-train length and echo time, thus improving image blurring, and reducing susceptibility artifacts and geometric distortion.[20] The technique also reduces the sensitivity to motion-induced phase errors. Using this technique allows higher spatial resolution for DWI in the body at field strengths of 3.0 T and beyond,[20–23] and has been successfully applied for the evaluation of tumors in the breast,[4,24–26] kidneys,[27] and the pelvis[28] (**Fig. 3**).

One study compared the use of readout-segmented versus conventional single-shot EPI techniques for evaluating breast cancer, and

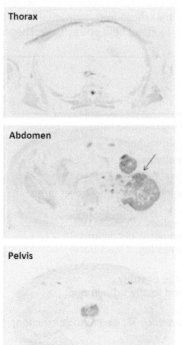

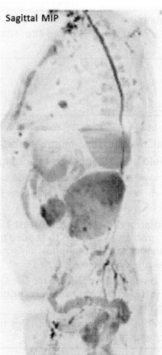

Fig. 2. A 46-year-old man with renal cell carcinoma. Examples of inverted grayscale b = 800s/mm² images acquired axially through the thorax, abdomen, and pelvis. Note the uniform fat suppression using advanced shimming and STIR fat suppression for image acquisition. The left renal tumor (*arrow*) and associated anterior peritoneal deposit show impeded diffusion on the image through the abdomen. The sagittal maximum intensity projection (MIP) shows good spinal alignment.

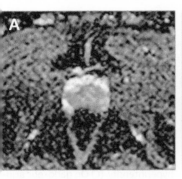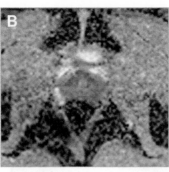

Fig. 3. Readout-segmented EPI DWI. ADC maps obtained using (*A*) conventional single-shot echo-planar DWI and (*B*) readout-segmented EPI DWI using similar imaging parameters. The ADC map obtained using the readout-segmented EPI technique shows less artifacts and geometric distortion compared with that acquired using the conventional EPI technique.

found the readout-segmented technique to be superior for structure distinction, lesion delineation, reduction in ghosting artifact, and overall image quality.[25] Another study compared readout-segmented with reduced-field-of-view DWI for the evaluation of breast cancers at 3.0 T. The image signal/noise, lesion conspicuity, and overall image quality were significantly higher for reduced-field-of-view EPI.[4] Depending on the specific scan parameters used, it may be difficult to generalize these observations. Nonetheless, this study emphasizes the need to optimize image signal/noise when using either the readout-segmented or reduced-field-of-view techniques across the body.

For the evaluation of pelvic tumors at 3.0 T, geometric distortion, imaging blurring, ghosting artifacts, lesion conspicuity, and the overall image quality were significantly better using readout-segmented echo-planar DWI compared with conventional single-shot echo-planar acquisitions.[28] Furthermore, the mean difference and the limits of agreement between the ADC values obtained from the two methods were 0.01 (−0.08, 0.10) × 10^{-3} mm^2/s,[28] suggesting good concordance in the ADC quantification compared with the conventional EPI technique.

CLINICAL APPLICATIONS OF BODY DIFFUSION-WEIGHTED IMAGING FOR ONCOLOGY AT 3.0 TESLA

In general, body DWI is easier to implement at 1.5 T and most clinical applications in oncology can be addressed on 1.5-T MR systems. However, imaging at 3.0 T has continued to improve and high-quality diffusion-weighted images can now be reliably attained at 3.0 T; ADC quantification in the body has also been shown to be reliable and repeatable.[29,30]

Disease Detection

One of the most widely used clinical application for DWI is for the detection of liver metastases. The application of a low–b-value diffusion-weighting effectively suppresses the signal from the intrahepatic vasculature, thus enhancing the detection of focal metastases. Although most liver MR studies are still performed at 1.5 T, imaging at 3.0 T is increasing. Many DWI studies at 1.5 T use a bipolar gradient scheme at image acquisition to optimize image quality. However, one study at 3.0 T found that imaging using a monopolar gradient scheme resulted in better image quality in the liver compared with a bipolar gradient.[31] Nonetheless, imaging optimization at 3.0 T can be challenging and to a significant extent depends on the vendor platform, hardware, and software available. A recent study at 3.0 T showed the value of DWI to confidently diagnose pseudolesions, which are typically invisible on DWI, in patients with liver cirrhosis[32] (**Fig. 4**).

The anatomic site where 3-T imaging has been shown to be of significant advantage compared with 1.5 T is the prostate gland. There is compelling evidence for the use of MR imaging for the detection of prostate cancer in patients with increased serum prostate-specific antigen (PSA) levels,[33] and to help localize disease for image-guided targeted biopsy.[34,35] The higher signal/noise at 3.0 T allows diffusion-weighted images with higher spatial resolution (using reduced-field-of-view or readout-segmented EPI techniques) and also can be used for obtaining images with ultrahigh b-values (≥1000 s/mm^2).

Because of the T2 shine-through from the normal peripheral zone of the prostate gland, the endogenous contrast between tumor and the normal gland may be reduced (at b-values <1000 s/mm^2), making it more difficult to identify disease on these images. However, imaging at 3.0 T affords a higher signal/noise, which allows ultrahigh–b-value images of 1500 to 2000 s/mm^2 to be acquired, thus overcoming the T2 shine-through effects.[36] One study showed that using a b-value of 2000 s/mm^2 improved cancer detection in the prostate gland in the peripheral zone, but

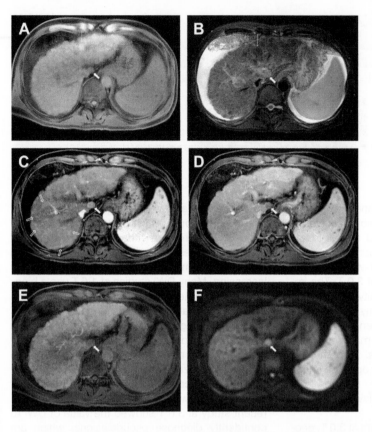

Fig. 4. Pseudolesions in the cirrhotic liver. A 56-year old man with hepatitis B–related liver cirrhosis. (A) Fat-suppressed T1-weighted image shows a hyperintense nodule in segment III (*thin arrow*) and a subtle hypointense nodule in segment I (*thick arrow*). Note surface irregularity of the liver, splenomegaly, and ascites. (B) On fat-suppressed T2-weighted image, the segment III nodule is hypointense and the segment I nodule subtly hyperintensity. (C) On gadoxetic acid–enhanced arterial-phase T1-weighted imaging, there are multiple arterially enhancing lesions in both lobes of the liver (*outline arrows*), including the segment I nodule. (D) In the portal venous phase, only the segment I nodule shows washout. (E) On the 20-minute delayed T1-weighted image, the segment I nodule is hypointense, with all the other arterial enhancing lesions isointense to liver. (F) On DWI with high b-value (b = 800), only the nodule in segment I shows hyperintensity. The lesion in segment I is consistent with a hepatocellular carcinoma. The other transient hypervascular lesions in the liver, which show no increased signal on DWI, are pseudolesions.

was unchanged for the transitional zone.[37] Where acquisition of ultrahigh b-value images may be impractical or noise limited, it may be possible to use computed ultrahigh–b-value images that are mathematically generated from images acquired at lower b-values (typically <1000 s/mm^2) to improve the diagnostic performance[37–39] (Fig. 5). Despite this high sensitivity of DWI for prostate cancer detection, lesions may still be missed. A recent study found that missed lesions at DWI using a b-value of 2000 s/mm^2 were typically small (mean diameter of 5 mm) but may contain a minor

Gleason grade 4 component.[40] In the postradiotherapy setting, DWI was superior to T2-weighted MR imaging for the detection of local disease recurrence in patients presenting with an increasing serum PSA level.[41]

DWI at 3.0 T has been applied to other anatomic sites for cancer detection and/or disease staging, including peritoneal disease,[42,43] renal tumors,[44] lymphoma,[45] gynecologic cancers,[46,47] and bladder tumors.[48] Of these, the application for the detection of peritoneal disease also seems highly promising for the staging of ovarian cancer,

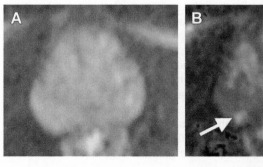
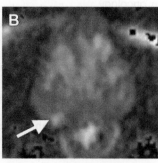

Fig. 5. Computed DWI for prostate cancer detection. A middle-aged man with prostate cancer. (A) DWI image acquired at b-value of 1000 s/mm^2 shows no definite lesion in the peripheral zone, because of T2 shine-through from the normal glandular peripheral zone. (B) Computed b = 2000 s/mm^2 image derived from ADC and images acquired at lower b-values clearly shows a focal lesion in the right peripheral zone (*arrow*).

Disease Characterization

The basis for disease characterization at 3.0 T is similar to that at 1.5 T, relying on the lesion signal on the high–b-value images and/or quantitative DWI parameters (eg, ADC) to discriminate between benign and malignant lesions. However, as at 1.5 T, there can be substantial overlap in the signal intensity appearances and ADC values of benign and malignant tumors. Thus, lesion characterization is best made by using a combination of morphologic imaging with DWI.

In patients with suspected prostate cancers, DWI at 3.0 T can help to characterize focal prostatic lesions as benign or malignant.[49] In one study,[49] the ADC values of malignant tissues were significantly lower than those of benign tissues in both the peripheral zone and the transitional zone, consistent with previous observations at 1.5 T.[50] Threshold cutoff values

of 1.67×10^{-3} mm^2/s in the peripheral zone and 1.61×10^{-3} mm^2/s in the transitional zone showed diagnostic sensitivities/specificities of 94%/91% and 90%/84% respectively for the detection of prostate cancer.[49]

Once a prostate cancer is diagnosed, DWI can inform on the biological aggressiveness of the tumor.[51] Inverse correlations have been shown between the ADC value derived from monoexponential data fitting with that of the Gleeson score[37,52] at 3.0 T. A recent study also found a negative correlation between the ADC value and the Ki-67 proliferative index, which reflects the proliferation rate of the cancer.[53]

As quantitative DWI becomes increasing important, there is interest in moving beyond simple ADC quantification for disease characterization. It is well recognized that the pattern of signal attenuation in tissues is nonexponential, including in prostate cancer. One study explored 4 different DWI signal attenuation models for prostate cancer for images acquired at 3.0 T, including monoexponential fit, biexponential fit, stretched exponential, and diffusion kurtosis models.[54] The study found that, overall, taking into account both measurement repeatability and model fitting, the diffusion kurtosis model resulted in the best fit of the acquired data with good intraclass correlation of the measurement repeatability for b-values up to 2000 s/mm^2.

Although the IVIM diffusion model has been widely explored at 1.5 T, its deployment at 3.0 T has been more limited, in part because of the poor measurement repeatability of the perfusion-sensitive parameters in various body organs. However, there is now considerable interest in exploring another nonmonoexponential diffusion model: the diffusion kurtosis model in prostate cancer,[39,54–56] which requires the acquisition of b-values typically greater than 1500 s/mm^2 for model fitting. Diffusion kurtosis imaging (DKI) results in quantification of diffusion kurtosis (K), which is a measure of the deviation of water diffusion from gaussian free diffusion and may provide unique insights into the behavior of intracellular versus extracellular water (Fig. 7). One study in prostate cancer suggested that the parameter K, derived using DKI, may better discriminate between benign and malignant prostate lesion compared with the monoexponentially derived ADC value.[55] Nonetheless, more research is needed in this area, particularly as to whether DKI may improve the identification of prostate cancer within the transitional zone of the prostate gland, as well as for characterizing tumor biological aggressiveness and the identification of significant prostate cancers.[55,56]

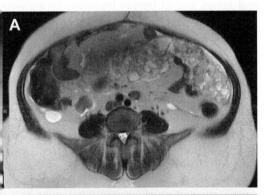

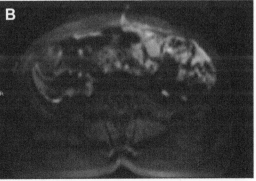

Fig. 6. Detection of peritoneal disease. A 71-year-old woman on follow-up for mucinous tumor of the appendix. (A) T2-weighted MR imaging shows mixed solid and cystic disease within the peritoneal cavity. (B) The extent of disease is well shown on the high (b = 500 s/mm^2) diffusion-weighted image acquired at 3.0 T.

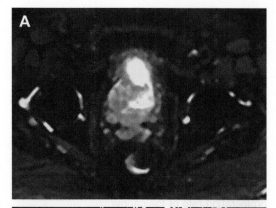

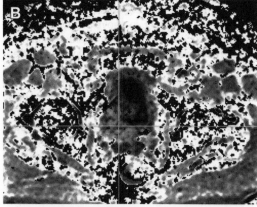

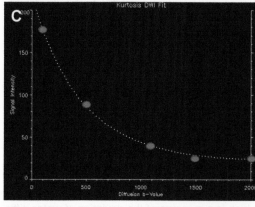

Fig. 7. Diffusion kurtosis. An elderly man with recurrent prostate cancer. (A) The b = 0 s/mm² DWI image shows an irregular mass towards the right bladder base. (B) Diffusion kurtosis map shows increased diffusion kurtosis in the tumor. Cross lines indicate position of (C) signal attenuation curve fitted using the diffusion kurtosis model in the tumor.

DWI at 3.0 T has also been applied for the characterization of tumors at other sites, including the kidneys,[57] peripheral nerve,[58,59] soft tissue, and skeletal lesions.[60] In addition, DKI has been used to provide additional discriminatory information for the characterization of nasopharyngeal carcinomas.[61]

Assessment of Tumor Response to Treatment

The anticipated ADC changes in responders to successful therapy should theoretically be similar at both 1.5 T and 3.0 T. DWI studies at 1.5 T have shown that the ADC values increases in responders to chemotherapy, radiotherapy, embolization treatment, and novel therapeutics.[62] There are currently only a few studies evaluating tumor response to treatment in the body at 3.0 T.[63] One study in rectal cancer[63] showed that there was a significant correlation between tumor volume reduction with the pretreatment ADC value and the change in ADC value after therapy (r = −0.352, r = 0.615). Furthermore, the pretreatment ADC of responders at histopathology was significantly lower than that of nonresponders. The change in ADC value of histopathologic responders was also significantly larger than that of nonresponders.

In a study of prostate cancer treated with radiotherapy,[64] the mean tumor ADC value after therapy was increased compared with the mean ADC value before therapy. After radiotherapy, the mean ADC values of benign peripheral zones and of benign transition zones were also significantly reduced. Before treatment, a significant difference of ADC values between the tumors and benign tissues was found (P<.001), whereas there was no significant difference in the ADC values between them after treatment (P>.1).

The repeatability and reproducibility of ADC measurements have been found to be robust at 1.5 T. A recent body DWI study conducted in healthy volunteers at both 1.5 T and 3.0 T using different MR vendor platforms showed that the measured ADC values of intra-abdominal organs[30] showed no significant differences at 1.5 T or at 3.0 T for any of the anatomic regions evaluated. In terms of measurement repeatability, the highest coefficient of variance (CV) was observed in the liver (CV = 27% in left lobe of the liver) and the lowest within the kidneys (CV = 7% in renal medulla). The ADC variation caused by vendor differences was reportedly 0% to 13.6%.[30] These results indicate that ADC quantification at 3.0 T is robust and the ADC values derived can be used for disease characterization and the assessment of treatment response. Note that for serial follow-up studies, it is still preferable to schedule patients, if possible, on the same MR scanner each time, to minimize ADC variations that can result across imaging platforms so that smaller changes in ADC values may be detected with confidence.

Whole-body Diffusion-weighted Imaging

High-quality multistation diffusion-weighted images of the body, including whole-body images, can now be acquired at 3.0 T. However, depending of the vendor system, careful imaging optimization is still recommended to ensure that the highest image quality is consistently achieved. There is significant interest within the oncologic community in using WB-DWI for the detection of malignancy in the at-risk population, for cancer staging and for the assessment of tumor response to treatment.

One major area of development of WB-DWI is for the assessment of metastatic bone disease. In high-risk patients with prostate and breast cancer, conventional bone scintigraphy is insensitive to disease confirmed to the bone marrow, because the technique is reliant on detecting bone reaction around metastases rather than direct visualization of the tumor. Recent studies have shown that WB-DWI is at least equivalent, if not superior, to skeletal scintigraphy for the detection of metastatic bone disease.[65,66]

Once diagnosed with metastatic bone disease, one of the current major unmet needs in oncologic imaging is the reliable assessment of the response of bone disease to treatment. Bone scintigraphy may erroneously diagnose disease progression as a result of the flare phenomenon, whereas treatment response is often difficult to appreciate by visual assessment of the radionuclide bone scan. Furthermore, bone disease not associated with significant soft tissue is deemed nonmeasurable by RECIST (Response Evaluation Criteria In Solid Tumors) size measurement criteria.[67]

DWI shows substantial promise as potential response biomarkers for bone metastases[68] and other diseases confined to the bone marrow, such as multiple myeloma.[69,70] Studies performed at 1.5 T have shown that ADC increase can be observed in bone metastases from prostate[71,72] and breast cancers[73] in response to hormonal, chemotherapy, or radiotherapy treatment. In addition, the high b-value diffusion-weighted images can be used for tumor segmentation, which enables quantification of the total tumor volume, as well as the associated global ADC value (Fig. 8). These quantities can be used to describe bone response to therapy.[74]

Another evolving application for whole-body DWI is for the evaluation of lymphoma.[75–77] One study of diffuse large B-cell lymphoma at 3.0 T found that the mean ADC value of nodal disease[78] was 0.68×10^{-3} mm^2/s at baseline; which increased by 89% after chemotherapy.

The change in ADC value was significantly correlated with the change in tumor volume ($r = 0.66$). The baseline ADC value also correlated inversely with the percentage change in ADC after treatment ($r = -0.62$).[78] Another study compared the staging of lymphoma at 1.5 T versus 3.0 T[45] and found excellent concordance between the site of nodal disease (intraclass correlation coefficient [ICC] = 0.995), organ involvement (ICC = 0.990), and Ann Arbor stages (kappa = 0.967).

DIFFUSION-WEIGHTED IMAGING ON A HYBRID PET–MR IMAGING SYSTEM

At present, there are 2 commercial whole-body hybrid PET-MR imaging systems, which integrate a 3.0-T MR system with solid-state PET photodetectors to enable synchronous acquisition of MR and PET images. This combination of technologies allows the high sensitivity and high specificity of molecular imaging to be combined with MR imaging, which provides exquisite soft tissue morphology, as well as integrating a range of functional MR imaging techniques (eg, DWI, dynamic contrast-enhanced MR imaging, arterial spin labeling, dynamic susceptibility contrast MR imaging, intrinsic susceptibility MR imaging, magnetization transfer), with each providing specific insight into particular aspects of tumor pathophysiology.

Most PET-MR imaging hybrid systems are currently installed in academic or university departments, where significant local support is often needed to optimize system performance, undertake quality control and assurance procedures, investigate new acquisition protocols, and define its role in clinical pathways and patient management.

Even for practitioners who are accustomed to operating at 3.0 T, translation of DWI onto a PET-MR imaging 3.0-T hybrid system may not be straightforward, because the combination of the two imaging technologies onto a single platform necessitates modifications, which can affect their individual performance. Nonetheless, this is a rapidly developing field and continued research and innovation will in time overcome current shortcomings.

The principles of optimizing image acquisition on a hybrid PET-MR imaging system remain similar to those of conventional MR systems. However, some of the advanced shimming options that are critical for high-quality multistation DWI at 3.0 T are not yet available on the PET-MR imaging system, which may affect the quality and robustness of the images achievable.

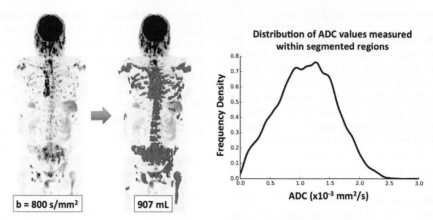

Fig. 8. (*Left*) A maximum intensity projection of whole body diffusion-weighted MR data acquired at a b-value of 800 s/mm². Regions of suspect malignancy are segmented (*center*) using a Markov random field approach resulting in estimation of disease volume (907 mL). The segmented regions are transferred to the ADC maps to determine the distribution of ADC values throughout the skeleton (*right*). Such an approach can be used to assess the response of bone metastases to treatment.

Nonetheless, a study evaluated the stability of ADC measurements on a hybrid PET-MR imaging system with and without simultaneous PET acquisition[79] and found no significant difference in the mean ADC values obtained in the myocardium, paraspinal muscle, liver, kidney, and lymph nodes whether the images were acquired with or without simultaneous PET acquisition, indicating that the ADC measurements were not affected by the synchronous image acquisition schemes.[79]

Using the PET-MR imaging hybrid system allows clinicians to corroborate the functional MR characteristics of tumors with their molecular imaging properties. In one study in patients with recurrent cervical cancer evaluated on a PET-MR imaging system, the maximum standardized uptake value (SUV$_{max}$) of [18F]-fluorodeoxyglucose (FDG) tracer was compared with the contemporaneous ADC values. In primary tumors and associated primary lymph node metastases, there was a significant and strong inverse correlation between SUV$_{max}$ and minimum ADC ($R = -0.692$; $P<.001$), whereas recurrent cancer lesions did not show a significant correlation. Similar observations of an inverse correlation between SUV and ADC values were made in studies of mixed primary cancers,[80] bone metastases,[81] and non–small cell lung cancer.[82] However, several studies failed to show any significant relationship between SUV measurements and the ADC or minimum ADC values.[83,84]

When using a hybrid PET-MR imaging system, it is important to consider how best to combine the individual techniques to their best advantage.

One study evaluated the value of DWI for diagnostic benefit when combined with a whole-body [18F]-FDG-PET–MR imaging protocol.[85] The study showed that all lesions were concordantly detected by [18F]-FDG-PET–MR imaging alone and [18F]-FDG-PET–MR imaging with DWI, suggesting that there is duplicity of information provided by both imaging techniques. In this regard, it may be advantageous to combine DWI with another PET imaging tracer (other than FDG) to maximize the information that can be derived from the PET-MR imaging examination.

The use of a PET-MR imaging system allows a multiparametric multimodal paradigm approach to be evaluated for enhancing patient management (Fig. 9). One of the most promising areas for its application is for the evaluation of primary prostate cancer. Multiparametric MR imaging is now the standard of care for evaluating prostate cancer, often at the higher field strength of 3.0 T. Multiparametric MR imaging shows high diagnostic accuracy for local disease staging, but assessment of nodal disease in high-risk patients remains suboptimal because MR imaging has low diagnostic sensitivity for detecting malignant nonenlarged pelvic lymph nodes. By combining multiparametric MR imaging with a highly specific prostate cancer imaging tracer (eg, prostate-specific membrane antigen), it may be possible to further improve the diagnostic accuracy for nodal disease, thus providing a 1-stop shop for the comprehensive evaluation of prostate cancer.

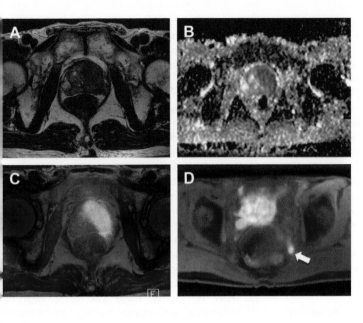

Fig. 9. An 81-year-old man with prostate cancer. (*A*) T2-weighted MR imaging shows the erased charcoal sign within the left prostate gland, in keeping a tumor in the left transitional zone. (*B*) The ADC map returns low ADC values from the same region. (*C*) Fused ^{18}F-choline PET and T2-weighted MR imaging image shows intense tracer uptake in the left transitional zone, which corresponds with the site of tumor. (*D*) The large-field-of-view PET-MR imaging fusion also shows a subcentimeter lymph node (*arrow*) at the left pelvic sidewall showing intense tracer uptake in keeping with nodal involvement. The PET-MR imaging examination provides excellent 1-stop staging of prostate cancer, which helps to overcome the insensitivity of MR imaging for detecting nodal disease in normal-sized lymph nodes.

SUMMARY

In the past decade, body DWI has significantly transformed the evaluation of patients with cancer, such that the technique is now routinely used in many radiological departments to improve diagnostic performance in oncology. Although many DWI examinations are still performed at 1.5 T, technological evolution in the last few years has enabled high-quality body DWI studies at 3.0 T. The imaging technology is now sufficiently mature to be recommended for clinical deployment at 3.0 T. Future use of DWI on a hybrid PET-MR imaging system will see this functional MR imaging technique provide synergistic information toward better understanding of tumor biology and for optimizing patient care in oncology.

ACKNOWLEDGMENT

Acknowledgement is made to the NIHR Biomedical Research Centre at the Royal Marsden Hospital, UK; and to the Cancer Research UK grant C7224/A13407

REFERENCES

1. Koh DM, Blackledge M, Padhani AR, et al. Whole-body diffusion-weighted MRI: tips, tricks, and pitfalls. AJR Am J Roentgenol 2012;199:252–62.
2. Koh DM, Collins DJ. Diffusion-weighted MRI in the body: applications and challenges in oncology. AJR Am J Roentgenol 2007;188:1622–35.
3. Koh DM, Takahara T, Imai Y, et al. Practical aspects of assessing tumors using clinical diffusion-weighted imaging in the body. Magn Reson Med Sci 2008;6:211–24.
4. Park JY, Shin HJ, Shin KC, et al. Comparison of readout segmented echo planar imaging (EPI) and EPI with reduced field-of-view diffusion-weighted imaging at 3t in patients with breast cancer. J Magn Reson Imaging 2015. [Epub ahead of print].
5. Barentsz MW, Taviani V, Chang JM, et al. Assessment of tumor morphology on diffusion-weighted (DWI) breast MRI: diagnostic value of reduced field of view DWI. J Magn Reson Imaging 2015. [Epub ahead of print].
6. Singer L, Wilmes LJ, Saritas EU, et al. High-resolution diffusion-weighted magnetic resonance imaging in patients with locally advanced breast cancer. Acad Radiol 2012;19:526–34.
7. Reischauer C, Wilm BJ, Froehlich JM, et al. High-resolution diffusion tensor imaging of prostate cancer using a reduced FOV technique. Eur J Radiol 2011;80:e34–41.
8. Thierfelder KM, Scherr MK, Notohamiprodjo M, et al. Diffusion-weighted MRI of the prostate: advantages of Zoomed EPI with parallel-transmit-accelerated 2D-selective excitation imaging. Eur Radiol 2014;24:3233–41.
9. Rosenkrantz AB, Chandarana H, Pfeuffer J, et al. Zoomed echo-planar imaging using parallel transmission: impact on image quality of diffusion-weighted imaging of the prostate at 3T. Abdom Imaging 2015;40:120–6.
10. Korn N, Kurhanewicz J, Banerjee S, et al. Reduced-FOV excitation decreases susceptibility artifact in

diffusion-weighted MRI with endorectal coil for prostate cancer detection. Magn Reson Imaging 2015; 33:56–62.

11. Wilm BJ, Svensson J, Henning A, et al. Reduced field-of-view MRI using outer volume suppression for spinal cord diffusion imaging. Magn Reson Med 2007;57:625–30.

12. Saritas EU, Lee D, Cukur T, et al. Hadamard slice encoding for reduced-FOV diffusion-weighted imaging. Magn Reson Med 2014;72:1277–90.

13. Andre JB, Zaharchuk G, Saritas E, et al. Clinical evaluation of reduced field-of-view diffusion-weighted imaging of the cervical and thoracic spine and spinal cord. AJNR Am J Neuroradiol 2012;33: 1860–6.

14. Zaharchuk G, Saritas EU, Andre JB, et al. Reduced field-of-view diffusion imaging of the human spinal cord: comparison with conventional single-shot echo-planar imaging. AJNR Am J Neuroradiol 2011;32:813–20.

15. Budzik JF, Verclytte S, Lefebvre G, et al. Assessment of reduced field of view in diffusion tensor imaging of the lumbar nerve roots at 3 T. Eur Radiol 2013;23: 1361–6.

16. Park JK, Kim SE, Trieman GS, et al. High-resolution diffusion-weighted imaging of neck lymph nodes using 2D-single-shot interleaved multiple inner volume imaging diffusion-weighted echo-planar imaging at 3T. AJNR Am J Neuroradiol 2011;32:1173–7.

17. Lu Y, Hatzoglou V, Banerjee S, et al. Repeatability investigation of reduced field-of-view diffusion-weighted magnetic resonance imaging on thyroid glands. J Comput Assist Tomogr 2015;39:334–9.

18. Taviani V, Nagala S, Priest AN, et al. 3T diffusion-weighted MRI of the thyroid gland with reduced distortion: preliminary results. Br J Radiol 2013;86: 20130022.

19. Rahbar H, Partridge SC, Demartini WB, et al. Improved B1 homogeneity of 3 Tesla breast MRI using dual-source parallel radiofrequency excitation. J Magn Reson Imaging 2012;35:1222–6.

20. Porter DA, Heidemann RM. High resolution diffusion-weighted imaging using readout-segmented echo-planar imaging, parallel imaging and a two-dimensional navigator-based reacquisition. Magn Reson Med 2009;62:468–75.

21. Holdsworth SJ, Skare S, Newbould RD, et al. Readout-segmented EPI for rapid high resolution diffusion imaging at 3 T. Eur J Radiol 2008;65:36–46.

22. Heidemann RM, Porter DA, Anwander A, et al. Diffusion imaging in humans at 7T using readout-segmented EPI and GRAPPA. Magn Reson Med 2010;64:9–14.

23. Holdsworth SJ, Skare S, Newbould RD, et al. Robust GRAPPA-accelerated diffusion-weighted readout-segmented (RS)-EPI. Magn Reson Med 2009;62: 1629–40.

24. Bogner W, Pinker-Domenig K, Bickel H, et al. Readout-segmented echo-planar imaging improves the diagnostic performance of diffusion-weighted MR breast examinations at 3.0 T. Radiology 2012; 263:64–76.

25. Kim YJ, Kim SH, Kang BJ, et al. Readout-segmented echo-planar imaging in diffusion-weighted MR imaging in breast cancer: comparison with single-shot echo-planar imaging in image quality. Korean J Radiol 2014;15:403–10.

26. Bogner W, Pinker K, Zaric O, et al. Bilateral diffusion-weighted MR imaging of breast tumors with submillimeter resolution using readout-segmented echo-planar imaging at 7 T. Radiology 2015;274: 74–84.

27. Friedli I, Crowe LA, Viallon M, et al. Improvement of renal diffusion-weighted magnetic resonance imaging with readout-segmented echo-planar imaging at 3T. Magn Reson Imaging 2015;33(6):701–8.

28. Thian YL, Xie W, Porter DA, et al. Readout-segmented echo-planar imaging for diffusion-weighted imaging in the pelvis at 3T–A feasibility study. Acad Radiol 2014;21:531–7.

29. Malyarenko D, Galban CJ, Londy FJ, et al. Multi-system repeatability and reproducibility of apparent diffusion coefficient measurement using an ice-water phantom. J Magn Reson Imaging 2013; 37(5):1238–46.

30. Donati OF, Chong D, Nanz D, et al. Diffusion-weighted MR imaging of upper abdominal organs: field strength and intervendor variability of apparent diffusion coefficients. Radiology 2014;270:454–63.

31. Azzedine B, Kahina MB, Dimitri P, et al. Whole-body diffusion-weighted MRI for staging lymphoma at 3.0T: comparative study with MR imaging at 1.5T. Clin Imaging 2015;39:104–9.

32. Fayad LM, Blakeley J, Plotkin S, et al. Whole body MRI at 3T with quantitative diffusion weighted imaging and contrast-enhanced sequences for the characterization of peripheral lesions in patients with neurofibromatosis Type 2 and Schwannomatosis. ISRN Radiol 2013;2013:627932.

33. Rosenkrantz AB, Geppert C, Kiritsy M, et al. Diffusion-weighted imaging of the liver: comparison of image quality between monopolar and bipolar acquisition schemes at 3T. Abdom Imaging 2015; 40:289–98.

34. Fruehwald-Pallamar J, Bastati-Huber N, Fakhrai N, et al. Confident non-invasive diagnosis of pseudolesions of the liver using diffusion-weighted imaging at 3T MRI. Eur J Radiol 2012;81:1353–9.

35. Miao H, Fukatsu H, Ishigaki T. Prostate cancer detection with 3-T MRI: comparison of diffusion-weighted and T2-weighted imaging. Eur J Radiol 2007;61:297–302.

36. Park BK, Lee HM, Kim CK, et al. Lesion localization in patients with a previous negative transrectal

ultrasound biopsy and persistently elevated prostate specific antigen level using diffusion-weighted imaging at three Tesla before rebiopsy. Invest Radiol 2008;43:789–93.

37. Kim CK, Park BK, Lee HM, et al. Value of diffusion-weighted imaging for the prediction of prostate cancer location at 3T using a phased-array coil: preliminary results. Invest Radiol 2007;42:842–7.

38. Metens T, Miranda D, Absil J, et al. What is the optimal b value in diffusion-weighted MR imaging to depict prostate cancer at 3T? Eur Radiol 2012; 22:703–9.

39. Kitajima K, Takahashi S, Ueno Y, et al. Clinical utility of apparent diffusion coefficient values obtained using high b-value when diagnosing prostate cancer using 3 tesla MRI: comparison between ultra-high b-value (2000 s/mm^2) and standard high b-value (1000 s/mm^2). J Magn Reson Imaging 2012;36(1): 198–205.

40. Bittencourt LK, Attenberger UI, Lima D, et al. Feasibility study of computed vs measured high b-value (1400 s/mm^2) diffusion-weighted MR images of the prostate. World J Radiol 2014;6:374–80.

41. Grant KB, Agarwal HK, Shih JH, et al. Comparison of calculated and acquired high b value diffusion-weighted imaging in prostate cancer. Abdom Imaging 2015;40:578–86.

42. Barral M, Cornud F, Neuzillet Y, et al. Characteristics of undetected prostate cancer on diffusion-weighted MR Imaging at 3-Tesla with a b-value of 2000 s/mm(2): Imaging-pathologic correlation. Diagn Interv Imaging 2015;96:923–9.

43. Kim CK, Park BK, Lee HM. Prediction of locally recurrent prostate cancer after radiation therapy: incremental value of 3T diffusion-weighted MRI. J Magn Reson Imaging 2009;29:391–7.

44. Iafrate F, Ciolina M, Sammartino P, et al. Peritoneal carcinomatosis: imaging with 64-MDCT and 3T MRI with diffusion-weighted imaging. Abdom Imaging 2012;37:616–27.

45. Michielsen K, Vergote I, Op de Beeck K, et al. Whole-body MRI with diffusion-weighted sequence for staging of patients with suspected ovarian cancer: a clinical feasibility study in comparison to CT and FDG-PET/CT. Eur Radiol 2014;24:889–901.

46. Mirka H, Korcakova E, Kastner J, et al. Diffusion-weighted imaging using 3.0 T MRI as a possible biomarker of renal tumors. Anticancer Res 2015; 35:2351–7.

47. Lin G, Ho KC, Wang JJ, et al. Detection of lymph node metastasis in cervical and uterine cancers by diffusion-weighted magnetic resonance imaging at 3T. J Magn Reson Imaging 2008;28:128–35.

48. Seo JM, Kim CK, Choi D, et al. Endometrial cancer: utility of diffusion-weighted magnetic resonance imaging with background body signal suppression at 3T. J Magn Reson Imaging 2013;37:1151–9.

49. Ohgiya Y, Suyama J, Sai S, et al. Preoperative T staging of urinary bladder cancer: efficacy of stalk detection and diagnostic performance of diffusion-weighted imaging at 3T. Magn Reson Med Sci 2014;13:175–81.

50. Kim CK, Park BK, Han JJ, et al. Diffusion-weighted imaging of the prostate at 3 T for differentiation of malignant and benign tissue in transition and peripheral zones: preliminary results. J Comput Assist Tomogr 2007;31:449–54.

51. Yamamura J, Salomon G, Buchert R, et al. MR imaging of prostate cancer: diffusion weighted imaging and (3D) hydrogen 1 (H) MR spectroscopy in comparison with histology. Radiol Res Pract 2011;2011: 616852.

52. Nagarajan R, Margolis D, Raman S, et al. Correlation of Gleason scores with diffusion-weighted imaging findings of prostate cancer. Adv Urol 2012;2012: 374805.

53. Rosenkrantz AB, Triolo MJ, Melamed J, et al. Whole-lesion apparent diffusion coefficient metrics as a marker of percentage Gleason 4 component within Gleason 7 prostate cancer at radical prostatectomy. J Magn Reson Imaging 2015;41:708–14.

54. Zhang J, Jing H, Han X, et al. Diffusion-weighted imaging of prostate cancer on 3T MR: relationship between apparent diffusion coefficient values and Ki-67 expression. Acad Radiol 2013;20:1535–41.

55. Jambor I, Merisaari H, Taimen P, et al. Evaluation of different mathematical models for diffusion-weighted imaging of normal prostate and prostate cancer using high b-values: a repeatability study. Magn Reson Med 2015;73:1988–98.

56. Rosenkrantz AB, Sigmund EE, Johnson G, et al. Prostate cancer: feasibility and preliminary experience of a diffusional kurtosis model for detection and assessment of aggressiveness of peripheral zone cancer. Radiology 2012;264:126–35.

57. Wang Q, Li H, Yan X, et al. Histogram analysis of diffusion kurtosis magnetic resonance imaging in differentiation of pathologic Gleason grade of prostate cancer. Urol Oncol 2015;33(8):337.e15–24.

58. Sasamori H, Saiki M, Suyama J, et al. Utility of apparent diffusion coefficients in the evaluation of solid renal tumors at 3T. Magn Reson Med Sci 2014;13:89–95.

59. Chhabra A, Thakkar RS, Andreisek G, et al. Anatomic MR imaging and functional diffusion tensor imaging of peripheral nerve tumors and tumorlike conditions. AJNR Am J Neuroradiol 2013; 34:802–7.

60. Ahlawat S, Khandheria P, Subhawong TK, et al. Differentiation of benign and malignant skeletal lesions with quantitative diffusion weighted MRI at 3T. Eur J Radiol 2015;84:1091–7.

61. Yuan J, Yeung DK, Mok GS, et al. Non-Gaussian analysis of diffusion weighted imaging in head and

neck at 3T: a pilot study in patients with nasopharyngeal carcinoma. PLoS One 2014;9:e87024.

62. Padhani AR, Koh DM. Diffusion MR imaging for monitoring of treatment response. Magn Reson Imaging Clin N Am 2011;19:181–209.

63. Jung SH, Heo SH, Kim JW, et al. Predicting response to neoadjuvant chemoradiation therapy in locally advanced rectal cancer: diffusion-weighted 3 Tesla MR imaging. J Magn Reson Imaging 2012;35:110–6.

64. Song I, Kim CK, Park BK, et al. Assessment of response to radiotherapy for prostate cancer: value of diffusion-weighted MRI at 3 T. AJR Am J Roentgenol 2010;194:W477–82.

65. Lecouvet FE, El Mouedden J, Collette L, et al. Can whole-body magnetic resonance imaging with diffusion-weighted imaging replace Tc 99m bone scanning and computed tomography for single-step detection of metastases in patients with high-risk prostate cancer? Eur Urol 2012;62:68–75.

66. Stecco A, Lombardi M, Leva L, et al. Diagnostic accuracy and agreement between whole-body diffusion MRI and bone scintigraphy in detecting bone metastases. Radiol Med 2013;118:465–75.

67. Eisenhauer EA, Therasse P, Bogaerts J, et al. New response evaluation criteria in solid tumours: revised RECIST guideline (version 1.1). Eur J Cancer 2009; 45:228–47.

68. Padhani AR, Makris A, Gall P, et al. Therapy monitoring of skeletal metastases with whole-body diffusion MRI. J Magn Reson Imaging 2014;39:1049–78.

69. Horger M, Weisel K, Horger W, et al. Whole-body diffusion-weighted MRI with apparent diffusion coefficient mapping for early response monitoring in multiple myeloma: preliminary results. AJR Am J Roentgenol 2011;196:W790–5.

70. Giles SL, Messiou C, Collins DJ, et al. Whole-body diffusion-weighted MR imaging for assessment of treatment response in myeloma. Radiology 2014; 271:785–94.

71. Messiou C, Collins DJ, Giles S, et al. Assessing response in bone metastases in prostate cancer with diffusion weighted MRI. Eur Radiol 2011;21: 2169–77.

72. Reischauer C, Froehlich JM, Koh DM, et al. Bone metastases from prostate cancer: assessing treatment response by using diffusion-weighted imaging and functional diffusion maps–initial observations. Radiology 2010;257:523–31.

73. Woolf DK, Padhani AR, Makris A. Assessing response to treatment of bone metastases from breast cancer: what should be the standard of care? Ann Oncol 2015;26(6):1048–57.

74. Blackledge MD, Collins DJ, Tunariu N, et al. Assessment of treatment response by total tumor volume and global apparent diffusion coefficient using diffusion-weighted MRI in patients with metastatic bone disease: a feasibility study. PLoS One 2014; 9:e91779.

75. Lin C, Itti E, Luciani A, et al. Whole-body diffusion-weighted imaging with apparent diffusion coefficient mapping for treatment response assessment in patients with diffuse large B-cell lymphoma: pilot study. Invest Radiol 2011;46:341–9.

76. Montoro J, Laszlo D, Zing NP, et al. Comparison of whole-body diffusion-weighted magnetic resonance and FDG-PET/CT in the assessment of Hodgkin's lymphoma for staging and treatment response. Ecancermedicalscience 2014;8:429.

77. Tsuji K, Kishi S, Tsuchida T, et al. Evaluation of staging and early response to chemotherapy with whole-body diffusion-weighted MRI in malignant lymphoma patients: a comparison with FDG-PET/CT. J Magn Reson Imaging 2015;41(6):1601–7.

78. Wu X, Nerisho S, Dastidar P, et al. Comparison of different MRI sequences in lesion detection and early response evaluation of diffuse large B-cell lymphoma–a whole-body MRI and diffusion-weighted imaging study. NMR Biomed 2013;26:1186–94.

79. Buchbender C, Hartung-Knemeyer V, Heusch P, et al. Does positron emission tomography data acquisition impact simultaneous diffusion-weighted imaging in a whole-body PET/MRI system? Eur J Radiol 2013;82:380–4.

80. Rakheja R, Chandarana H, DeMello L, et al. Correlation between standardized uptake value and apparent diffusion coefficient of neoplastic lesions evaluated with whole-body simultaneous hybrid PET/MRI. AJR Am J Roentgenol 2013;201:1115–9.

81. Wetter A, Lipponer C, Nensa F, et al. Quantitative evaluation of bone metastases from prostate cancer with simultaneous [18F] choline PET/MRI: combined SUV and ADC analysis. Ann Nucl Med 2014;28:405–10.

82. Schaarschmidt BM, Buchbender C, Nensa F, et al. Correlation of the apparent diffusion coefficient (ADC) with the standardized uptake value (SUV) in lymph node metastases of non-small cell lung cancer (NSCLC) patients using hybrid 18F-FDG PET/MRI. PLoS One 2015;10:e0116277.

83. Heacock L, Weissbrot J, Raad R, et al. PET/MRI for the evaluation of patients with lymphoma: initial observations. AJR Am J Roentgenol 2015;204:842–8.

84. Wetter A, Nensa F, Schenck M, et al. Combined PET imaging and diffusion-weighted imaging of intermediate and high-risk primary prostate carcinomas with simultaneous [18F] choline PET/MRI. PLoS One 2014;9:e101571.

85. Buchbender C, Hartung-Knemeyer V, Beiderwellen K, et al. Diffusion-weighted imaging as part of hybrid PET/MRI protocols for whole-body cancer staging: does it benefit lesion detection? Eur J Radiol 2013; 82:877–82.

Assessment of Tumor Angiogenesis
Dynamic Contrast-enhanced MR Imaging and Beyond

Ahmed Salem, MB ChB, FRCR,
James P.B. O'Connor, PhD, FRCR*

KEYWORDS

• Angiogenesis • Biomarker • Clinical trials • DCE-MR imaging • Diagnosis • Quantitative imaging

KEY POINTS

• Dynamic contrast-enhanced (DCE) MR imaging methods track the passage of a contrast agent bolus through tumor microvessels, thus enabling estimation of blood flow, blood volume, and permeability.
• DCE-MR imaging has some limited practical applications in clinical medicine that include screening for disease, lesion localization and characterization, and monitoring response to therapy.
• DCE-MR imaging has a well-established role in go/no-go decision-making tools in early-phase trials of angiogenesis inhibitors.
• Further prospective studies with adequate power are required to determine whether DCE-MR imaging and other imaging techniques have a role as prognostic biomarkers or predictive indicators to specific antiangiogenic therapies.
• Imaging techniques such as DCE-MR imaging have been hampered by a lack of validation and addressing this shortfall is an area of intense current research.

INTRODUCTION

Over the last 30 years there has been much interest in using imaging to identify, quantify, and monitor change in the vascular architecture and function of tumors, particularly in tracking response to antiangiogenic therapy. Although the term angiogenesis dates back to 1971 with the seminal publication by Folkman,[1] initial computed tomography (CT), MR imaging, or PET studies evaluating angiogenesis in preclinical models of cancer and in patients were not published until the late 1980s.[2,3] Following a steady increase in publications to around 200 per year, interest in imaging angiogenesis pathways and therapeutic inhibition was further fueled in the early 2000s, when the modest survival advantage of vascular endothelial growth factor (VEGF) inhibition became clear in renal,[4] colorectal,[5] non–small cell lung,[6] hepatocellular,[7] ovarian,[8] and other cancers. From 2004 until the present date, more than 400 journal articles covering imaging and angiogenesis in cancer have been published yearly and this trend continues to increase.

Imaging studies can probe tumor angiogenesis in various different ways. PET tracers can show

Disclosure: The authors have nothing to disclose.
Cancer Research UK and EPSRC Cancer Imaging Centre, University of Manchester, Oxford Road, Manchester M13 9PT, UK
* Corresponding author. Department of Radiology, The Christie Hospital NHS Trust Wilmslow Road, Withington M20 4BX, UK.
E-mail address: james.o'connor@manchester.ac.uk

Magn Reson Imaging Clin N Am 24 (2016) 45–56
http://dx.doi.org/10.1016/j.mric.2015.08.010
1064-9689/16/$ – see front matter © 2016 Elsevier Inc. All rights reserved.

proof of mechanism by mapping and quantifying the in vivo distribution of drug targets, including VEGF receptors[9] and α_v integrins.[10] Clinical studies have mapped and quantified drug-target interaction for VEGF inhibitors[11] and α_v integrin–targeted agents.[12] This research not only shows proof of mechanism but also helps to map the variation in drug target expression. For example, the uptake of ^{18}F-galacto-RGD peptide ($\alpha_v\beta_3$-selective PET tracer) showed substantial spatial variation between individual patients with breast cancer and also between primary and metastatic lesions in the same individuals.[13] These molecular imaging studies are expensive and limited to specialist centers, but provide clear mechanistic data to facilitate drug development.

In contrast, most studies that image angiogenesis quantify and map aspects of the microenvironment at the phenotypic level, rather than the molecular level.[14,15] These methods are also expensive and require investment of time from both patients and scientists. This article focuses on the role of T_1-weighted dynamic contrast-enhanced (DCE) MR imaging as a method of evaluating tumor angiogenic

signatures and response to therapy in the clinic and in research applications. It summarizes the major strengths and limitations and provides examples, with particular focus on how DCE-MR imaging has altered decision making. The benefits of DCE-MR imaging are then contextualized with other competitor methods (imaging and nonimaging) and the unmet needs and future directions of angiogenesis imaging are discussed.

KEY METHODOLOGICAL DECISIONS

The term DCE-MR imaging represents a family of related methods, all of which image the passage of low-molecular-weight gadolinium-based contrast agents as they traverse the tumor vasculature. All methods require a T_1-weighted sequence to be performed and serial images are collected so that the differences in contrast agent concentration within the tumor can be visually interpreted (qualitative assessment by radiologist) or measured (semiquantitative or truly quantitative assessment by imaging scientists)[15,16] (Fig. 1). In general, scan quality (determined by spatial resolution) is sacrificed for

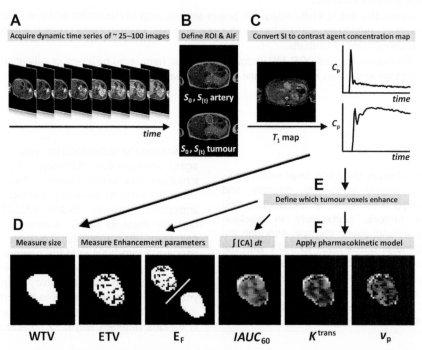

Fig. 1. Overview of DCE-MR imaging data acquisition and analysis. (*A*) Multiple images (approximately 25–100) are acquired before and then after a bolus of gadolinium-based contrast agent (CA) passes through tissue capillaries. (*B*) The region of interest (ROI) for a tumor and the feeding vessel arterial input function (AIF) are defined. (*C*) Signal intensity (SI) values for each voxel are converted into CA concentration by calculating the longitudinal relaxation (T_1) values, to allow plots of contrast agent concentration in plasma (C_p). These steps allow calculation of (*D*) whole-tumor volume (WTV). (*E*) Next, the voxels that enhance are used to calculate enhancing fraction (E_F), from which the $IAUC_{60}$ can be defined. In addition, in (*F*) tracer kinetic models may be applied to derive parameters such as K^{trans} and plasma volume (v_p). ETV, Enhancing tumor volume. (*From* O'Connor JP, Jackson A, Parker GJ, et al. Dynamic contrast-enhanced MRI in clinical trials of antivascular therapies. Nat Rev Clin Oncol 2012;9:169, with permission.)

speed of repeated acquisitions (to enable high temporal resolution, to track passage of the contrast agent bolus), markedly so in the case of quantitative DCE-MR imaging.

DCE-MR imaging data analysis requires several key decision-making steps, which in turn impose requirements on data acquisition strategies. These steps are outlined in detail elsewhere (references are cited later), but key questions are:

1. Will data analysis be based on signal intensity changes only, or will an attempt be made to turn measured signal changes into dynamic alteration in contrast agent concentration? The former approach is used widely in clinical decision making where the overall shape of the enhancement curve may distinguish benign and malignant disease (eg, breast cancer[17]) or where the presence of a hot spot may indicate tumor location (eg, prostate cancer[18]). However, this approach is not useful in therapeutic trials.[19]

2. How will T_1 be mapped? If semiquantitative or quantitative data are required, then signal intensity changes must be converted to dynamic flux in contrast agent concentration. Consensus recommendations require mapping of the T_1 values in a tumor to achieve this.[20] However, several different approaches exist to produce a T_1 map,[21] with differences in their time constraints and accuracy.

3. Will an input function be measured? Some parameters are derived from DCE-MR imaging by applying a tracer kinetic model to describe the relationship between the feeding vessel (usually a large artery, such as aorta, femoral, or carotid, but occasionally a cerebral vein) and the tumor. However, measuring the input function is difficult[22] and so many investigators use either a mathematical approximation[23,24] or an averaged function derived from patient data collected previously.[25]

4. Will a tracer kinetic model be applied to the data? Semiquantitative data may be analyzed by defining a parameter such as uptake slope, or by measuring the area under the enhancement curve at a given time, such as 60 or 90 seconds after contrast agent injection.[26] Alternatively, the data may be modeled to attempt to derive physiologic parameters of varying sophistication. If modeling is used, then there are several different models of increasing complexity that may be applied.[27] Modeling sounds attractive, but requires specialist image analysis software or reliance on vendor packages that may not describe the data appropriately.[28] As models become

increasingly complex they generate more parameters that seem, superficially, to better describe pathophysiologic processes such as flow and permeability, but are increasingly unstable and prone to fit errors.[15,27]

5. Will the tumor be analyzed on a voxel-by-voxel basis? Tumors are biologically heterogeneous and this can be quantified by imaging.[29] There is some evidence that measuring the overall degree of heterogeneity (eg, the histogram distribution of DCE-MR imaging values in glioma[30]) or identifying specific tumor subregions (eg, viable vs necrotic regions in preclinical data[31]) may detect important biological features of tumors that are masked by simple average-value analyses. However, some DCE-MR imaging analyses only measure the median or mean parameter value for a tumor.

Thus, acquisition and analysis approaches vary considerably, not only between clinical and research applications but also between individual hospital institutions and laboratories. This variation has important consequences. Studies may seem to derive equivalent biomarkers, such as the bulk volume transfer coefficient (K^{trans}), but the meaning and numerical value of this parameter varies between studies depending on T_1 mapping, use of input function (or not), model choice, and other factors.[32] This variation has some effect on comparing data from studies in which reductions in parameter are measured (eg, percentage change in K^{trans}). However, lack of method standardization prevents multicentre comparison of raw values of K^{trans} (eg, as a prognostic or predictive test) because a 5-fold difference in parameter value could be caused by methodology differences rather than disease characteristic; this is a stark difference from well-established tests such as systolic blood pressure, full blood count, cancer antigen 125 (CA 125), or echo-derived left ventricular ejection fraction, in which biologically relevant small differences in measurement can be detected between different clinics or laboratories. This issue has limited application of DCE-MR imaging in some aspects of clinical medicine and so standardization and harmonization of parameters such as K^{trans} have become major priorities for imagers, seen within groups such as the Radiological Society of North America sponsored Quantitative Imaging Biomarkers Alliance initiative.[33]

CLINICAL APPLICATIONS

In most clinical applications, DCE-MR imaging is performed in nonspecialist centers and analysis is tailored to describing simple qualitative metrics such as curve shape or rapidity of enhancement and washout. It is rare to perform tracer kinetic modeling in the clinic. Most often, DCE-MR imaging is used to characterize lesions as malignant or not and is used as part of a wider MR imaging examination, including anatomic and other advanced techniques, such as diffusion-weighted imaging (DWI). DCE-MR imaging data interpretation is qualitative and subjective in the clinical setting and reliant on an expert opinion by a highly trained radiologist on a per-patient basis. Two important clinical applications (breast cancer and prostate cancer) are discussed later, but qualitative DCE-MR imaging is also used to solve other clinical questions; for example, in distinguishing benign liver lesions from metastases and in targeting primary brain tumor biopsy sites in some centers.

Imaging Primary Breast Tumors

Breast cancer is the most frequently diagnosed cancer worldwide and is the leading cause of cancer death in women. It accounts for nearly one-quarter of all new cancer cases and accounted for 14% of all cancer deaths in 2008.[34] Most patients with breast cancer undergo triple assessment (clinical, x-ray mammography, and ultrasonography with option of a biopsy) without the need for MR imaging. However, indications for using MR imaging in general and DCE-MR imaging in particular have increased over the last decade.

Technical issues surrounding image acquisition at 1.5 and 3 T are reviewed elsewhere.[17] In brief, breast MR imaging is performed with a dedicated coil, with the patient prone and the breasts lying centrally within the receiver apparatus. This setup is designed to control patient motion, optimize patient comfort, and provide breast support. Typically, three-dimensional DCE-MR imaging sequences are acquired with a temporal resolution of around 20 to 30 seconds, near-isotropic resolution, and excellent uniform fat/water suppression throughout the volume of interest. At 1.5 T some compromise must be made between requirements for acceptable temporal resolution, high spatial resolution, and high signal/noise ratio, but at 3 T these difficulties are largely overcome and it is now routine to acquire high-quality volumetric images through both breasts simultaneously at around 1 volume every 15 seconds.[35]

Many radiologists use simple visual inspection of signal intensity (SI) curves to define enhancement rate and SI curve shape. This work (eg, as reported by Kuhl and colleagues[36]) is simple to perform with a region of interest drawn on a series of images with or without correction for motion. This method has proved extremely useful in distinguishing benign from malignant lesions (Fig. 2) and is still used daily by experienced radiologists in evaluation of breast lesions. Vendor packages offer the option of performing advanced analysis (pharmacokinetic modeling) as well as routine curve analysis.

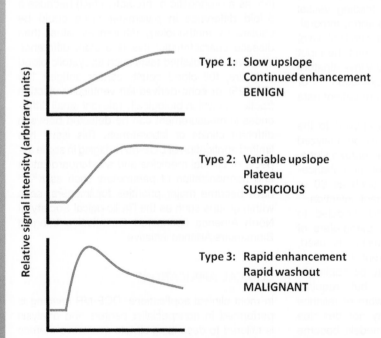

Type 1: Slow upslope
Continued enhancement
BENIGN

Type 2: Variable upslope
Plateau
SUSPICIOUS

Type 3: Rapid enhancement
Rapid washout
MALIGNANT

Relative signal intensity (arbitrary units)

Fig. 2. Example of simple SI curves used to characterize breast lesions. Most (but not all) malignant lesions are characterized by rapid arterial enhancement and rapid washout. These features are used in clinical practice in conjunction with other morphologic MR imaging to determine the index of suspicion for malignancy.

Malignant breast lesion detection with dynamic contrast-enhanced MR imaging

Since the 1990s, DCE-MR imaging has been used to characterize malignant breast lesions. In general terms, malignant lesions were found to have washout of contrast agent after initial rapid enhancement, reflecting greater microvessel density[37] and greater microvascular permeability.[38] Over time, the relative values of various features, such as rim enhancement and lesion spiculation, have been realized and incorporated into scoring systems. The American College of Radiology BI-RADS-MRI Lexicon classification system provides a simple method of reporting likelihood of malignancy in a breast lesion.[39] Multiple studies suggest that the area under the curve for receiver operator characteristic (ROC) curve analysis to distinguish benign from malignant disease is typically 0.8 to 0.9 depending on each study analysis.[40] In practice, most patients still undergo ultrasonography or x-ray mammographic assessment and DCE-MR imaging is reserved for problem solving of cases that remain equivocal. Therefore, the true positive predictive value for this technique as used in clinical practice may be lower than the data discussed earlier imply.

Screening in high-risk populations with dynamic contrast-enhanced MR imaging

Several gene mutations have been identified that predispose women to higher risk of developing breast cancer. Mutations in the BRCA1 and BRCA2 genes result in a cumulative risk of breast cancer by the age of 70 years of 39% to 87% and 26% to 91%, respectively,[41] and in many cases these women develop cancer at an early age. Some rarer gene mutations, such as TP53, also confer high risks, and evidence is growing of further mutations in a range of genes that singly cause a small increase in risk, but may increase breast cancer risk in some women by acting together.[42] These women with increased risk of breast cancer can be identified by performing genetic testing for breast cancer predisposition mutations typically triggered following evaluation of family history. Because many of these patients are young, there is a need for appropriate screening methods[43] for these subpopulations at high risk of developing breast cancer.

X-ray mammography is an effective screening method in the normal population in women in their late 40s and older. It is less effective in younger high-risk women, in whom the higher proportion of breast parenchyma to fat can result in dense mammograms that are hard to interpret. Several large multicentre studies have evaluated the role of DCE-MR imaging in screening for cancers in women with a high genetic risk of breast cancer.[44,45] Results are consistent: DCE-MR imaging is the most sensitive method for detecting cancer in women with strong familial risk of breast cancer, despite the differences in the age range of patients and in the percentage risk for developing breast cancer relative to the normal population required for entry into each study. For example, in the MR Imaging in Breast Cancer Screening (MARIBS) study,[45] a standardized acquisition and analysis approach was used in 22 centers, following training to ensure compliance. Prescriptive analyses were followed, using both morphology (well or poorly defined, spiculation), enhancement pattern (homogeneous, heterogeneous, rimlike), simple quantification of enhancement upslope, and washout pattern (based on the grading system of Kuhl and colleagues[36]). This system allowed lesions to be graded as malignant, suspicious, or benign. This study and other similar studies have shown the sensitivity of DCE-MR imaging to be approximately twice that of x-ray mammography (75%–90% vs 40%). Combined with mammography, DCE-MR imaging has a sensitivity of more than 90%, with a recall rate of around 10%. The additional benefit was largely from detection of small, node-negative tumors. The strength of these results has enabled guidelines to be issued regarding the high-risk groups who may benefit from annual breast screening using DCE-MR imaging.[46]

Dynamic contrast-enhanced MR imaging–based early assessment of response to chemotherapy

Around 5% of patients with breast cancer receive cytotoxic neoadjuvant chemotherapy (NAC). Because approximately one-third respond poorly to this therapy, there is interest in using advanced imaging techniques to identify those patients who are responding to NAC as soon as possible. Several independent studies have reported a statistically significant reduction in K^{trans} or similar parameters in breast cancer at or around 2 completed cycles of therapy in patients treated with a variety of different cytotoxic regimens. These small studies suggest that larger reductions in K^{trans} indicate subsequent favorable response.[47–49] This finding is consistent with preliminary evidence from 62 patients (120 evaluable DCE-MR imaging scans) that suggested that those with persistent higher K^{trans} values after around 2 cycles of treatment with NAC have a significantly worse overall survival compared with those with a lower/reduced K^{trans} value, using multivariate analysis that included other imaging and nonimaging indicators of prognosis.[50] Further studies are required to test whether these findings are repeatable, robust, and can be translated into altered treatment selection and improving outcomes for those patients who show early indicators of poor response to NAC.

Imaging Tumor Foci Within the Prostate Gland

Prostate cancer is a major health concern because there is around 8% cumulative risk of men developing the disease by 75 years of age, making it the second most frequently diagnosed cancer worldwide and accounting for 14% of all cancer deaths.[34] Diagnosis is made by ultrasonography-guided random biopsies, following prostate-specific antigen measurement and digital rectal examination. Nearly all patients then undergo MR imaging for staging assessment. There is considerable variation in MR imaging technique in examining the prostate, particularly in field strength and in the use of body or endorectal coil. Few studies have examined these issues in detail and at present the value of high field strength and use of an endorectal coil have not been proved.[18]

The marked variation seen in prostate DCE-MR imaging, diffusion-weighted, and spectroscopy protocols and their adoption in multiparametric imaging has prompted attempts to define consensus recommendations for use in imaging in prostate cancer.[51] However, these guidelines are not universally accepted.[52] Thus, the value of DCE-MR imaging in assessment of prostate cancer is yet to be fully determined despite the considerable promise shown to date.

Lesion detection and localization with dynamic contrast-enhanced MR imaging

Primary tumors are difficult to identify accurately within the prostate gland using conventional T_1-weighted and T_2-weighted MR imaging. DCE-MR

imaging parameters such as flow are increased in prostate cancer relative to the normal glandular tissue,[53] which has prompted interest in how DCE-MR imaging, DWI, and other techniques might be used to aid prostate cancer diagnosis and monitoring.[18] At present, DCE-MR imaging, along with DWI and MR spectroscopy, are used widely but inconsistently across specialist cancer centers[52] (Fig. 3).

Initial work suggests that DCE-MR imaging may increase detection accuracy in prostate cancer, but this benefit is likely to be as part of a multiparametric approach.[18] There is well-documented and striking spatial heterogeneity across the tumor in functional image parameters such as K^{trans}, making definition of tumor margins difficult.[54] Consequently, the ability of functional techniques to accurately define tumor margins is poor. ROC curve analysis is approximately 0.65 for perfusion-based parameters (similar to DWI).[55] However, combination of DCE-MR imaging, DWI, and anatomic T_1-weighted and T_2-weighted sequences improves sensitivity of cancer detection in the peripheral zone, from around 63% to 80%.[56] In addition, combination of DCE-MR imaging with DWI improves localization accuracy, with a sensitivity of approximately 80% using functional imaging (compared with 70% for anatomic sequences alone),[57] helping to improve local staging.

Targeting biopsy and dose painting with functional imaging

Gleason score (the grading system used in prostate cancer) is a key prognostic determinant in prostate cancer, but has a high sampling error in ultrasonography-guided biopsy.[18] This sampling error can lead to undertreatment and overtreatment

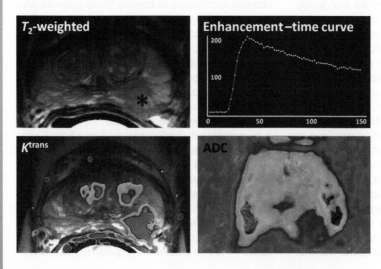

Fig. 3. Multiparametric images in a 62-year-old man with T3a Gleason 4 + 3 prostatic adenocarcinoma. T_2-weighted image shows an ill-defined low-signal nodule in the left peripheral zone (denoted by the asterisk). The DCE-MR imaging enhancement-time curve over the nodule shows rapid enhancement followed by washout, indicating malignancy. K^{trans} and apparent diffusion coefficient (ADC) maps show the tumor extent, with early extracapsular infiltration into surrounding periprostatic fat. (Courtesy of Dr Thomas Hambrock, Department of Radiology, University Medical Center, Nijmegen.)

of lesions assigned an incorrect Gleason score. Initial studies with functional MR imaging have shown correlations between image parameters and Gleason grade at prostatectomy.[58] This work requires further evaluation in large prospective studies to determine specificity, but such methods show promise in targeting tumor biopsy, akin to regional cerebral blood volume mapping used in neuroradiology. Based on a similar principle, the value of DCE-MR imaging, in addition to DWI and spectroscopy, in delineating prostate gross tumor volume is currently being studied in a single-blind randomized phase III trial that is investigating the benefit of an integrated radiotherapy dose painting boost (up to a total dose of 95 Gy) in patients with prostate cancer.[59]

RESEARCH APPLICATIONS

DCE-MR imaging research is a large and growing field, in which the technique is used to quantify vascular characteristics such as blood flow, blood volume, and vessel permeability. DCE-MR imaging parameters are used as biological markers (termed biomarkers) that are objectively measured and evaluated as indicators of normal biological processes, pathogenic processes, or pharmacologic responses to a therapeutic intervention.[60] Biomarkers have multiple uses, including monitoring response once therapy has begun (pharmacologic biomarkers) and predicting response regardless of the specific therapy (prognostic biomarkers) or for a specific given therapy (predictive biomarkers).

Showing Proof of Mechanism with Dynamic Contrast-enhanced MR Imaging

More than 100 studies have used MR imaging–based measurement of tumor perfusion to evaluate drugs with proposed antivascular mechanisms of action.[19] These compounds include anti-VEGF antibodies, tyrosine kinase receptor inhibitors (of VEGF and other growth factors that mediate tumor angiogenesis), and vascular disrupting agents.

Most studies have used T_1-weighted DCE-MR imaging as a method of evaluating perfusion and have calculated either the area under the contrast agent concentration–time curve at 60 seconds ($IAUC_{60}$), or K^{trans}. There is compelling evidence that $IAUC_{60}$, K^{trans}, and related parameters (K_i, k_{ep}, and permeability surface area product) are consistently reduced following administration of several antivascular compounds with proven antivascular mechanisms of action. For example, statistically significant reductions in K^{trans} have been reported in 9 published DCE-MR imaging studies of bevacizumab monotherapy with pooled data from 162 patients[61–69] (eg, the parameter maps shown in **Fig. 4**). This finding is consistent across multiple patient populations, at various time points between 4 hours and 28 days and is congruent with data from CT perfusion studies of bevacizumab-treated patients.[70] These findings support the notion that VEGF blockade causes rapid and sustained antivascular effects that evolve during a single cycle of anti-VEGF therapy.[63] Comparable results have been reported in studies of patients with solid tumors with clinically

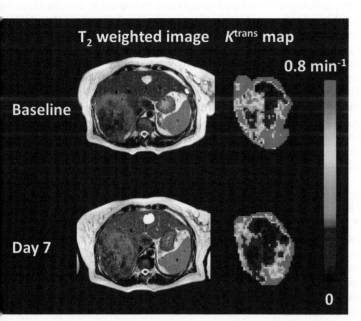

Fig. 4. Baseline anatomic images and K^{trans} maps of a liver metastasis in a patient with colorectal cancer reveal a highly vascular tumor. Substantial antivascular effects are seen after 7 days of therapy with 10 mg/kg of the monoclonal antibody to VEGF, bevacizumab, as indicated by reduction in tumor K^{trans}. (*From* O'Connor JP. Imaging angiogenesis: role in measuring response to treatment. In: Basu B, Biswas S, Pacey S, editors. Clinical insights: antiangiogenesis in cancer therapy. London: Future Medicine, 2014:29–48; with permission.)

effective tyrosine kinase inhibitors, including multiple studies of cediranib,[71–73] sorafenib,[74,75] sunitinib,[76,77] and pazopanib.[78] Consistent reduction in $IAUC_{60}$ or K^{trans} between 4 hours and 5 days has also been reported with the antitubulin agent fosbretabulin.[79–81]

In order for the biomarker to be regarded as a true pharmacologic indicator of drug efficacy, change in the biomarker should be accompanied by change in plasma or tumor drug pharmacokinetics (PK). Vascular response (reduction in $IAUC_{60}$ or K^{trans} from baseline) has been shown to have clear dose-dependent relationship with cediranib,[71] vatalanib,[82] sorafenib,[74] and pazopanib[83] in clinical trials. In many of these and other phase I studies, PK data show that active drug concentrations are reached within individual patients' plasma. The area under the plasma concentration–time curve at a steady state or the maximum drug concentration in the plasma have correlated significantly with change in $IAUC_{60}$ or K^{trans} following cediranib,[71] vatalanib,[82,84,85] pazopanib,[83] and brivanib.[86]

Dynamic Contrast-enhanced MR Imaging as a Decision-making Tool in the Phase I and II Arena

It is important to emphasize that DCE-MR imaging biomarkers can alter decision making in drug development,[87] despite reservations of the oncology and pharmaceutical communities.[88] Parameters derived from DCE-MR imaging can be used to select optimum drug dose and schedule for future studies. In 4 unrelated studies of the antitubulin agent fosbretabulin, vascular response was observed at 45 mg/m² or greater, defining a therapeutic window between the biologically active dose and the clinical maximum tolerated dose of 68 mg/m².[79–81,89] In a study of brivanib[86] that evaluated different dose schedules in multiple cohorts with 12 to 15 patients per cohort, the optimum schedule for subsequent phase II studies was determined using DCE-MR imaging. Statistically significant reductions in $IAUC_{60}$ and K^{trans} were seen with brivanib either 400 mg twice daily or 800 mg once daily in continuous daily dosing, but not with 800 mg intermittent dosing or at lower dose levels.

It is crucial to note that many drugs with little demonstrable clinical benefit show little or no significant reduction in $IAUC_{60}$ or K^{trans}. For example, studies of semaxanib[90] and vandetanib showed negligible reduction in tumor $IAUC_{60}$ or K^{trans} and these drugs were discontinued because of lack of efficacy.[91] However, this significant reduction in biomarkers in active compounds and lack of change in biomarkers in ineffectual compounds

is not seen so clearly in all studies. Reductions in K^{trans} seen in studies of vatalanib[82,84,85] were comparable with those seen with bevacizumab, cediranib, sorafenib, and fosbretabulin, but vatalanib failed to show a survival benefit at phase III testing in colorectal cancer when used in combination with cytotoxic agents.[92] Thus antivascular activity does not guarantee phase III success.[93] Statistically significant change in MR imaging–based perfusion biomarkers seems necessary but does not provide sufficient evidence of clinically significant antivascular efficacy.

In addition, DCE-MR imaging biomarkers have helped make no-go decisions. The antivascular agent ZD6126 disrupts the endothelial tubulin cytoskeleton and causes selective occlusion of the tumor vasculature. This drug had been shown to have antivascular effects that were detected by significant reductions in $IAUC_{60}$ in mouse models of cancer and in patients.[94] At phase I these changes were shown at doses of 56 mg/kg and greater, but these dose levels exceeded the maximum tolerated dose, at which patients developed significant cardiotoxicity.[95] The combination of information on biologically active dose (DCE-MR imaging) and toxicity contributed to the cessation of development of this drug.

Prognostic and Predictive Dynamic Contrast-enhanced MR Imaging Biomarkers: Indicators of Outcome

There is considerable current interest in evaluating how imaging biomarkers may be used to inform clinical outcome irrespective of the treatment prescribed (prognostic indicator) or directly because of a specific therapy (predictive indicator).[96] Both baseline parameters and early PK changes in a parameter have been investigated to this end; for example, as reviewed earlier.

An example is found in studies of anti-VEGF monotherapy in patients with metastatic renal clear cell cancer (RCC), with multiple studies evaluating image biomarkers of tumor vascularity measured both before treatment and between 3 and 12 weeks following therapy. Two independent studies of patients with metastatic RCC treated with sorafenib have reported that high baseline values of K^{trans} were associated with longer progression-free survival (PFS).[74,75] In one of these studies, higher baseline plasma volume was also related to a longer PFS.[74] An equivalent relationship between K^{trans} and PFS has been shown in a study of sunitinib in metastatic RCC.[97] Because K^{trans} is a composite parameter reflecting flow and permeability, it is not possible to determine exactly which biological correlate relates to outcome. In addition, there is evidence that early reduction in perfusion parameters may relate to outcome. K^{trans} reduction following sorafenib therapy has shown a statistically significant relationship to progression in 1 small study[75] but not in another larger study with more tightly controlled imaging protocols.[74]

There is, therefore, some weak evidence that high baseline perfusion and rapid early reduction in perfusion may relate to beneficial outcome following anti-VEGF therapy. Because all of these studies are small and many are retrospective, conclusions from such data have to be interpreted with caution.[96] Further data are required to determine whether these findings are predictive or, more likely, simply prognostic of outcome.

SUMMARY

DCE-MR imaging assessment of tumor angiogenesis has several applications in both routine oncologic practice and in the research arena. In clinical practice, DCE-MR imaging is typically used along with morphologic imaging and DWI. In this context, DCE-MR imaging has already found a role as part of a multiparametric approach to lesion characterization, delineation, and identification of aggressive tumor foci. Research applications, centered on the evaluation of novel antivascular therapies, have driven a desire for parameter quantification using pharmacokinetic modeling and by doing so enable other applications, such as whether baseline values of perfusion are prognostic of outcome, to be applied to clinical data sets, as in breast cancer. However, the role of perfusion MR imaging in prediction and prognosis is still unclear.

ACKNOWLEDGMENTS

The authors are grateful to Dr Thomas Hambrock for supplying the images used in Fig. 3.

REFERENCES

1. Folkman J. Tumor angiogenesis: therapeutic implications. N Engl J Med 1971;285:1182–6.
2. Zagzag D, Goldenberg M, Brem S. Angiogenesis and blood-brain barrier breakdown modulate CT contrast enhancement: an experimental study in a rabbit brain-tumor model. AJR Am J Roentgenol 1989;153:141–6.
3. Kallinowski F, Schlenger KH, Runkel S, et al. Blood flow, metabolism, cellular microenvironment, and growth rate of human tumor xenografts. Cancer Res 1989;49:3759–64.
4. Yang JC, Haworth L, Sherry RM, et al. A randomized trial of bevacizumab, an anti-vascular endothelial growth factor antibody, for metastatic renal cancer. N Engl J Med 2003;349:427–34.
5. Hurwitz H, Fehrenbacher L, Novotny W, et al. Bevacizumab plus irinotecan, fluorouracil, and leucovorin for metastatic colorectal cancer. N Engl J Med 2004; 350:2335–42.
6. Sandler A, Gray R, Perry MC, et al. Paclitaxel-carboplatin alone or with bevacizumab for non-small-cell lung cancer. N Engl J Med 2006;355:2542–50.
7. Llovet JM, Ricci S, Mazzaferro V, et al. Sorafenib in advanced hepatocellular carcinoma. N Engl J Med 2008;359:378–90.
8. Burger RA, Brady MF, Bookman MA, et al. Incorporation of bevacizumab in the primary treatment of ovarian cancer. N Engl J Med 2011;365:2473–83.
9. Chen K, Cai W, Li ZB, et al. Quantitative PET imaging of VEGF receptor expression. Mol Imaging Biol 2009;11:15–22.
10. Chen X, Liu S, Hou Y, et al. MicroPET imaging of breast cancer alphav-integrin expression with 64Cu-labeled dimeric RGD peptides. Mol Imaging Biol 2004;6:350–9.
11. Jayson GC, Zweit J, Jackson A, et al. Molecular imaging and biological evaluation of HuMV833 anti-VEGF antibody: implications for trial design of antiangiogenic antibodies. J Natl Cancer Inst 2002; 94:1484–93.
12. Beer AJ, Haubner R, Goebel M, et al. Biodistribution and pharmacokinetics of the alphavbeta3-selective tracer 18F-galacto-RGD in cancer patients. J Nucl Med 2005;46:1333–41.
13. Beer AJ, Niemeyer M, Carlsen J, et al. Patterns of alphavbeta3 expression in primary and metastatic human breast cancer as shown by 18F-Galacto-RGD PET. J Nucl Med 2008;49:255–9.
14. Gillies RJ, Anderson AR, Gatenby RA, et al. The biology underlying molecular imaging in oncology: from genome to anatome and back again. Clin Radiol 2010;65:517–21.
15. O'Connor JP, Jackson A, Asselin MC, et al. Quantitative imaging biomarkers in the clinical development of targeted therapeutics: current and future perspectives. Lancet Oncol 2008;9:766–76.
16. Padhani AR. Dynamic contrast-enhanced MRI in clinical oncology: current status and future directions. J Magn Reson Imaging 2002;16:407–22.
17. Turnbull LW. Dynamic contrast-enhanced MRI in the diagnosis and management of breast cancer. NMR Biomed 2009;22:28–39.
18. Hoeks CM, Barentsz JO, Hambrock T, et al. Prostate cancer: multiparametric MR imaging for detection, localization, and staging. Radiology 2011;261:46–66.
19. O'Connor JP, Jackson A, Parker GJ, et al. Dynamic contrast-enhanced MRI in clinical trials of antivascular therapies. Nat Rev Clin Oncol 2012;9:167–77.
20. Leach MO, Brindle KM, Evelhoch JL, et al. The assessment of antiangiogenic and antivascular

therapies in early-stage clinical trials using magnetic resonance imaging: issues and recommendations. Br J Cancer 2005;92:1599–610.

21. Fram EK, Herfkens RJ, Johnson GA, et al. Rapid calculation of T1 using variable flip angle gradient refocused imaging. Magn Reson Imaging 1987;5: 201–8.

22. Khalifa F, Soliman A, El-Baz A, et al. Models and methods for analyzing DCE-MRI: a review. Med Phys 2014;41:124301.

23. Weinmann HJ, Laniado M, Mutzel W. Pharmacokinetics of GdDTPA/dimeglumine after intravenous injection into healthy volunteers. Physiol Chem Phys Med NMR 1984;16:167–72.

24. Fritz-Hansen T, Rostrup E, Larsson HB, et al. Measurement of the arterial concentration of Gd-DTPA using MRI: a step toward quantitative perfusion imaging. Magn Reson Med 1996;36:225–31.

25. Parker GJ, Roberts C, Macdonald A, et al. Experimentally-derived functional form for a population-averaged high-temporal-resolution arterial input function for dynamic contrast-enhanced MRI. Magn Reson Med 2006;56:993–1000.

26. Evelhoch JL. Key factors in the acquisition of contrast kinetic data for oncology. J Magn Reson Imaging 1999;10:254–9.

27. Sourbron SP, Buckley DL. Tracer kinetic modelling in MRI: estimating perfusion and capillary permeability. Phys Med Biol 2012;57:R1–33.

28. Buckley DL. Are measurements from two commercial software packages interchangeable? Possibly, if like is compared with like. Radiology 2008;246:642.

29. O'Connor JP, Rose CJ, Waterton JC, et al. Imaging intratumor heterogeneity: role in therapy response, resistance, and clinical outcome. Clin Cancer Res 2015;21:249–57.

30. Tofts PS, Benton CE, Weil RS, et al. Quantitative analysis of whole-tumor Gd enhancement histograms predicts malignant transformation in low-grade gliomas. J Magn Reson Imaging 2007;25: 208–14.

31. Berry LR, Barck KH, Go MA, et al. Quantification of viable tumor microvascular characteristics by multispectral analysis. Magn Reson Med 2008;60:64–72.

32. Sourbron SP, Buckley DL. On the scope and interpretation of the Tofts models for DCE-MRI. Magn Reson Med 2011;66:735–45.

33. Buckler AJ, Bresolin L, Dunnick NR, et al. A collaborative enterprise for multi-stakeholder participation in the advancement of quantitative imaging. Radiology 2011;258:906–14.

34. Jemal A, Bray F, Center MM, et al. Global cancer statistics. CA Cancer J Clin 2011;61:69–90.

35. Henderson E, Rutt BK, Lee TY. Temporal sampling requirements for the tracer kinetics modeling of breast disease. Magn Reson Imaging 1998;16: 1057–73.

36. Kuhl CK, Mielcareck P, Klaschik S, et al. Dynamic breast MR imaging: are signal intensity time course data useful for differential diagnosis of enhancing lesions? Radiology 1999;211:101–10.

37. Buckley DL, Drew PJ, Mussurakis S, et al. Microvessel density of invasive breast cancer assessed by dynamic Gd-DTPA enhanced MRI. J Magn Reson Imaging 1997;7:461–4.

38. Knopp MV, Weiss E, Sinn HP, et al. Pathophysiologic basis of contrast enhancement in breast tumors. J Magn Reson Imaging 1999;10:260–6.

39. Erguvan-Dogan B, Whitman GJ, Kushwaha AC, et al. BI-RADS-MRI: a primer. AJR Am J Roentgenol 2006;187:W152–60.

40. El Khouli RH, Macura KJ, Jacobs MA, et al. Dynamic contrast-enhanced MRI of the breast: quantitative method for kinetic curve type assessment. AJR Am J Roentgenol 2009;193:W295–300.

41. Robson M, Offit K. Clinical practice. Management of an inherited predisposition to breast cancer. N Engl J Med 2007;357:154–62.

42. Easton DF, Pooley KA, Dunning AM, et al. Genome-wide association study identifies novel breast cancer susceptibility loci. Nature 2007;447:1087–93.

43. Leach MO. Breast cancer screening in women at high risk using MRI. NMR Biomed 2009;22:17–27.

44. Kriege M, Brekelmans CT, Boetes C, et al. Efficacy of MRI and mammography for breast-cancer screening in women with a familial or genetic predisposition. N Engl J Med 2004;351:427–37.

45. Leach MO, Boggis CR, Dixon AK, et al. Screening with magnetic resonance imaging and mammography of a UK population at high familial risk of breast cancer: a prospective multicentre cohort study (MARIBS). Lancet 2005;365:1769–78.

46. National Institute for Clinical Excellence. Familial breast cancer: classification and care of people at risk of familial breast cancer and management of breast cancer and related risks in people with a family history of breast cancer. London: National Institute for Clinical Excellence; 2013. Available at: http://www.nice.org.uk/guidance/cg164. Accessed June 3, 2015.

47. Hayes C, Padhani AR, Leach MO. Assessing changes in tumour vascular function using dynamic contrast-enhanced magnetic resonance imaging. NMR Biomed 2002;15:154–63.

48. Martincich L, Montemurro F, De Rosa G, et al. Monitoring response to primary chemotherapy in breast cancer using dynamic contrast-enhanced magnetic resonance imaging. Breast Cancer Res Treat 2004; 83:67–76.

49. Baar J, Silverman P, Lyons J, et al. A vasculature-targeting regimen of preoperative docetaxel with or without bevacizumab for locally advanced breast cancer: impact on angiogenic biomarkers. Clin Cancer Res 2009;15:3583–90.

50. Li SP, Makris A, Beresford MJ, et al. Use of dynamic contrast-enhanced MR imaging to predict survival in patients with primary breast cancer undergoing neoadjuvant chemotherapy. Radiology 2011;260:68–78.

51. Dickinson L, Ahmed HU, Allen C, et al. Magnetic resonance imaging for the detection, localisation, and characterisation of prostate cancer: recommendations from a European consensus meeting. Eur Urol 2011;59:477–94.

52. deSouza NM, Sala E. Imaging: standardizing the use of functional MRI in prostate cancer. Nat Rev Urol 2011;8:127–9.

53. Buckley DL, Roberts C, Parker GJ, et al. Prostate cancer: evaluation of vascular characteristics with dynamic contrast-enhanced T1-weighted MR imaging–initial experience. Radiology 2004;233:709–15.

54. Riches SF, Payne GS, Morgan VA, et al. MRI in the detection of prostate cancer: combined apparent diffusion coefficient, metabolite ratio, and vascular parameters. AJR Am J Roentgenol 2009;193:1583–91.

55. Langer DL, van der Kwast TH, Evans AJ, et al. Prostate cancer detection with multi-parametric MRI: logistic regression analysis of quantitative T2, diffusion-weighted imaging, and dynamic contrast-enhanced MRI. J Magn Reson Imaging 2009;30:327–34.

56. Delongchamps NB, Rouanne M, Flam T, et al. Multiparametric magnetic resonance imaging for the detection and localization of prostate cancer: combination of T2-weighted, dynamic contrast-enhanced and diffusion-weighted imaging. BJU Int 2011;107:1411–8.

57. Futterer JJ, Heijmink SW, Scheenen TW, et al. Prostate cancer localization with dynamic contrast-enhanced MR imaging and proton MR spectroscopic imaging. Radiology 2006;241:449–58.

58. Hambrock T, Somford DM, Huisman HJ, et al. Relationship between apparent diffusion coefficients at 3.0-T MR imaging and Gleason grade in peripheral zone prostate cancer. Radiology 2011;259:453–61.

59. Lips IM, van der Heide UA, Haustermans K, et al. Single blind randomized phase III trial to investigate the benefit of a focal lesion ablative microboost in prostate cancer (FLAME-trial): study protocol for a randomized controlled trial. Trials 2011;12:255.

60. Biomarkers Definitions Working Group. Biomarkers and surrogate endpoints: preferred definitions and conceptual framework. Clin Pharmacol Ther 2001;69:89–95.

61. Wedam SB, Low JA, Yang SX, et al. Antiangiogenic and antitumor effects of bevacizumab in patients with inflammatory and locally advanced breast cancer. J Clin Oncol 2006;24:769–77.

62. Li SP, Taylor NJ, Mehta S, et al. Evaluating the early effects of anti-angiogenic treatment in human breast cancer with intrinsic susceptibility-weighted and diffusion-weighted MRI: initial observations. Proc ISMRM 2011;19:342.

63. O'Connor JP, Carano RA, Clamp AR, et al. Quantifying antivascular effects of monoclonal antibodies to vascular endothelial growth factor: insights from imaging. Clin Cancer Res 2009;15:6674–82.

64. Barboriak DP, DesJardins A, Rich J, et al. Treatment of recurrent glioblastoma multiforme with bevacizumab and irinotecan leads to rapid decreases in tumor plasma volume and Ktrans. RSNA 2007;93. SST09–05.

65. Gutin PH, Iwamoto FM, Beal K, et al. Safety and efficacy of bevacizumab with hypofractionated stereotactic irradiation for recurrent malignant gliomas. Int J Radiat Oncol Biol Phys 2009;75:156–63.

66. Zhang W, Kreisl TN, Solomon J, et al. Acute effects of bevacizumab on glioblastoma vascularity assessed with DCE-MRI and relation to patient survival. Proc ISMRM 2009;17:282.

67. Gururangan S, Chi SN, Young Poussaint T, et al. Lack of efficacy of bevacizumab plus irinotecan in children with recurrent malignant glioma and diffuse brainstem glioma: a Pediatric Brain Tumor Consortium study. J Clin Oncol 2010;28:3069–75.

68. Kreisl TN, Zhang W, Odia Y, et al. A phase II trial of single-agent bevacizumab in patients with recurrent anaplastic glioma. Neuro Oncol 2011;13:1143–50.

69. Siegel AB, Cohen EI, Ocean A, et al. Phase II trial evaluating the clinical and biologic effects of bevacizumab in unresectable hepatocellular carcinoma. J Clin Oncol 2008;26:2992–8.

70. Willett CG, Duda DG, di Tomaso E, et al. Efficacy, safety, and biomarkers of neoadjuvant bevacizumab, radiation therapy, and fluorouracil in rectal cancer: a multidisciplinary phase II study. J Clin Oncol 2009;27:3020–6.

71. Drevs J, Siegert P, Medinger M, et al. Phase I clinical study of AZD2171, an oral vascular endothelial growth factor signaling inhibitor, in patients with advanced solid tumors. J Clin Oncol 2007;25:3045–54.

72. Batchelor TT, Sorensen AG, di Tomaso E, et al. AZD2171, a pan-VEGF receptor tyrosine kinase inhibitor, normalizes tumor vasculature and alleviates edema in glioblastoma patients. Cancer Cell 2007;11:83–95.

73. Mitchell CL, O'Connor JP, Roberts C, et al. A two-part phase II study of cediranib in patients with advanced solid tumours: the effect of food on single-dose pharmacokinetics and an evaluation of safety, efficacy and imaging pharmacodynamics. Cancer Chemother Pharmacol 2011;68:631–41.

74. Hahn OM, Yang C, Medved M, et al. Dynamic contrast-enhanced magnetic resonance imaging pharmacodynamic biomarker study of sorafenib in metastatic renal carcinoma. J Clin Oncol 2008;26:4572–8.

75. Flaherty KT, Rosen MA, Heitjan DF, et al. Pilot study of DCE-MRI to predict progression-free survival with sorafenib therapy in renal cell carcinoma. Cancer Biol Ther 2008;7:496–501.

76. Zhu AX, Sahani DV, Duda DG, et al. Efficacy, safety, and potential biomarkers of sunitinib monotherapy in advanced hepatocellular carcinoma: a phase II study. J Clin Oncol 2009;27:3027–35.

77. Machiels JP, Henry S, Zanetta S, et al. Phase II study of sunitinib in recurrent or metastatic squamous cell carcinoma of the head and neck: GORTEC 2006-01. J Clin Oncol 2010;28:21–8.

78. Hurwitz HI, Dowlati A, Saini S, et al. Phase I trial of pazopanib in patients with advanced cancer. Clin Cancer Res 2009;15:4220–7.

79. Galbraith SM, Maxwell RJ, Lodge MA, et al. Combretastatin A4 phosphate has tumor antivascular activity in rat and man as demonstrated by dynamic magnetic resonance imaging. J Clin Oncol 2003; 21:2831–42.

80. Stevenson JP, Rosen M, Sun W, et al. Phase I trial of the antivascular agent combretastatin A4 phosphate on a 5-day schedule to patients with cancer: magnetic resonance imaging evidence for altered tumor blood flow. J Clin Oncol 2003;21:4428–38.

81. Nathan P, Zweifel M, Padhani AR, et al. Phase I trial of combretastatin A4 phosphate (CA4P) in combination with bevacizumab in patients with advanced cancer. Clin Cancer Res 2012;18:3428–39.

82. Morgan B, Thomas AL, Drevs J, et al. Dynamic contrast-enhanced magnetic resonance imaging as a biomarker for the pharmacological response of PTK787/ZK 222584, an inhibitor of the vascular endothelial growth factor receptor tyrosine kinases, in patients with advanced colorectal cancer and liver metastases: results from two phase I studies. J Clin Oncol 2003;21:3955–64.

83. Murphy PS, Roberts C, Whitcher B, et al. Vascular response of hepatocellular carcinoma to pazopanib measured by dynamic contrast-enhanced MRI: pharmacokinetic and clinical activity correlations. Proc ISMRM 2010;18:2720.

84. Mross K, Drevs J, Muller M, et al. Phase I clinical and pharmacokinetic study of PTK/ZK, a multiple VEGF receptor inhibitor, in patients with liver metastases from solid tumours. Eur J Cancer 2005;41:1291–9.

85. Thomas AL, Morgan B, Horsfield MA, et al. Phase I study of the safety, tolerability, pharmacokinetics, and pharmacodynamics of PTK787/ZK 222584 administered twice daily in patients with advanced cancer. J Clin Oncol 2005;23:4162–71.

86. Jonker DJ, Rosen LS, Sawyer MB, et al. A phase I study to determine the safety, pharmacokinetics and pharmacodynamics of a dual VEGFR and FGFR inhibitor, brivanib, in patients with advanced or metastatic solid tumors. Ann Oncol 2011;22: 1413–9.

87. Zweifel M, Padhani AR. Perfusion MRI in the early clinical development of antivascular drugs: decorations or decision making tools? Eur J Nucl Med Mol Imaging 2010;37:S164–82.

88. Collins JM. Functional imaging in phase I studies: decorations or decision making? J Clin Oncol 2003;21:2807–9.

89. Akerley WL, Schabel M, Morrell G, et al. A randomized phase 2 trial of combretatstatin A4 phosphate (CA4P) in combination with paclitaxel and carboplatin to evaluate safety and efficacy in subjects with advanced imageable malignancies. J Clin Oncol (Meetings Abstracts) 2007;25(18S): 14060.

90. O'Donnell A, Padhani A, Hayes C, et al. A phase study of the angiogenesis inhibitor SU5416 (semaxanib) in solid tumours, incorporating dynamic contrast MR pharmacodynamic end points. Br J Cancer 2005;93:876–83.

91. Miller KD, Trigo JM, Wheeler C, et al. A multicenter phase II trial of ZD6474, a vascular endothelial growth factor receptor-2 and epidermal growth factor receptor tyrosine kinase inhibitor, in patients with previously treated metastatic breast cancer. Clin Cancer Res 2005;11:3369–76.

92. Hecht JR, Trarbach T, Hainsworth JD, et al. Randomized, placebo-controlled, phase III study of first-line oxaliplatin-based chemotherapy plus PTK787/ZK 222584, an oral vascular endothelial growth factor receptor inhibitor, in patients with metastatic colorectal adenocarcinoma. J Clin Oncol 2011;29: 1997–2003.

93. Ellis LM. Antiangiogenic therapy: more promise and yet again, more questions. J Clin Oncol 2003;21: 3897–9.

94. Evelhoch JL, LoRusso PM, He Z, et al. Magnetic resonance imaging measurements of the response of murine and human tumors to the vascular-targeting agent ZD6126. Clin Cancer Res 2004;10: 3650–7.

95. LoRusso PM, Gadgeel SM, Wozniak A, et al. Phase clinical evaluation of ZD6126, a novel vascular-targeting agent, in patients with solid tumors. Invest New Drugs 2008;26:159–67.

96. O'Connor JP, Jayson GC. Do imaging biomarkers relate to outcome in patients treated with VEGF inhibitors? Clin Cancer Res 2012;18:6588–98.

97. Bjarnason GA, Williams R, Hudson JM, et al. Microbubble ultrasound (DCE-US) compared to DCE-MRI and DCE-CT for the assessment of vascular response to sunitinib in renal cell carcinoma (RCC). J Clin Oncol (Meetings Abstracts) 2011; 29(S):4627.

Clinical Imaging of Tumor Metabolism with [1]H Magnetic Resonance Spectroscopy

Teodoro Martín Noguerol, MD[a],*, Javier Sánchez-González, PhD[b],
José Pablo Martínez Barbero, MD[a], Roberto García-Figueiras, MD, PhD[c],
Sandra Baleato-González, MD, PhD[c], Antonio Luna, MD[d,e]

KEYWORDS

- [1]H magnetic resonance spectroscopy metabolites • Choline
- Magnetic resonance spectroscopic imaging • Brain tumor • Prostate cancer • Breast cancer
- Hepatocellular carcinoma

KEY POINTS

- Magnetic resonance spectroscopy (MRS) is able to determine the tissue chemical composition of a certain tissue, providing clinical valuable information for oncologic molecular imaging.
- Clinical MRS is mainly based on ^{1}H protons, which is technically challenging and needs robust quality control of sequence design, acquisition including artifact identification and postprocessing, and quantification steps for clinical implementation.
- MRS increases the overall diagnostic accuracy in multiparametric evaluation of brain tumors and is a key tool especially for lesion characterization, tumor grading, and assessment of local extension, as well as for treatment monitoring.
- MRS has been included in routine clinical MR imaging protocols for prostate cancer assessment for years, although its role is now under debate because of limited reproducibility, complex interpretation, and long acquisition time.
- Choline has emerged as a metabolic hallmark of malignancy in tumors of breast, the musculoskeletal system, and other abdominopelvic organs.

INTRODUCTION

Magnetic resonance spectroscopy (MRS) creates a specific spectral curve of the area of interest, because of its ability to depict the tissue chemical composition and analyze the radiofrequency signals generated by the precession frequency of different active molecules in an external magnetic field (B_0). In recent years, MRS has gradually been introduced into clinical practice. The capability of MRS to noninvasively determine the concentration of different metabolites in a certain tissue provides powerful biological information not given by other

J. Sánchez-González is a clinical scientist at Philips Healthcare Iberia, Spain. Drs T. Martín Noguerol, J.P. Martínez Barbero, R. García-Figueiras, S. Baleato-González, and A. Luna have nothing to disclose.
[a] Neuroradiology Section, Health – Time, Jaén, Spain; [b] Philips Healthcare Iberia, Madrid, Spain; [c] Department of Radiology, Hospital Clínico Universitario de Santiago de Compostela, Santiago de Compostela, Spain; [d] Department of Radiology, Health Time, Carmelo Torres 2, Jaén 23006, Spain; [e] Department of Radiology, University Hospitals of Cleveland, Case Western Reserve University, 11100 Euclid Ave, 44106 Cleveland, Ohio, USA
* Corresponding author.
E-mail address: t.martin.f@htime.org

functional techniques performed with MR imaging, such as diffusion-weighted imaging (DWI) or dynamic contrast-enhanced (DCE) MR imaging. MRS can study different endogenous metabolites, such as phosphorus (^{31}P), carbon (^{13}C), sodium (^{23}Na), fluor (^{19}F), or hydrogen (^{1}H) protons. However, because of the high ^{1}H concentration in the human body and the absence of need for additional hardware, ^{1}H is the preferred option for most clinical applications, which also provides a higher signal-to-noise ratio (SNR).

The characterization and posttreatment follow-up of tumors in different regions is the most common clinical application of ^{1}H MRS. ^{1}H MRS has been used for tumor assessment of the central nervous system (CNS) for years, integrated as part of a multiparametric MR imaging protocol; in some clinical scenarios, it is the only tool with discriminative value.[1] Recent technical advances have favored the spread of ^{1}H MRS outside the brain. However, this technique has been integrated in clinical settings only in selected anatomic features, such as the prostate, where MRS has been successfully performed for cancer assessment.[2] This slow expansion is mainly because of technical difficulties that limit reproducibility between different centers. The use of MRS for evaluation of other anatomic areas, such as the breast or the musculoskeletal system, is emerging strongly but is still limited to a few centers with sufficient expertise. The implementation of MRS for evaluation of other abdominopelvic organs is progressing even more slowly, because this technique is prone to motion artifacts, but progress is steady and there have been promising results. For all these reasons, MRS has to be considered in the battery of functional MR imaging techniques for evaluation of cancer, because it provides unique biochemical information and can create a specific metabolic fingerprint of different malignancies.

In this review, the focus is on the principles and technical adjustments necessary to perform ^{1}H MRS in different organs; the clinical experience for the assessment of cancer in the brain and body is also analyzed.

Physical Bases

MRS is based on the same MR principle as conventional MR imaging and can excite and acquire information from nuclei with spin equal to half during the relaxation process. Unlike conventional MR imaging, in which frequency information of the received signal is used for imaging encoding, in MRS, this information is sensitive to the magnetic field shielding of the electron surrounding the nucleus. This property allows MRS to distinguish between different molecular bonds, and therefore, between different chemical compounds. MRS can use this capability to observe in vivo several metabolites, which provides biochemical information from living tissues.

A nucleus inside a molecular bond fills a magnetic field shielding, resulting in the combination of external magnetic field and the molecular bond electron shielding, which can be expressed as:

$$\omega_i = \gamma(1 - \sigma_i)B_o \qquad (1)$$

where ω_i represents the MR frequency of a specific molecular bond, σ_i is the electron shielding of a this bond, γ represents the gyromagnetic ratio, and B_o represents the external magnetic field.

From Equation 1, it can be observed that the direct comparison of peak position inside MRS spectra depends on the external magnetic field, making it difficult to compare spectra results acquired at different magnetic field strengths. To overcome this limitation, a new scale called parts per million (ppm) (Equation 2) allows direct comparison of the electron shielding, avoiding any dependency with the external magnetic field.

$$\text{ppm} = \frac{\omega - \omega_0}{\omega_0} \times 10^6 = \frac{\sigma - \sigma_0}{1 - \sigma_0} \times 10^6 \qquad (2)$$

Information from MRS is normally represented as a spectroscopic signal (**Fig. 1**) with different peaks located in a specific frequency position (or ppm) that are associated with a particular molecular bond, and therefore, with a determined metabolite. **Fig. 1A** shows a conventional ^{1}H spectrum of the brain of a healthy volunteer, in which different peaks associated with defined metabolites can be distinguished.

Clinical Information

MRS is able to obtain information from metabolites that are present at the cellular level with millimolar concentrations ($\sim 1e^{-4}$ times less concentration than water). Those metabolites that have less than millimolar concentration are difficult to be detected in a conventional MRS experiment due to their decrease in signal in the noise range. Lack of MRS signal, due to low concentration of the metabolites, needs to be compensated during MRS acquisition, limiting the minimum voxel size or increasing the number of repetitions to average the signal to reduce noise contamination.

Most of the relevant proton metabolites that can be found in a conventional MR spectrum are described in **Table 1**.

A   **B**

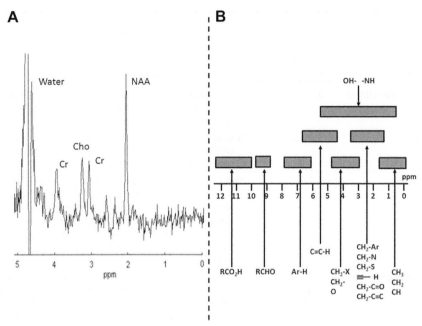

Fig. 1. (*A*) Example of conventional MR spectrum from the brain of a healthy volunteer, in whom different peaks corresponding to different metabolites are observed. (*B*) ppm position of the ^{1}H proton MRS peaks according to the corresponding molecular bond.

ACQUISITION PREPARATION

MRS signal has very low SNR as a result of low metabolite concentration. In addition, several important peaks in clinical practice are located close and tend to overlap because of limited chemical shift dispersion and J-coupling. The use of higher field strength magnets improves both chemical shift separation and SNR. To acquire a good-quality spectrum, coil selection and positioning are critical steps during patient preparation. Special mention is required for prostate and breast applications. Although coil technology allows clinical prostate MRS data to be acquired using phased-array surface coils with adequate SNR, the combination of these surface elements with an endorectal one greatly increases MRS signal, allowing smaller voxel size or faster scans by using parallel acquisition techniques.[3,4] In breast applications, MRS requires proper selection of coil elements that cover only the studied breast and switching off the elements from the contralateral breast to reduce noise contamination.

During the acquisition, the first requisite to acquire high-quality spectroscopic data is to improve magnetic field homogeneity inside the studied volume. Magnetic field shimming is required to concentrate all the signal provided from a metabolite in a limited frequency window, obtaining high and narrow spectroscopic peaks,

and therefore, improving SNR. To understand the degree of homogeneity required inside the acquired volume, it is worth performing a frequency analysis from a 1.5-T brain spectrum, in which all spectral information falls in a frequency window of 5 ppm, equivalent to 320 Hz. Using the gyromagnetic constant for the ^{1}H proton (γ = 42.577 MHz/T), this frequency window is equivalent to a magnetic field variation lower than 10^{-6} T to avoid the spread of the MR signal of each metabolite along the whole frequency range. Good spectrum quality is achieved with a line width of the water peak of 7 Hz inside the studied volume. This restriction requires a magnetic field variation inside the studied volume in the range of 10^{-8} T to avoid signal spread along different frequency components and losing the signal in the noise level. **Fig. 2** shows the importance of magnetic field shimming conditions during MRS acquisition.

This sensitivity to potential sources of magnetic field variations makes it necessary to avoid positioning the volume of interest (VOI) close to high susceptibility areas such as hemorrhage, air, calcification, or metallic devices and also to eliminate potential homogeneity distortions caused by motion, which are critical in body acquisitions.

On ^{1}H proton MRS, the difference in concentration between water and the rest of the metabolites requires an additional preparation phase to reduce

Table 1
Summary of the most representative metabolites that can be found in a ¹H MRS spectrum

Metabolite Name	Resonance Peaks (ppm)	Functional Description
N-Acetylaspartate (NAA)	2,02 and 2.52	Its metabolic function is still unclear but it seems to be a good neuronal marker. Only (functional) neurons contain this substance
Creatine (Cr)	3.02 and 3.94	It is the sum of Cr and its phosphorylated form, phosphocreatine. Phosphocreatine probably has the role of an energy buffer
Choline (Cho)	3.22	The Cho peak is a peak consisting of free Cho, phosphocholine, and glycerophosphocholine. These compounds are important intermediates of lipid metabolism. Abnormal cell growth can be accompanied by an increase in intermediates of lipid metabolism. It is the most important metabolic biomarker of malignancy in body tumors
Glutamate-glutamine (Glx)	2.06, 2.10, and 2.36	The resonances of glutamine and glutamate, 2 similar compounds, are overlapping. Glutamine is the nitrogen donor in some important metabolic pathways, such as the purine and pyrimidine synthesis. In the brain, glutamate is a precursor of γ-aminobutyric acid (GABA). Glutamate and GABA are both involved in regulating nerve transmissions
Myoinositol (ml)	3.54 y 4.06	ml is an alcohol, related to the diphosphorylated and triphosphorylated forms of ml (DPI and TPI), that plays an important role in the cell as second messenger for many hormonal signals
Lactate (Lac)	1.33	Lactic acid is the breakdown product of anaerobic glycolysis
Lipids (Lip)	0.9 and 1.3	The Lip signal in the spectrum is originated from a pool of relatively mobile lipids, fatty acid, and triglycerides

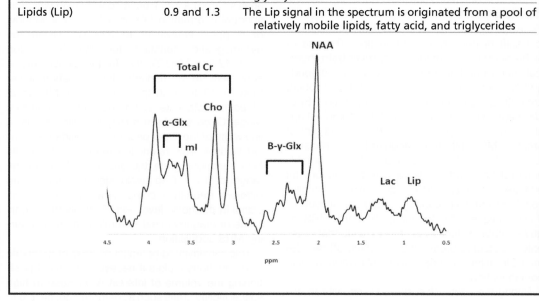

the signal of the water peak in the spectrum (**Fig. 3**).[5] No water suppression spectrum has a maximum signal intensity greater than 100 arbitrary units (au), whereas the water suppression spectrum has a maximum signal around 0.06 au, making a signal difference between both spectra of 10^{-4} time difference. To suppress the water signal before volume excitation, a water

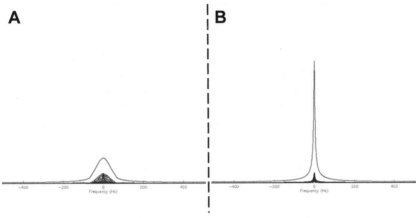

Fig. 2. The result of a water spectrum acquired with poor (*A*) and high (*B*) magnetic field shimming. Both MRS data are presented with equivalent intensity scale. The red line represents the reference frequency at the established magnetic field strength. Blue lines represent the effect of magnetic field variations in the peak positioning in the spectrum. The green line represents the addition of all the blue lines. In A, the information from the resonance peak (*red peak*) is shifted in the frequency domain because of magnetic field variation in the excited MRS volume (*blue lines*); as a result, the average spectrum (*green line*) is spread among different frequencies. On the contrary, in B, with none magnetic field variation, the whole volume is contributing to the same frequency. As a result, the average peak presents higher signal intensity compared with the A spectrum.

suppression pulse is applied. This pulse is tuned to the water frequency band to avoid saturation of any other metabolite close to the water peak.

In addition to water suppression, in specific anatomies such as breast or prostate MRS, it is also necessary to suppress fat signal. Saturation bands are placed surrounding the VOI to eliminate fat contamination from surrounding tissue (eg, prostate MRS). Also, this suppression is obtained by a frequency selective technique, such as spectrally adiabatic inversion recovery or chemical shift selective (CHESS) pulses, tuned to the fat frequency bandwidth and fat inversion time.

SPATIAL ENCODING

MRS studies can be acquired from a single spatial position, using single-voxel (SV) excitation techniques, or combining spectral information with spatial metabolite distribution by the MR spectroscopic imaging (MRSI) technique, also known as chemical shift imaging or multivoxel (MV) MRS (Table 2).

In the SV technique, slice selection gradients are applied in 3 orthogonal spatial directions. The combination of the 3 slice selection gradients excites a single volume in the space. The most established

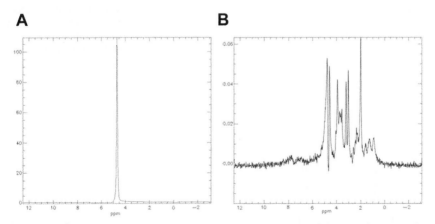

Fig. 3. A shows a brain ¹H MRS without applying any water suppression technique, whereas B shows the same spectra acquired with a water suppression technique. Nonwater suppression spectrum of A shows a single peak corresponding to ¹H protons from water, whereas in a water suppression spectrum (*B*), the rest of the metabolites can be clearly identified in the frequency window between 5 and 0 ppm.

Table 2
Comparison between SV and MV sequences for MRS

	SV (MRS)	MV (MRSI)
Technique	PRESS or STEAM	Chemical shift imaging (CSI)
TE	Usually short	Usually long
Information area	Limited to target	Tumor and peritumoral tissue
Metabolic information	Limited to target lesion	Assess tumor heterogeneity and margin infiltration
Acquisition time	Shorter	Longer
Spectral resolution	Higher	Lower
Brain	++++	+++
Breast	+++	+
Prostate	+	++++
Abdominal organs	+++	+
Musculoskeletal system	+++	+

The clinical usefulness of each type of ^1H MRS sequences at each anatomical region is graded from + to ++++, in a growing manner, according to reported experience.

SV excitation techniques are point-resolved spectroscopy (PRESS),[6] in which the last 2 excitation pulses are of 180°, or stimulated-echo acquisition mode (STEAM),[7] in which all pulses are of 90° (**Fig. 4**). PRESS has more signal compared with STEAM for equivalent echo time (TE), whereas STEAM achieves a shorter TE, because the spins do not undergo T2 relaxation during the mixing time (TM) between the latest 2 90° pulses of the sequence (**Table 3**).

Contrary to conventional MR imaging, in MRSI, frequency is used to obtain the information between different metabolites, limiting the use of gradients during signal readout. For this reason, in MRSI experiments, spatial encoding is obtained by a phase-encoding step, making the acquisition of MRSI longer than conventional MR imaging sequences (**Fig. 5**). This phase encoding can be performed in 1 dimension, 2 dimensions, or 3 dimensions (3D), just adding extra phase-encoding steps in the acquisition, and therefore, increasing acquisition time.

Both spatial encoding strategies can be combined. SV excitation is applied to select a voxel that is later spatially encoded with a reduced field of view to obtain spatial distribution of a limited region.

ACQUISITION PARAMETERS

In the MRS signal, each metabolite has different T1 and T2 relaxation constants, making the selection

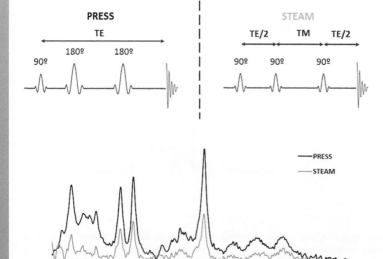

Fig. 4. SV excitation sequence schemes using PRESS and STEAM techniques (*upper row*) and the comparative result obtained with both techniques from the same voxel and same sequence parameters in normal brain (*lower row*). TM, mixing time.

Table 3
Comparison between PRESS and STEAM sequences for MRS

	PRESS	STEAM
Voxel technique supported	SV and MV	SV
Physical basis	1 × 90° and 2 × 180° pulses	3 × 90° pulses
TE	Short and long TE	Short TE
SNR	Higher	Lower
Water suppression	Acceptable	Optimal
Motion artifact	Less susceptibility	High susceptibility
Clinical use	Common	Limited to high field magnets

of sequence parameters important, such as repetition time (TR) and TE (Table 4). MR spectroscopic experiments are normally acquired with long TR to avoid T1 signal saturation caused by the application of very close excitation pulses. Once the TR is fixed, the values of TE completely defined the metabolites that can be seen in an MRS study (Fig. 6). With short TE acquisitions,

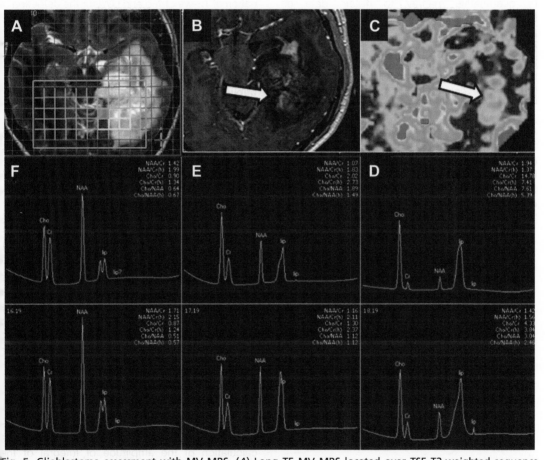

Fig. 5. Glioblastoma assessment with MV MRS. (A) Long TE MV MRS located over TSE T2-weighted sequence demonstrating a large left temporal lobe infiltrating lesion with heterogeneous enhancement (arrows) on post-contrast Spoiled Gradient Echo T1-weighted image (B) and high relative cerebral blood volume on T2* perfusion map (C). MV MRS located as shown in the yellow box on (A) shows the distribution of Cho, NAA, and Lip in the tumor burden, showing a good correlation of areas with more aggressive behavior (D, right voxels) with enhancing areas. Central voxels (E) show high Cho/Cr despite the absence of enhancement, consistent with tumor infiltration without blood-brain barrier leakage. Left voxels (F), out of the apparent burden of the lesion, show a decreased Cho/Cr ratio with normal NAA peak. MRS was used to perform a targeted biopsy.

Table 4
Summary of acquisition recommendations for ¹H MRS in different anatomies

Anatomic Region	TE	Water/Fat Suppression	SV/MRSI
Brain	Shortest possible TE = 144 ms to allow fully lactate inversion	Water suppression Lipid signal can be used for necrosis assessment	Normally, an SV acquisition within the lesion and another in the contralateral normal brain are used It can be combined with two-dimensional MRSI encoding scheme to analyze tumor heterogeneity or diffuse disease
Prostate	Normally TE = 120 ms is applied for proper evolution of Cit peak	Water and fat suppression to avoid contamination of periprostatic fat	Combination of PRESS with 3D MRSI encoding to cover the whole gland
Breast	Long TE (normally around 288 ms) to avoid fat contamination	Water and fat suppression	Normally, SV acquisition on the lesion for Cho peak assessment
Liver	Shortest possible TE for adequate assessment of water and fat peaks For other metabolites (like Cho) a TE = 144 ms is applied	For fat infiltration assessment nonsuppression is applied. For Cho detection in tumor, both lipid and water suppression techniques need to be applied	Normally breath-hold or respiratory triggered SV technique

most of the metabolites can be detected, even those with a short T2 constant, like the lipids (Lip) or myoinositol (mI). On the other hand, for longer TE sequences, the signal from those metabolites with short T2 relaxation disappears and only the signal from those metabolites with longer T2 relaxation values is detectable (see **Fig. 6**).

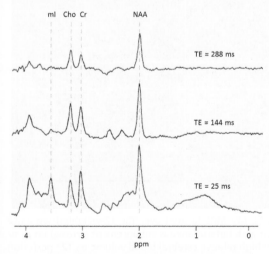

Fig. 6. MRS data acquired with different TE maintaining fixed the rest of acquisition parameters in a normal brain. Notice how myo-inositol is better depicted on short TE acquisition, and the changes in peak height of the rest of metabolites with different TEs.

An additional limitation on the TE is imposing by the J-coupling systems, like lactate (Lac) peak Phase cycling for this J-coupling system is modulated by the sequence TE and this parameter is normally chosen to improve its signal visualization. For in vivo MRS, a TE of 144 milliseconds is used in brain MRS for Lac peak detection and in prostate MRS normally a TE of 120 milliseconds is recommended to optimize depiction of the Citrate (Cit) peak.

Another important parameter is the number of repetitions during the acquisition to reduce noise contamination in the MRS data. This parameter basically depends on the excited voxel. The smaller the voxel, the more repetitions are required to compensate for the lack of signal.

MAGNETIC RESONANCE SPECTROSCOPY SIGNAL QUANTIFICATION

Clinically, MR spectra are read qualitatively, identifying only the presence or absence of a metabolite. A semiquantitative approach needs the calculation of the amplitude or integral of the metabolite peaks or use of a metabolite ratio Also, quantitative data from MRS examinations may be obtained as the area under each peak. This area is related to metabolite concentration, and normally, the results are normalized by a defined metabolite or the unsuppressed water signal acquired in a separate scan.

Different steps are required to perform a proper MRS analysis (**Fig. 7**). In the first step, residual water signal needs to be removed from the spectrum for better visualization of the metabolite signal. Although water suppression is applied during the acquisition, some residual water can be presented in the final acquired spectrum (see **Fig. 7A**). This residual water signal can be removed by digital low pass filters tuned to the water signal (see **Fig. 7B**). After suppression of the residual water, the spectrum phase is corrected to place most of the area of each peak over baseline (see **Fig. 7C**). After phase correction, the peaks are fitted following a Lorentzian or Gaussian shape in the frequency domain (red lines in **Fig. 7D**). After this fitting, the area for each metabolite is obtained from fitted peak parameters to generate the final report (see **Fig. 7E**). Final values are normally reported as ratios with a reference peak like nonsuppression water spectrum. These steps can be performed on the original signal in the time domain or after Fourier transform in the frequency domain, obtaining equivalent results.[8]

A different MRS quantification technique relies on a linear combination of a database of a pure metabolite spectrum acquired with the same sequence parameters as the analyzed MR spectrum.[9] Because database metabolites have a known concentration, these values can be used as a reference to provide absolute quantification.

For MRSI, the same procedure is repeated for every voxel. The final image is generated with the area of each metabolite per each voxel, generating the so-called metabolic maps.

A basic knowledge of the physical basis of MRS would allow us to identify and determine if the spectrum obtained has sufficient quality for clinical diagnostic purposes[10] (**Box 1**).

CLINICAL APPLICATIONS IN ONCOLOGY
^{1}H Magnetic Resonance Spectroscopy of the Central Nervous System in a Clinical Setting

Technical considerations in brain spectroscopy
The use of MRS for tumor evaluation in the CNS is based on proton ^{1}H imaging.[11] MRS has to be considered as a complementary tool for brain tumor assessment, along with other morphologic and functional techniques, such as DWI and T1-weighted DCE-MR imaging or T2*-weighted dynamic susceptibility perfusion MR imaging, in a multiparametric approach. The biochemical information that provides MRS has been shown to boost the overall accuracy for both lesion detection and characterization.[12]

Several technical considerations and adjustments are necessary when an MRS of the brain is performed, as SV or MV acquisitions can be performed (**Table 5**).

Voxel positioning may be a challenge, especially when the SV approach is used.[13] To obtain a diagnostic spectrum of adequate quality, almost every structure that could induce an inhomogeneity of the magnetic field (bone, air, blood products, fat, or necrosis) should be avoided. It is recommended to place the voxel at the hyperenhanced area within the tumor excluding adjacent tissue, to reduce volume partial effects, and thus, false-negative results.[14]

The selection of an appropriate TE is crucial to obtain the expected results. The use of short TE

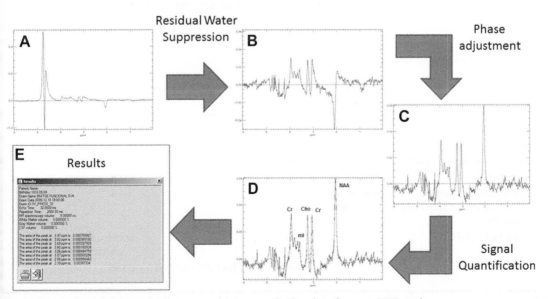

Fig. 7. Description of the required steps to obtain quantitative data from an MRS study.

(20–40 milliseconds) provides a better SNR with representation of almost all metabolite peaks. If a large TE is applied (135–144 milliseconds), information for small peaks may be lost, but better and robust discrimination of the main metabolites (N-acetylaspartate [NAA], choline [Cho], and creatine [Cr]) is shown. The inversion of the Lac peak occurs only at long TE, which is used to separate classic Lip-Lac overlapping, which helps in the assessment of inflammatory processes and other tumor lesions such as lymphoma. In clinical practice, short TE acquisitions are preferred, although both (short and long) TE can be acquired to get complementary data.[15]

Physiopathology and clinical relevance of the main spectra metabolites The clinical meaning of

the different metabolites obtained by MRS is closely related to its physiopathologic origin. These metabolites can be considered as real biomarkers of health and disease and are useful for diagnosis, therapy monitoring, and prediction of response to treatment of brain tumors.[16] **Box 2** summarizes the meaning of the main metabolites used in ¹H MRS of the brain[1,14,17–24] and **Table 6** analyzes the main metabolic characteristic of brain tumors. **Figs. 8–14** are examples of MRS in the assessment of brain tumors.

Surgical planning, prognosis, and therapeutic considerations Before tumor treatment planning, it is important to evaluate not only the metabolic characteristics of the main tumor lesion but also the area of altered signal intensity on T2-weighted images that surrounds the tumor. This area usually does not enhance on postcontrast series, but it is not uncommonly infiltrated by malignant cells in case of gliomas.[25] The use of MRS, especially with an MV approach, can detect high levels of Cho in infiltrated tissue beyond hyperenhancing areas.[26] This issue allows the real extension of tumoral infiltration to be assessed, which helps to select candidates for surgery, better delimitates the area of surgical excision, and predicts the possible recurrence pathways in successive controls.[27] In a similar manner, MRS may be used as a guide for biopsy of brain tumors, selecting the most metabolically active regions (see **Fig. 5**). As discussed earlier, in some clinical scenarios, the most aggressive tumor component does not correlate with the hyperenhancing area.[28] Thus, biopsy should be directed at those areas with highest Cho level and lowest NAA level, to avoid false-negative results, which may occur if necrotic or gliotic tissue or posttreatment changes are sampled.[29]

Table 5
Comparison of SV and MV MRS for brain tumor assessment

	SV and MV Techniques for Tumor Brain Evaluation	
	SV	MV
Reproducibility	++	+
Spatial resolution	++	+
Water suppression quality	++	+
Scan time	+	+++
Assessment of tumor heterogeneity and infiltration of surrounding tissue in gliomas	+	+++
Data obtained	Spectrum	Spectrum and metabolic distribution map
TE	Mainly short (but also long is possible)	Long

The usefulness of each acquisition technique is graded from + to +++ in a growing manner.

Box 2
Meaning of the main metabolites in the brain

Meaning of MRS metabolites in the CNS

N-acetylaspartate (NAA) 2.02 ppm

- Most specific metabolite for normal (both gray and white matter) brain
- Marker of axonal integrity, sensitive to neural damage
- Low NAA peak is found in almost every CNS disease also including brain tumors
- Not present in extraneural lesions, as metastasis or meningiomas (see Fig. 8)
- A reduced NAA/Cr ratio is usually detected in glial tumors

Choline (Cho) 3.22 ppm

- Main biomarker of cellular membrane turnover
- The increase of Cho peak indicates increase cellular proliferation, related to malignant lesions
- Cho levels are used for glioma grading
- In high-grade tumors, a false-negative result is possible if necrosis is included in the region of interest

Creatine (Cr) 3.02 ppm

- One of the most constant metabolic peaks
- Usually used as an internal reference for metabolic ratios as NAA/Cr or Cho/Cr

Lactate (Lac) 1.33 ppm

- Shows a doublet that can be inverted if a long TE acquisition is applied
- Related to anaerobic metabolism
- Present in necrotic high-grade glial tumors and also in other inflammatory and infectious conditions
- May also be present in lymphoma and metastasis
- Complementary role in glioma grading
- May be found, physiologically, on pediatric age spectra

Lipids (Lip) 1.3 ppm

- Main cellular membrane component
- High levels are closely related to necrosis in high-grade gliomas
- Complementary role in glioma grading
- In therapy monitoring of gliomas, an increase in the Lip peak and the Cho/Cr ratio, a tumoral turn to high grade can be suggest (see Fig. 9)
- May be found in other brain malignancies such as metastasis (absence of NAA combined with high Cho and Lip/Lac)

Myoinositol (mI) 3.54–4.06 ppm

- Related to gliosis or astrocytosis
- Increases typically more in low-grade gliomas than in high-grade ones, which helps to characterize as low-grade astrocytomas, tumors with normal Cho/Cr ratios (see Fig. 10)

Alanine (Ala) 1.48 ppm

- Only detectable using short TE
- May appear inverted at long TE
- Closely related to Lip/Lac peak
- Increased at meningiomas (see Fig. 11)

Taurine (Tau) 3.3 ppm

- Only detectable using short TE
- May appear inverted at long TE

- Great specificity for medulloblastoma (see Fig. 12)
- Along with high Cho levels, helps in the differential with other pediatrics tumors at posterior fossa as astrocytoma

Glutamine and glutamate (Glx) 2.05–2.5 ppm

- Small group of metabolites with scarce clinical relevance for brain tumor diagnosis
- An increase of Glx peak, along with low NAA and high Cho peak, has shown high accuracy in the diagnosis of tumefactive pseudotumoral demyelinizing lesions (see Fig. 13)

A comprehensive MR imaging protocol of a brain tumor includes both morphologic and functional data (DCE-MR imaging, DWI, and MRS).[30] In the case of functional sequences, each has been shown to predict patient outcome and prognosis.[31] In MRS, various studies have proved the accuracy of different metabolites as biomarkers of patient outcome. High Lip values have been correlated with low survival.[32] Other studies reported similar results if an increased Cho/NAA ratio was present.[33]

One of the workhorses of every neuroradiologist is the evaluation and follow-up of brain tumors after treatment has been established. The use of new antiangiogenic drugs, as well as concomitant radiation therapy, completely changes the behavior of the tumor and its surrounding tissue.[34,35] Morphologic sequences show large involvement of the tumor bed and neighboring gray and white matter on T2-weighted and fluid-attenuated inversion recovery sequences, and it is difficult to discriminate between edema, gliosis, or even tumoral infiltration.[36] On the other hand, postcontrast T1-weighted images may show a wide range of enhancement patterns that do not allow differentiation between disease persistence, radionecrosis, progression, or pseudoprogression.[37] MRS may help (along with perfusion and DWI) in this challenging task. When, despite an increase of gadolinium uptake or global lesion volume, there are no significant metabolic changes (specially increase of Cho/Cr ratio) on MRS, pseudoprogression has to be suspected (see Fig. 14). The increase of Cho/Cr or Cho/NAA ratios and decrease of NAA/Cr ratio in a treated area suggests with high confidence tumor recurrence rather than radionecrosis, especially for the Cho/NAA ratio.[38] Other investigators support these data, even in previously treated patients.[39]

However, in clinical practice, it is not uncommon for both viable tumor and necrosis-induced changes to coexist in the same area. In this scenario, MRS may not result as accurate as expected. Moreover, NAA levels decrease in postradiation changes because of cell damage which also occurs in treated brain tumors. The same cell-induced damage by radiation could lead to a slight increase in Cho levels that may be misinterpreted as tumor recurrence. In addition, the presence of hemorrhage products makes voxel positioning difficult and supposes a loss of magnetic field homogeneity, leading to a poor SNR ratio and spectra quality. For posttherapeutic tumor evaluation, a multiparametric approach is recommended to increase the overall accuracy of the MR imaging studies.[40]

Table 6
Metabolic fingerprint of main brain tumors

	NAA	Cho	Cr	Lip-Lac	mI	Ratios
Normal tissue	↑	↓	↑	↓↓	↓	Cho/Cr ↓, Cho/NAA ↑
Malignant glial tumor	↓	↑	↓	↑	↑	Cho/Cr ↑, Cho/NAA ↓
Low-grade glioma	↓	↑	↓	↑	↑↑	Cho/Cr↑ Cho/NAA↑, Myo/Cr ↑↑
High-grade glioma	↓↓	↑↑	↓↓	↑↑	↑	Cho/Cr↑↑ Cho/NAA ↑↑ Myo/Cr ↓
Intra-axial neoplasms	↓	↑↑	↓↓	↑↑	↑	Cho/Cr ↑, Cho/NAA ↓
Extra-axial lesions (and metastases)	—	↑↑	↓	↑↑	↑	Cho/Cr ↑, Cho/NAA ↓↓
Progression after treatment	↓↓	↑↑	↓↓	↑↑	—	Cho/Cr ↑↑, Cho/NAA ↓↓
Response to therapy	↓↓	↓↓	↓↓	↑↑	—	Cho/Cr ↓↓, Cho/NAA ↓↓

Changes at each metabolite and ratios are graded from severe decrease (↓↓) to severe increase (↑↑).

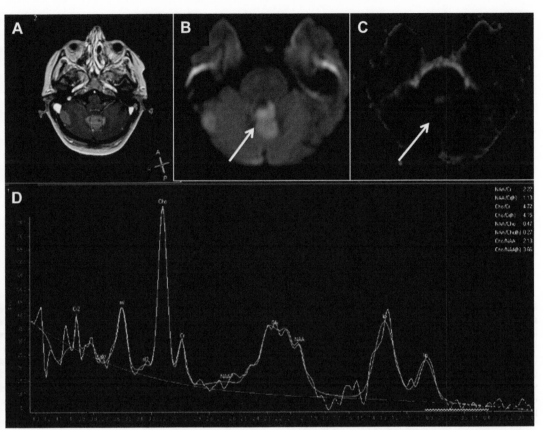

Fig. 8. Brain MRS in a 58-year-old woman with breast cancer and multiple enhancing lesions in posterior fossa identified on (A) axial postcontrast spoiled gradient echo T1-weighted sequence. (B, C) Axial DWI with a b value of 1000 s/mm^2 and apparent diffusion coefficient map show severe restriction of diffusion of all these lesions (red box in A, and arrows in B and C). (D) SV MRS with short TE at the most prominent vermian lesion confirmed the malignant origin of these metastases, with increased Cho and Lip peaks and decreased levels of NAA.

Oncologic Applications of ^{1}H Magnetic Resonance Spectroscopy Outside the Brain

The acquisition of MR spectra in other anatomic areas than the brain implies several technical and physiopathologic peculiarities. The major drawback in body applications of ^{1}H MRS is related to motion artifacts, especially in the abdominal organs. As reviewed in the technical section of this article, different technical strategies based on acquisition of cardiac or respiratory synchronism have been developed, with successful results,[41] allowing a slow translation of this technique to the clinical setting for the assessment of several body malignancies. In addition, MRS is acquired using nonspecific coils, which allow a good, but sometimes not optimal, spectrum to be obtained.[42] Body MRS has been performed most commonly with 1.5 T, although, as in the brain, it largely benefits from the use of higher field strength magnets.

Outside the brain, the range of metabolites that can be shown on a spectrum is lower than in a brain MRS (Table 7). This phenomenon may be caused by the less complex metabolic environment of nonneural tissue, but most likely, it is related to inner technical limitations and above all, to the limited clinical experience in abdominopelvic malignancies compared with the widely studied brain diseases using MRS. Nevertheless, several metabolites have been shown in several studies and clinical trials to be real biomarkers of different malignancies and normal tissue.

Cho is considered the main metabolic biomarker of several malignant body tumors. Cho is essential in the synthesis of phospholipids in the membrane cell turnover process. Most cancers show an activated phosphocholine metabolism activated by oncogenic signaling, producing increased levels of phosphocholine and total Cho (tCho)-containing compounds.[43] Higher levels of Cho have been found

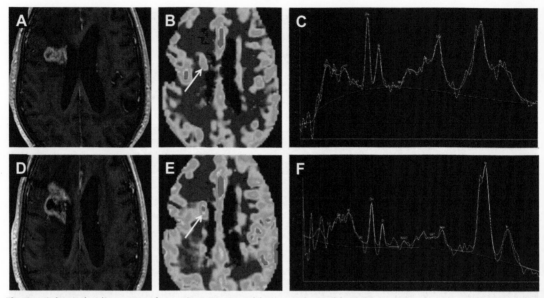

Fig. 9. High-grade glioma transformation. 54-year-old man with World Health Organization grade III glioma presents at baseline MR imaging (*A–C*) with a hyperenhancing lesion located at the right frontal lobe (*A*) with increased values of relative cerebral blood volume (*arrow* in *B*). (*C*) SV MRS performed with short TE shows an increase of Cho/Cr ratio, but with a relative preservation of NAA peak and a high Lip peak caused by necrosis. (*D–F*) 4-month follow-up MR imaging after chemo and radiotherapy shows tumor growth with central necrosis (*D*) and higher relative cerebral blood volume values compared to previous MR study (*arrow* in *E*). Spectra (*F*) show a change of the metabolic profile with a higher Lip/Lac doublet peak due to increased necrosis, and increased Cho/Cr ratio as a manifestation of increased cellular turnover, metabollic changes consistent with malignant degeneration.

in proliferative malignant lesions of several organs, such as lung, prostate, breast, colon, cervix, or adnexa as a result of an overexpression of various Cho transporters in the cell membrane, compared with normal parenchyma.[43–45] In vivo ^{1}H MRS is not able to measure the different compounds of Cho because of limited spectra resolution, and due to overlap of the signal of free Cho, phosphocholine, and glycerophosphocholine between 3.2 and 3.3 ppm. tCho is usually depicted, and its increased

levels have shown high accuracy for the detection and characterization of malignant lesions.[46–49] Moreover, changes in tCho levels after treatment are useful in therapy monitoring and detection of recurrence. Several methods have been used for Cho assessment, which covers from a qualitative evaluation of its peak height to the most extended ratios with other metabolites, such as NAA, Cr, or even Lip, in order to have an internal reference. The use of cutoff points of those ratios has been

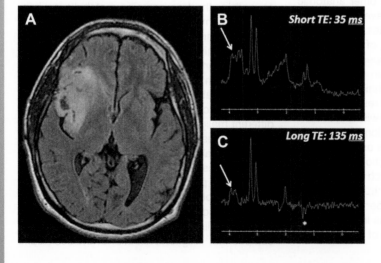

Fig. 10. 33-year-old man with migraines. (*A*) Axial fluid-attenuated inversion recovery shows a large ill-defined hyperintense tumefactive lesion at right opercular frontal area. (*B*) SV MRS with short TE shows high Cho level with relative reduction of NAA peak and a small Lip-Lac peak, consistent with malignant origin. However, an increased mI peak (*arrow*) suggests a low-grade lesion. (*C*) SV MRS with long TE shows similar findings, including the persistence of mI peak (*arrow*). Note the inverted Lip-Lac doublet on long TE MRS (*asterisk*). Biopsy results confirm a diffuse astrocytoma grade II. (*Courtesy of* Dr Jorge Pastor Rull, Complejo Hospitalario de Granada, Granada, Spain.)

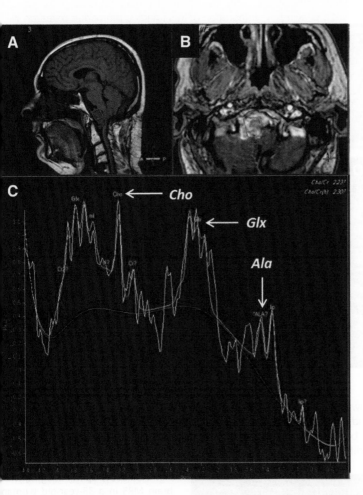

Fig. 11. 59-year-old man with fora-men magnum mass. *Red box* in *A* (sagittal turbo spin echo T1-weighted sequence) and *B* (post-contrast axial fast field echo T1-weighted image) shows the positioning of the VOI of the MRS in a large hyperenhancing lesion with mass effect against medulla. (*C*) MRS shows high Cho and Glx peaks as well as the presence of an Ala peak (*arrows* in *C*). This metabolic pattern is consistent with meningioma.

proposed to discriminate between normal tissue and cancer (eg, in prostate cancer [Pca]), but the use of numeric references may be variable between different centers because of different field strengths, sequence design, and postprocessing. Other investigators propose quantification using absolute tCho level; however, this approach, which requires complex postprocessing methods, is not always feasible

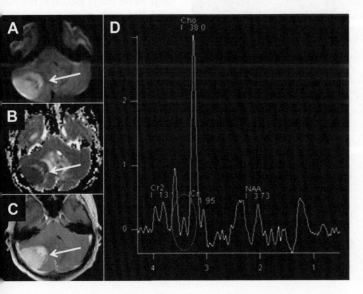

Fig. 12. Brain MRS in an 8-year-old boy with a posterior fossa tumor. (*A*) Axial DWI with high b value shows a large right cerebellar hemispheric mass (*arrow* from *A* to *C*) with severe restricted diffusion on apparent diffusion coefficient map (*B*) and intense enhancement on (*C*) axial postcontrast turbo spin echo T1-weighted sequence. (*D*) SV MRS with short TE showed a large Cho peak with severe reduction of NAA and a small peak at 3.3 ppm (*red circle*) representing Taurine. These findings are consistent with medulloblastoma, surgically confirmed. (*Courtesy of* Dr Laura Oleaga, Hospital Clinic, Barcelona, Spain.)

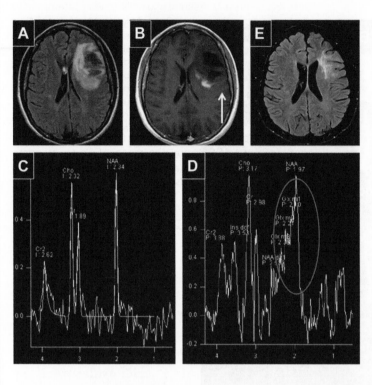

Fig. 13. Brain MRS of pseudotumoral demyelinating lesion in a 27-year-old woman with right-sided progressive weakness. (A) Axial fluid-attenuated inversion recovery sequence shows a large left frontal lesion with mass effect. (B) On axial turbo spin echo T1-weighted an area with nodular enhancement (arrow) is identified at the posterior aspect of the lesion. (C) SV MRS with long TE shows a high Cho peak with preserved NAA, findings that may suggest low-grade glioma. (D) SV MRS with short TE showed 3 intermediate peaks of Glx between 2.30 and 2.10 ppm (red circle), which supports a more likely diagnosis of a pseudotumoral demyelinating lesion. (E) Axial fluid-attenuated inversion recovery of the 3-month follow-up MR imaging showed a marked reduction of lesion size and mass effect, consistent with demyelinating origin. (Courtesy of Dr Joan Carreres Polo, Hospital Universitari Politècnic La Fe, Valencia, Spain.)

in clinical practice.[50] Cho is not always a reliable marker of malignant disease. Depending on the targeted anatomic region, Cho may be part of the normal physiologic metabolism of different tissues and benign lesions. For example, a gradient of Cho concentration has been found between head/neck and tail of the pancreas, and lower Cho values have been found in pancreatic cancer than in normal

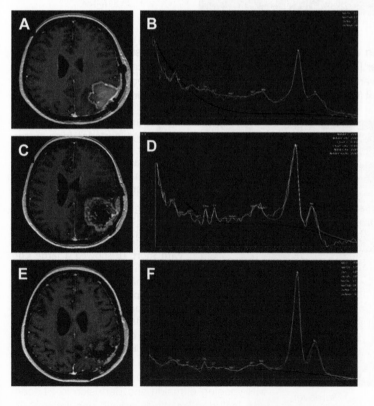

Fig. 14. Follow-up MR imaging with brain MRS in a 38-year-old woman with surgically resected frontoparietal glioblastoma in treatment with temozolamide (TMZ). (A) Axial contrast-enhanced Spoiled Gradient Echo T1-weighted image showed a large hemorrhagic loculus at the surgical bed with minimal peripheral enhancement. (B) SV MRS with short TE only shows a large Lip peak caused by necrosis. (C–D) 4-month follow-up MR imaging after TMZ treatment showed (C) intense nodular peripheral enhancement suggesting recurrence but (D) no significant metabolic abnormalities apart from necrosis were shown on MRS. (E–F) A new MR imaging was performed 3 months later after finishing the treatment with TMZ, showing scarce enhancement with mass volume reduction. (F) MRS confirmed again no abnormalities except for the presence of a Lip peak. Findings are consistent with pseudoprogression on the second study, and final proper response.

Table 7
Metabolic hallmarks in abdominal MRS

	Metabolic Origin	Biological Meaning	Clinical Application
Cho	Membrane cell turnover	High cellular proliferation	High levels in tumors increase specificity for malignant diagnosis Low Cho peaks in testes suggest spermatogenesis inhibition or testes infiltration
Lip	Membrane degradation	Necrosis	High levels support diagnosis of malignant lesions with necrotic areas
Cit	Normal epithelial prostate cells	Normal prostate gland function	Low levels increase specificity for prostate cancer

pancreas.[51] Also, Cho is part of a physiologic process of pubertal maturation and spermatogenesis.[52] Thus, high Cho levels in testicles must be considered a biomarker of healthy tissue and normal function, whereas a decrease in Cho levels is suspicious of malignancy. Moreover, the inner renal metabolism, which is responsible for the excretion of metabolites, includes Cho and has to be taken into account when its levels are analyzed.[53]

Lip has emerged as the other potential metabolic biomarker of malignancy in body tumors. The presence of Lip on a spectrum is highly suggestive of necrosis and membrane degradation products.[54] Necrosis is usually linked to rapid cell growth and presence of hypovascular and necrotic areas as a result of nonefficient vascular support and hypoxia. Malignant lesions show large necrotic areas, which may be reflected on the MR spectrum as a high Lip peak.[49] Moreover, Lip signal has been related to drug resistance in various human tumors.[55] However, as occurs with Cho, Lip are part of the physiologic structures of several organs, and high Lip levels can be found, for example, in breast normal tissue or even in benign adnexal lesions.[56] Moreover, Lip are complex chemical molecules that may resonate at different points in the spectra. Lip signal appears in the spectra mainly at 1.3 and 0.9 ppm, representing methylene and methyl groups, respectively. Lac signal overlaps at 1.3 ppm, although it can be separated with dedicated postprocessing. Polyunsaturated fatty acyl chains resonate at 5.3 to 5.4 ppm. Therefore, long and short fatty acid chains, cholesterol, triglycerides, or isolated methyl groups can be detected with distinct metabolic and clinical relevance.

Prostate magnetic resonance spectroscopy

^{1}H MRS has been largely investigated for assessment of PCa, which is the fifth most common cancer worldwide,[57] causing up to 6% of deaths in men. ^{1}H MRS is able to explore the metabolic insights of the prostate gland and to accurately differentiate between PCa and normal prostatic tissue, which has proved useful for PCa assessment in different clinical scenarios.[2] Despite these potential applications, its use in clinical setting is under debate because of limited reproducibility and technical difficulties in its acquisition.[47]

Technique Box 3 summarizes the main technical characteristics of a typical PCa sequence. A 3D MV sequence covering the whole gland is usually performed,[58] using long TE (120 milliseconds) because of better depiction of the tCho peak, although short TE acquisitions (32 milliseconds) may improve detection of Cit and polyamines

---

Box 3
Summary of technical characteristic of prostate MRS

Main technical characteristic of prostate MRS sequence

- 3D MV sequence covering the whole gland
- Combination of PRESS and 3D chemical shift imaging
- Lip and water suppression[58]
- Long TE (120 milliseconds)
- Voxel size inferior to 0.5 cm^3
- Saturation bands around prostate
- Automatic, manual, and higher-order shimming
- Performance 8 weeks after biopsy to reduce artifacts from postbiopsy hemorrhage
- 3 T improves SNR
- Endorectal coil is recommended on 1.5-T units, and considered optional on 3-T devices
- Acquisition time: 10 to 15 minutes approximately

(spermine).[59] ^{1}H MRS is usually acquired after morphologic multiplane T2-weighted sequences, which are used as a survey to locate the MRS volume in an axial or axial-oblique plane. Rectum wall and seminal vesicles should be excluded from the acquisition volume using saturation bands around the gland, which also help to reduce contamination from periprostatic fat. It is necessary to optimize acquisition with automatic and sometimes manual and higher-order shimming to optimize B_0 homogeneity, which is critical for adequate Lip and water suppression.[58] ^{1}H MRS is usually performed at least 8 weeks after biopsy to reduce susceptibility artifacts from postbiopsy hemorrhage.[60]

The use of an endorectal coil is recommended on 1.5-T units and considered optional on 3-T devices.[61] Independently of the field strength used, integrated ^{1}H MRS acquisition using endorectal and phased-array coils improves spectra quality and reduces the voxel size, increasing spatial resolution significantly. On the other hand, the use of an endorectal coil is not necessary for the rest of the multiparametric MR imaging protocol of PCa; it causes discomfort to patients and is expensive and time consuming. Thus, the necessity until recently of an endorectal coil for an accurate ^{1}H MRS acquisition is probably one of the main causes of the decline in the use of this technique in the detection of PCa.

Metabolites Cho and Cit are the most used metabolic biomarkers to detect PCa. Normal prostate tissue in the peripheral zone shows high levels of Cit and low content of Cho[62,63] (**Fig. 15**). Cit is also present in prostatic fluid.[63] In central and transition zones, the content in Cit diminishes, reflecting a decrease in glandular cell content. This decrease is even more evident in periurethral tissue and the anterior fibrostromal band, because these areas have no glandular content.[58] Conversely, in PCa, Cho, a marker of membrane turnover, is increased and Cit is decreased, reflecting loss of normal cellular function (**Fig. 16**). Cho is normally increased in tissue surrounding the ejaculatory ducts, urethra, and seminal vesicles, because of high levels of glycerolphosphocholine in the fluid of these structures, which is a potential cause of false-positive results.

The peak of Cho located at 3.2 ppm overlaps with the Cr peak (3.0 ppm), which is present in normal prostatic tissue and cancer.[64] The use of a 3-T magnet allows their accurate differentiation and also allows the detection of the polyamine peak, which is a broad spike, located between the Cr and Cho peaks. In PCa, polyamines, such as spermine, decrease significantly.[58,65]

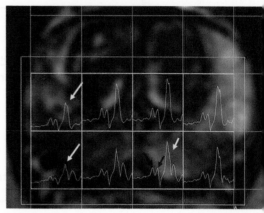

Fig. 15. A 72 year-old man with increased prostate-specific antigen levels (6.4 ng/mL). MV MRS presented over turbo spin echo T2-weighted image shows normal spectra (Cit [*white arrow*], Cr [*gray arrow*], and Cho [*black arrow*]) of left and central peripheral zone. However, a slight decreased of Cit without Cho increase (Cho + Cr/Cit ratio: 1.1) in right voxels (long white *arrows*) in a diffuse area of low signal intensity on T2-weighted image is consistent with chronic prostatitis, as confirmed in transrectal ultrasound guided biopsy.

Absolute quantification of the different peaks is complicated and rarely used in clinical practice. Thus, the use of metabolite ratios to identify abnormal metabolic patterns has become popular for the assessment of PCa. To accurately use these ratios, internal quality control is necessary to discard clinically uninterpretable spectra and to apply frequency and phase shifts corrections. Different commercial software allows for consistent estimation of the spectral baseline and phase corrections, and further manual adjustments are possible if necessary.[58] Also, a purely qualitative interpretation of the spectra has been shown to be valid, with similar results to a semiquantitative approach.[66]

Cho/Cit or Cho + Cr/Cit ratios are the most commonly used. Differences of 2 or 3 standard deviations of Cho + Cr/Cit ratio in the peripheral zone are considered as possible malignancy or highly suggestive of cancer, respectively.[67] The use of a numeric threshold for these ratios is not advisable because of differences between type of sequences applied, field strength (1.5-T vs 3-T magnets), and manufacturers. The greater the increase in Cho and the decrease in Cit, the more chances of a clinically significant PCa (see **Fig. 16**). In addition, in PCa, the Cho peak is superior to the polyamine peak, which can also be used as a clinical ratio for its depiction. The use of a standardized scoring system for the reading of spectra is accurate and increases interobserver agreement.[68,69]

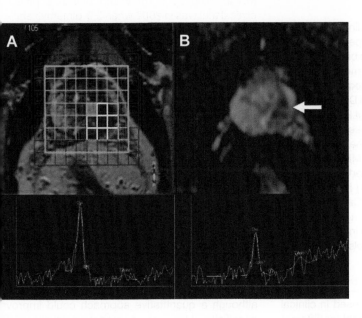

Fig. 16. MRS of PCa in a 65-year-old male. Low signal intensity lesion on axial TSE T2-weighted image (A) and with restriction of diffusion (B, ADC map) located on left peripheral zone is suspicious for malignancy. MV MRS (*bottom images*) show increased Cho peak with absence of visualization of both polyamine (Spm) and Cit caused by infiltration/substitution of normal prostatic tissue. This lesions corresponded to a prostatic carcinoma Gleason 6.

^{1}H MRS should always be integrated in a multiparametric MR imaging protocol, including other morphologic and functional sequences.[61] Using an integrated reading, it is possible to reduce false-positive results in MRS caused by stromal benign prostatic hyperplasia in the central gland or prostatitis in the peripheral zone, because both can show similar metabolic patterns to PCa.[2,70]

^{1}H MRS has been shown to improve PCa detection when added to an MR imaging protocol in several studies,[71–75] with a combined sensitivity and specificity on a patient level of 82% and 88%, respectively.[76] However, in a multicenter prospective trial,[65] the ACRIN (American College of Radiology Imaging Network) initiative reported absence of added benefit in the use of ^{1}H MRS compared with morphologic MR imaging in the localization of PCa using the prostatectomy specimens as reference. This result could be caused by either limited reproducibility of ^{1}H MRS between different centers or inherent limitations in sensitivity for PCa. Other potential applications in which MRS has shown to be of benefit are estimation of tumor volume, staging (extracapsular extension), tumor grading, and therapy monitoring of PCa[62,77–80] (Fig. 17).

The role of MR imaging in the management of PCa is a hot topic. Recent guidelines have accepted multiparametric MR imaging as a useful tool to localize

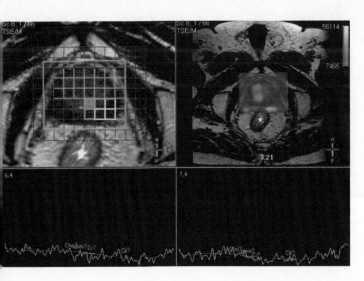

Fig. 17. Follow-up MRS of the previous patient, 5 months after radiotherapy. A diffuse decrease of signal intensity on axial T2-weighted images is identified related to radiation-induced changes. MV MRS at the location of previous malignant nodule shows a diffuse pattern of metabolic atrophy without clear identification of any metabolite peaks, consistent with adequate metabolic response.

and target biopsy in patients with clinical suspicion (persistent increased prostate-specific antigen levels) of PCa and previous negative biopsy.[81] Multi-parametric MR imaging combines morphologic information from T2-weighted sequences and functional information from DWI and DCE-MR imaging, with molecular characteristics of PCa, performing ^{1}H MRS. Although ^{1}H MRS has been shown to be useful, the most recent version of the standardized scoring system for multiparametric MR imaging, PI-RADS (Prostate Imaging and Reporting and Data System) version 2, has excluded ^{1}H MRS from the recommended protocol to detect PCa.[82] Therefore, ^{1}H MRS may soon be confined to a few research centers as an ancillary technique to increase specificity of multiparametric MR protocols.

Breast magnetic resonance spectroscopy

MR imaging is already commonly used in clinical practice for breast cancer assessment for different clinical indications. The vascular characteristics of breast lesions are explored using DCE-MR imaging sequences. Functional information has been obtained in clinical protocols with the introduction of DWI and true perfusion sequences (with high temporal resolution).[83] MR imaging has shown great sensitivity for breast cancer detection, but with reduced specificity. In this scenario, ^{1}H MRS, which is able to assess the biochemical behavior of breast lesions and helps in the differentiation between benign and malignant tumors,[48] has been proposed to increased specificity of breast MR imaging.[84,85]

The hallmark metabolite of malignancy in breast spectroscopy imaging is Cho. A Cho peak can be detected in normal breast tissue and benign lesions, but it increases in malignant lesions, related to the turnover of membranes (Fig. 18).[48] Measures of increased total Cho (tCho SNR>2) suppose a proper biomarker for malignant disease detection with good sensitivity and better specificity.[86] In clinical practice, a qualitative or semi-quantitative assessment of the Cho peak is used although a quantitative approach could improve specificity. However, a recent meta-analysis[86] did not find differences in lesion diagnosis with the different approaches to Cho evaluation.

Several technical considerations have to be taken in breast MR imaging, which are

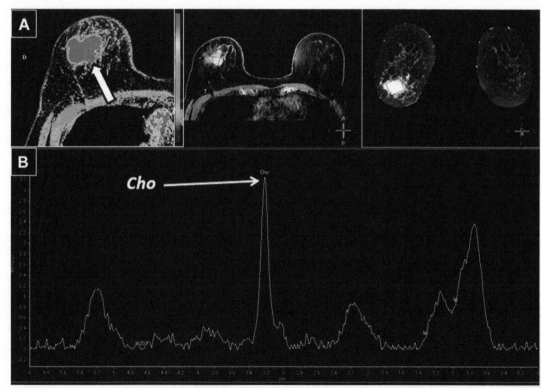

Fig. 18. Breast MRS in a 67-year-old woman with a suspicious right breast lesion (*solid arrow* in *A*) that shows high vascularization in (*A*) maximum relative enhancement parametric map and maximum intensity projection images derived from DCE-MR imaging, (*B*) SV MRS shows a marked Cho peak, both findings consistent with malignant origin. Notice the positioning of the VOI in *A* (middle and right images). Papillary breast carcinoma was confirmed on core biopsy.

summarized in **Box 4**. The use of 3-T and specific multiphase array coils of higher sensitivity improves SNR and spectral resolution.[87] The dominant physiological metabolite in the breast is Lip, and thus, a robust Lip suppression must be performed to obtain proper quality spectra. Most commonly, long TE acquisitions are used to detect Cho resonance, in an attempt to cancel any other peaks.[88] Most of the accumulated clinical experience has been with SV MRS (**Fig. 18**). Limitations in size and positioning of the sample voxel are challenging questions.[87] In addition, SV MRS limits normal MR imaging work flow, because an experienced radiologist is needed on site to place the voxel within doubtful enhancing lesions after the DCE-MR imaging sequence. The ^{1}H MRS sequence increased examination time between 5 and 10 minutes, with an overall MR imaging scan time of 45 minutes. Recently, MV sequences may have resolved some of these limitations, and they enable expanded coverage at the expense of longer acquisition time and lower SNR.[87] This approach can open new fields for breast MRS, such as breast cancer screening or local staging of breast cancer tissue.

Breast MRS can also be performed for tumor grading, therapy monitoring, and predicting response to treatment. Cho levels are related to histologic grade and biological aggressiveness.[89] In treated lesions, an early decrease of Cho levels, after the initial cycle of chemotherapy, is consistent with tumor response and is even more sensitive than morphologic and other functional criteria.[90,91] In addition, an increase of Cho concentration in patients with local recurrence has been shown.[89] Cho has been proposed as a potential biomarker for prediction of treatment response, because its levels are increased in breast cancer with adequate response to treatment compared with tumors with low Cho levels before treatment. In addition, patients with breast cancer demonstrating high pretreatment Cho levels show long-survival (>5 years). Malignant tumors with a high proliferative rate (and thus, high Cho levels) would be more sensitive to the effects of chemotherapy.[92]

Clinical experience with ^{1}H magnetic resonance spectroscopy in abdominal tumors

MRS application in upper abdominal organs is underdeveloped because of several technical drawbacks, mainly related to breathing and intestinal bowel motion. Thus, it should be considered an investigational technique confined to a few research centers. Specific MR imaging sequences with respiratory synchronization have to be applied to obtain acceptable quality spectra.[41,51,93,94] SV PRESS approaches are usually performed in the assessment of abdominal malignancies. 3 T magnets improve results, and the use of a torso phased-array coil is mandatory. Water suppression using a CHESS technique with short TE between 20 and 30 milliseconds is usually recommended. Local shimming ensures a uniform magnetic field and a more robust quality spectrum. Voxel placement with the solid component of the suspicious lesion avoiding vessels or parenchyma contamination is also critical. As in the breast, SV MRS is limited in the assessment of small lesions, because typical voxel size is between 10 and 30 mm^3.

MRS in the liver has increased substantially in its application to the characterization of diffuse hepatic disease, mostly fatty infiltration.[95] However, the evaluation of focal liver lesions with this technique is still in its firs steps. The presence of a large amount of Lip in liver makes it difficult to obtain an adequate isolated Cho peak.[96] Preliminary reports found a significant increase of Cho levels in hepatocellular carcinoma (HCC) compared with healthy liver tissue or benign lesions, which showed lower values.[97] Posteriorly, the increased Cho resonates in HCC and other malignant liver lesions have been confirmed (**Fig. 19**), although the use of Cho/Lip ratio to differentiate HCC from normal liver parenchyma remains controversial.[98,99] Conversely, the series by Fischbach and colleagues[100] did not report differences in Cho levels between malignant tumor and liver tissue. There is a reduced experience in focal liver lesion characterization with MRS, and different results may be caused by

---

Box 4

Summary of technical characteristic of breast MRS

Technical considerations in breast MRS

- SV technique

- Long TE acquisition

- Lip (and water) suppression

- 3-T magnets preferred over 1.5-T devices

- Specific multiphase array coils improve SNR and spectral resolution[93]

- Good shimming is critical to reduce B_0 field inhomogeneities

- Limitations in evaluation of lesions <10 mm

- Limitations in work flow because of SV positioning

- Acquisition time: 5–10 minutes

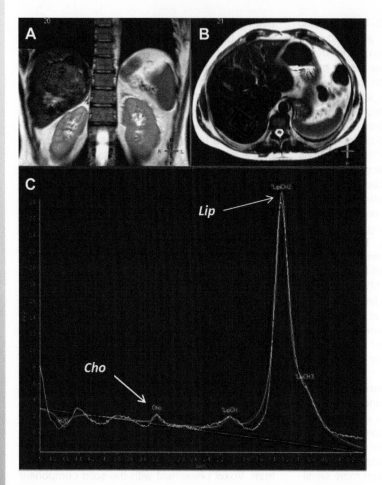

Fig. 19. Liver MRS of a focal lesion in a 56-year-old man with cirrhosis. (A and B) Coronal and axial TSE T2-weighted images show an ill-defined hyperintense lesion (red box in A and B, corresponding to the positioning of the VOI of MRS). (C) MRS SV shows a high Lip peak and a small Cho peak consistent with malignant origin. Well-differentiated HCC was surgically confirmed.

different sequences and postprocessing and reading methods, and the use of tCho (instead of its different compounds) to evaluate hepatic malignancies. Responding HCC after transcatheter arterial chemoembolization showed an early decrease in Cho levels, which creates a role for MRS in the therapy monitoring of HCC.[98,101] However, further studies have to be developed to improve both acquisition and spectra interpretation of MRS in liver.

Clinical pancreatic MRS is reduced to a few reports and presents similar limitations to liver MRS, but with another drawback, the physiologic presence of Cho in normal pancreatic tissue, with increased levels compared with pancreatic cancer. In this scenario, unsaturated fatty acids (located at 5.4 ppm) and Lip have been proposed as an alternative surrogate metabolic biomarker of pancreatic cancer, because there are significantly different levels in tumor tissue from those found in normal pancreas.[51,102]

Also, there is limited experience in the assessment of primary malignancies of the kidney with MRS. Significant differences in Lip content, rather than in Cho levels, can be detected with MRS between metastatic renal cell carcinoma (RCC) and normal tissue[53,103] (Fig. 20). In addition to problems derived from respiratory motion, the SV approach is limited in the assessment of tumor heterogeneity of large RCC.

^1H magnetic resonance spectroscopy in gynecologic malignancies

Several studies have reported that detection of increased levels of Cho and Cho/Cr ratios within an adnexal mass is suggestive of malignant origin with high sensitivity and specificity.[49] The presence of Lac peaks has been linked to malignancy. Other metabolites present in normal spectra have been used in the differential diagnosis of ovarian masses. For example, the presence of NAA is highly related to a mucinous component within a suspicious lesion, or the detection of a high Lip peak is specific of stromal cell tumors, like fibrothecoma.[56]

Cervical and endometrial carcinoma show increased Lip and Cho peaks. SV MRS or MRSI have been tested in experienced centers for

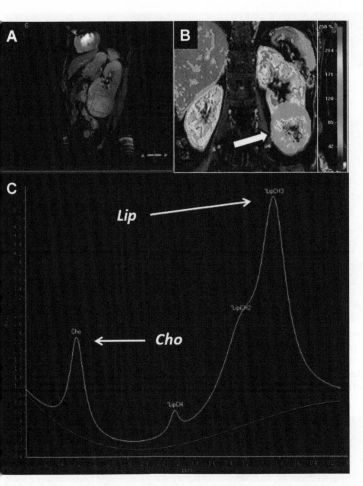

Fig. 20. MRS in a 37-year-old man with a left renal mass. (*A*) Sagittal balanced fast field-echo sequence (*red box*) and (*B*) coronal relative enhancement map from DCE-MR imaging sequence confirmed a large left renal mass (*arrow*) with intense peripheral enhancement and necrotic central area. (*C*) SV MRS showed increases in both Cho and Lip peaks, consistent with a malignant lesion with associated necrosis. A clear cell RCC was surgically confirmed.

evaluation of the uterus; however, the performance of high-quality spectra in the cervix is challenging.[104–106] Thus, MRS can differentiate between benign and malignant endometrial and myometrial lesions. Lip and Cho are metabolic biomarkers of endometrial carcinoma and help in its differentiation from benign lesions. In addition, Cho level increases with FIGO (International Federation of Gynecology and Obstetrics) tumor stage and size. Also, Lip can differentiate uterine sarcomas from leiomyomas.[104,105,107]

¹H magnetic resonance spectroscopy of testicular tumors

The biochemical evaluation of testicular function has been made classically through hormonal serum level or even spermiogram analysis. MRS provides a new insight in functional evaluation of the testicles. The spermatogenesis process implies an increase of cellular activity, and thus, increasing Cho peaks may be identified at spectra and considered as a biomarker of normal testicular

function.[52] Almost every clinical scenario featuring impaired testicular normal activity shows decreased levels of Cho peak, as it occurs in sterility or in focal testicular lesions (**Fig. 21**). The local infiltration or invasion of testicular parenchyma by tumor cells may lead to a lower Cho level than expected from normal testicular function.

¹H magnetic resonance spectroscopy of colorectal cancer

With the clinical use of 3-T magnets, it is possible to evaluate rectal cancer with phased-array coils. The evaluation of colorectal cancer using MRS is technically demanding, not only for bowel movement but also for the presence of multiple interfaces between air, fat, and rectal wall that may result in an inhomogeneous magnetic field and poor spectra quality. Although limited to investigational settings, MRS can show increases of Cho and Lip in colorectal cancer, and these metabolites have also been proposed as potential biomarkers of response to treatment[108] (**Fig. 22**). In

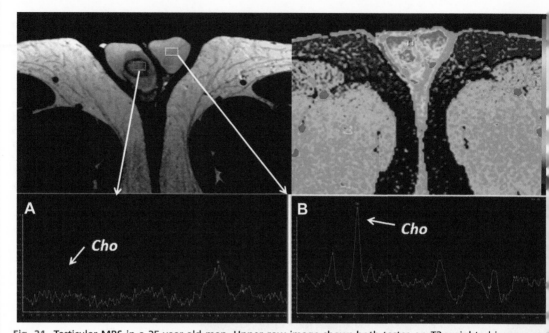

Fig. 21. Testicular MRS in a 25-year-old man. Upper row image shows both testes on T2-weighted images and DCE-MR imaging derived parametric map. (*B*) SV MRS of normal left testicle shows large Cho peak consistent with spermatogenesis and testicular function preserved. (*A*) SV MRS of right testicle located over an upper pole hypointense lesion on T2-weighted sequence shows a lower Cho peak caused by parenchymal substitution by tumoral cells. Surgical excision confirmed a right testicular seminoma.

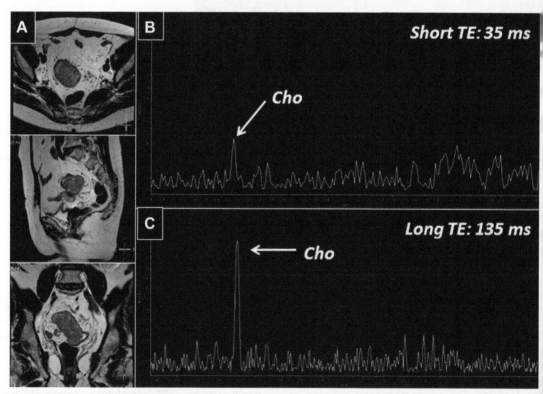

Fig. 22. MRS in a 67-year-old woman with a suspicious mass in the sigmoid colon (*A*) as shown in the 3 planes TSE T2-weighted images used for SV positioning. (*B*) SV short TE MRS spectra show a small Cho peak that becomes more evident on (*C*) long TE acquisition. This Cho peak is consistent with high cellular proliferation and thus, with malignant origin. Mucinous carcinoma was confirmed by endorectal biopsy.

patients who underwent chemotherapy and radio-therapy, a significant decrease of Cho level was found, whereas Lip levels remained unchanged.[109] ¹H MRS has also been found of interest in the assessment of postsurgical recurrence of rectal cancer, because an increase of residual Lip peaks in the postsurgical bed suggests tumor recurrence, and lower Lip peaks are present in scarring postoperative fibrosis.[110]

¹H magnetic resonance spectroscopy of soft tissue and bone tumors

Long-echo time SV MRS is most commonly used, but an MV approach can also be performed. Acquisitions include water suppression, although if metabolic quantification using water as reference is applied, a second acquisition without water suppression is recommended.[111] It is necessary to position the VOI in the solid area of the tumors, avoiding regions of hemorrhage, calcification, and necrosis. Local shimming, mostly manual, is necessary to ensure a homogeneous local magnetic field. The use of 3-T magnets and smaller surface coils improves results.

Malignant bone and soft tissue tumors show increased levels of tCho or its equivalent metabolite trimethylamine (TMA) (**Fig. 23**). However, the presence of Cho is not enough to characterize a musculoskeletal lesion as malignant, because it is also present in metabolically active benign lesions and abscesses.[112] In this setting, quantitative assessment of Cho shows a high negative predictive value, with specificity higher than 90%, which is of help in the characterization of indeterminate musculoskeletal lesions.[113] A negative MRS reduces dramatically the chance of a musculoskeletal lesion being malignant.

Another common peak in musculoskeletal lesions is Lip, which may present in abscess walls, malignant masses, and treated tumors.[114] Most of the reported experience with Lip peak has centered on bone marrow, because Lip/water ratio can differentiate normal bone marrow from that infiltrated by leukemia[115] and can help in the therapy monitoring of multiple myeloma.[116]

Moreover, preliminary reports suggest a potential role of MRS in therapy monitoring of bone and soft tissue sarcoma. The objective of chemotherapy is to produce massive necrosis within the lesion, which may be depicted as a decline of Cho to negligible levels.[117] In recurrent tumor after surgery or treatment, a Cho peak is usually present.[118] All these oncologic applications of MRS in the musculoskeletal system should be fully explored in multicenter trials, including the added value of its inclusion in a multiparametric protocol.

¹H magnetic resonance spectroscopy of head and neck tumors

Head and neck tumors have classically shown a poorer spectra quality when compared to other locations. Performing 1 H-MRS has always been a challenge in terms of its technical requisites, probably due to breathing and swallowing movements, susceptibility artifacts and heterogeneity of the target lesions. Nevertheless, some studies have shown increased Cho/Cr ratios in head and neck neoplastic lesions such as squamous cell carcinoma, but also in lesions with increased cell proliferation like schwanommas.[119] Recently, increased succinate levels have been described in neck succinate dehydrogenase related paragangliomas, while in other paragangliomas and tumors this metabolite was absent.[120]

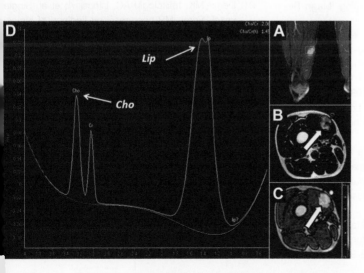

Fig. 23. MRS in a 28-year-old man with a right thigh palpable lump. (A) Coronal fat-suppressed turbo spin echo T2-weighted sequence shows an ill-defined hyperintense lesion at the vastus medialis (red box in A). (B) Fused axial turbo spin echo T2-weighted and DWI with high b value (1000 s/mm²) showed high cellularity within the lesion. (C) DCE-MR imaging shows an intense uptake on relative enhancement map. (D) SV MRS of the lesion shows a high Cho peak with large Lip peak (white arrows in D) consistent with metabolic aggressiveness of the lesion. Intramuscular lymphoma was confirmed by core biopsy.

SUMMARY

MRS is the single molecular MR imaging technique that provides in vivo biochemical information of different tissues. Clinical MRS is mainly based on the ^{1}H proton, which has been routinely used for brain tumor evaluation and treatment follow-up, as an essential piece of the multiparametric MR imaging assessment of the CNS, along with perfusion and DWI. MRS has overcome the limitations secondary to motion artifacts in the body and has been exported to other anatomic areas with successful clinical results, as in the case of PCa, increasing the overall specificity of a multiparametric MR imaging approach. However, its clinical role in prostate MR imaging is now under debate because of limited reproducibility. In malignancies of other locations, such as breast, several abdominopelvic organs, or the musculoskeletal system, Cho or Lip are used as biomarkers of malignancy, increasing the specificity of multiparametric MR imaging. However, clinical experience in these regions is limited to research centers and further investigation is needed for the expansion of this technique.

REFERENCES

1. Hollingworth W, Medina LS, Lenkinski RE, et al. A systematic literature review of magnetic resonance spectroscopy for the characterization of brain tumors. AJNR Am J Neuroradiol 2006;27(7):1404–11.

2. Murphy G, Haider M, Ghai S, et al. The expanding role of MRI in prostate cancer. AJR Am J Roentgenol 2013;201(6):1229–38.

3. Sánchez-González J, Tsao J, Dydak U, et al. Minimum-norm reconstruction for sensitivity-encoded magnetic resonance spectroscopic imaging. Magn Reson Med 2006;55(2):287–95.

4. Dydak U, Weiger M, Pruessmann KP, et al. Sensitivity-encoded spectroscopic imaging. Magn Reson Med 2001;46(4):713–22.

5. Haase A, Frahm J, Hänicke W, et al. 1H NMR chemical shift selective (CHESS) imaging. Phys Med Biol 1985;30(4):341–4.

6. Bottomley PA. Spatial localization in NMR spectroscopy in vivo. Ann N Y Acad Sci 1987;508:333–48.

7. Frahm J, Bruhn H, Merboldt K-D. Localized proton spectroscopy using stimulated echoes. Magn Reson Med 1987;72:502–8.

8. Van den Boogaart A, Ala-Korpela M, Jokisaari J, et al. Time and frequency domain analysis of NMR data compared: an application to 1D 1H spectra of lipoproteins. Magn Reson Med 1994; 31(4):347–58.

9. Provencher SW. Estimation of metabolite concentrations from localized in vivo proton NMR spectra. Magn Reson Med 1993;30(6):672–9.

10. Kreis R. Issues of spectral quality in clinical 1H-magnetic resonance spectroscopy and a gallery of artifacts. NMR Biomed 2004;17(6):361–81.

11. Galanaud D, Nicoli F, Chinot O, et al. Noninvasive diagnostic assessment of brain tumors using combined in vivo MR imaging and spectroscopy. Magn Reson Med 2006;55:1236–45.

12. Horská A, Barker PB. Imaging of brain tumors: MR spectroscopy and metabolic imaging. Neuroimaging Clin North Am 2010;20(3):293–310.

13. Fayed N, Olmos S, Morales H, et al. Physical basis of magnetic resonance spectroscopy and its application to central nervous system diseases. Am J Appl Sci 2006;3(5):1836–45.

14. Bertholdo D, Watcharakorn A. Brain proton magnetic resonance spectroscopy: introduction and overview. Neuroimaging Clin North Am 2013; 23(3):359–80.

15. Majos C, Julia-Sape M, Alonso J, et al. Brain tumor classification by proton MR spectroscopy: comparison of diagnostic accuracy at short and long TE. AJNR Am J Neuroradiol 2004;25(10):1696–704.

16. Soares DP, Law M. Magnetic resonance spectroscopy of the brain: review of metabolites and clinical applications. Clin Radiol 2009;64(1):12–21.

17. Zeng Q, Liu H, Zhang K, et al. Noninvasive evaluation of cerebral glioma grade by using multivoxel 3D proton MR spectroscopy. Magn Reson Imaging 2011;29(1):25–31.

18. Bulik M, Jancalek R, Vanicek J, et al. Potential of MR spectroscopy for assessment of glioma grading. Clin Neurol Neurosurg 2013;115(2):146–53.

19. Grand S, Passaro G, Ziegler A, et al. Necrotic tumor versus brain abscess: importance of amino acids detected at 1H MR spectroscopy–initial results. Radiology 1999;213(3):785–93.

20. Castillo M, Smith JK, Kwock L. Correlation of myo-inositol levels and grading of cerebral astrocytomas. Am J Neuroradiol 2000;21(9):1645–9.

21. Demir MK, Iplikcioglu AC, Dincer A, et al. Single voxel proton MR spectroscopy findings of typical and atypical intracranial meningiomas. Eur J Radiol 2006;60(1):48–55.

22. Moreno-Torres Á, Martínez-Pérez I, Baquero M, et al. Taurine detection by proton magnetic resonance spectroscopy in medulloblastoma: contribution to noninvasive differential diagnosis with cerebellar astrocytoma. Neurosurgery 2004;55(4):824–9.

23. Cianfoni A, Niku S, Imbesi SG. Metabolite findings in tumefactive demyelinating lesions utilizing short echo time proton magnetic resonance spectroscopy. Am J Neuroradiol 2007;28(2):272–7.

24. Brandão LA, Castillo M. Adult brain tumors: clinical applications of magnetic resonance spectroscopy. Neuroimaging Clin North Am 2013;23(3):527–55.

25. Stadlbauer A, Nimsky C, Buslei R, et al. Proton magnetic resonance spectroscopic imaging in

the border zone of gliomas: correlation of metabolic and histological changes at low tumor infiltration–initial results. Invest Radiol 2007;42(4):218–23.

26. McKnight TR, von dem Bussche MH, Vigneron DB, et al. Histopathological validation of a three-dimensional magnetic resonance spectroscopy index as a predictor of tumor presence. J Neurosurg 2002;97(4):794–802.

27. Pirzkall A, McKnight TR, Graves EE, et al. MR-spectroscopy guided target delineation for high-grade gliomas. Int J Radiat Oncol Biol Phys 2001; 50(4):915–28.

28. Hall WA, Martin A, Liu H, et al. Improving diagnostic yield in brain biopsy: coupling spectroscopic targeting with real-time needle placement. J Magn Reson Imaging 2001;13(1):12–5.

29. Hermann EJ, Hattingen E, Krauss JK, et al. Stereotactic biopsy in gliomas guided by 3-tesla 1H-chemical- shift imaging of choline. Stereotact Funct Neurosurg 2008;86(5):300–7.

30. Brandão LA, Shiroishi MS, Law M. Brain tumors. A multimodality approach with diffusion-weighted imaging, diffusion tensor imaging, magnetic resonance spectroscopy, dynamic susceptibility contrast and dynamic contrast-enhanced magnetic resonance imaging. Magn Reson Imaging Clin North Am 2013;21(2):199–239.

31. Wilson M, Cummins CL, MacPherson L, et al. Magnetic resonance spectroscopy metabolite profiles predict survival in paediatric brain tumours. Eur J Cancer 2013;49(2):457–64.

32. Majós C, Bruna J, Julià-Sapé M, et al. Proton MR spectroscopy provides relevant prognostic information in high-grade astrocytomas. Am J Neuroradiol 2011;32(1):74–80.

33. Li X, Jin H, Lu Y, et al. Identification of MRI and 1H MRSI parameters that may predict survival for patients with malignant gliomas. NMR Biomed 2004; 17(1):10–20.

34. Murphy PS, Viviers L, Abson C, et al. Monitoring temozolomide treatment of low-grade glioma with proton magnetic resonance spectroscopy. Br J Cancer 2004;90(4):781–6.

35. Shah R, Vattoth S, Jacob R, et al. Radiation necrosis in the brain: imaging features and differentiation from tumor recurrence. Radiographics 2012;32(5): 1343–59.

36. Bobek-Billewicz B, Stasik-Pres G, Majchrzak H, et al. Differentiation between brain tumor recurrence and radiation injury using perfusion, diffusion-weighted imaging and MR spectroscopy. Folia Neuropathol 2010;48(2):81–92.

37. Zhang H, Ma L, Wang Q, et al. Role of magnetic resonance spectroscopy for the differentiation of recurrent glioma from radiation necrosis: a systematic review and meta-analysis. Eur J Radiol 2014; 83(12):2181–9.

38. Smith EA, Carlos RC, Junck LR, et al. Developing a clinical decision model: MR spectroscopy to differentiate between recurrent tumor and radiation change in patients with new contrast-enhancing lesions. AJR Am J Roentgenol 2009;192(2):W45–52.

39. Elias AE, Carlos RC, Smith EA, et al. MR spectroscopy using normalized and non-normalized metabolite ratios for differentiating recurrent brain tumor from radiation injury. Acad Radiol 2011;18(9):1101–8.

40. Matsusue E, Fink JR, Rockhill JK, et al. Distinction between glioma progression and post-radiation change by combined physiologic MR imaging. Neuroradiology 2010;52(4):297–306.

41. Katz-Brull R, Rofsky NM, Lenkinski RE. Breathhold abdominal and thoracic proton MR spectroscopy at 3T. Magn Reson Med 2003;50(3):461–7.

42. Scheenen TWJ, Heijmink SWTPJ, Roell SA, et al. Three-dimensional proton MR spectroscopy of human prostate at 3 T without endorectal coil: feasibility. Radiology 2007;245(2):507–16.

43. Glunde K, Bhujwalla ZM, Ronen SM. Choline metabolism in malignant transformation. Nat Rev Cancer 2011;11(12):835–48.

44. Glunde K, Jie C, Bhujwalla ZM. Molecular causes of the aberrant choline phospholipid metabolism in breast cancer. Cancer Res 2004;64(12):4270–6.

45. Marchan R, Lesjak MS, Stewart JD, et al. Choline-releasing glycerophosphodiesterase EDI3 links the tumor metabolome to signaling network activities. Cell Cycle 2012;11(24):4499–506.

46. Awwad HM, Geisel J, Obeid R. The role of choline in prostate cancer. Clin Biochem 2012;45(18): 1548–53.

47. Weinreb JC, Blume JD, Coakley FV, et al. Prostate cancer: sextant localization at MR imaging and MR spectroscopic imaging before prostatectomy–results of ACRIN prospective multi-institutional clinicopathologic study. Radiology 2009;251(1):122–33.

48. Birdwell RL, Mountford CE, Iglehart JD. Molecular imaging of the breast. Radiol Clin North Am 2010; 48(5):1075–88.

49. Cho SW, Cho SG, Lee JH, et al. In-vivo proton magnetic resonance spectroscopy in adnexal lesions. Korean J Radiol 2002;3(2):105–12.

50. Vendrell MJ. Enhancing nonmass lesions in the breast: evaluation with proton (1H) MR spectroscopy. Breast Dis 2008;19(2):138–9.

51. Yao X, Zeng M, Wang H, et al. Metabolite detection of pancreatic carcinoma by in vivo proton MR spectroscopy at 3T: initial results. Radiol Med 2012;117(5):780–8.

52. Firat AK, Uğraş M, Karakaş HM, et al. 1H magnetic resonance spectroscopy of the normal testis: preliminary findings. Magn Reson Imaging 2008;26(2):215–20. Available at: http://www.scopus.com/inward/record.url?eid=2-s2.0-38349094164&partnerID=40&md5=3c3fdc6e5ed5020752fce38e64a1d1e1.

53. Katz-Brull R, Rofsky NM, Morrin MM, et al. Decreases in free cholesterol and fatty acid unsaturation in renal cell carcinoma demonstrated by breath-hold magnetic resonance spectroscopy. Am J Physiol Renal Physiol 2005;288(4):F637–41.

54. Ackerstaff E, Glunde K, Bhujwalla ZM. Choline phospholipid metabolism: a target in cancer cells? J Cell Biochem 2003;90(3):525–33.

55. Rizwan A, Glunde K. Imaging of tumor metabolism: MR spectroscopy. In: Luna A, Vilanova JC, Hygino Da Cruz LC Jr, et al, editors. Functional imaging in oncology, vol., 1st edition. Berlin; Heidelberg (Germany): Springer-Verlag; 2014;1(2) p. 147–80.

56. Ma FH, Qiang JW, Cai SQ, et al. MR spectroscopy for differentiating benign from malignant solid adnexal tumors. Am J Roentgenol 2015;204(6): W724–30.

57. Ferlay J, Shin HR, Bray F, et al. Estimates of worldwide burden of cancer in 2008: GLOBOCAN 2008. Int J Cancer 2010;127(12):2893–917.

58. Verma S, Rajesh A, Fütterer JJ, et al. Prostate MRI and 3D MR spectroscopy: how we do it. Am J Roentgenol 2010;194(6):1414–26.

59. Basharat M, Payne GS, Morgan VA. TE = 32 ms vs TE = 100 ms echo-time 1 H-magnetic resonance spectroscopy in prostate cancer: tumor metabolite depiction and absolute concentrations in tumors and adjacent tissues. J Magn Reson Imaging 2015. http://dx.doi.org/10.1002/jmri.24875.

60. Qayyum A, Coakley FV, Lu Y, et al. Organ-confined prostate cancer: effect of prior transrectal biopsy on endorectal MRI and MR spectroscopic imaging. Am J Roentgenol 2004;183(4):1079–83.

61. Barentsz JO, Richenberg J, Clements R, et al. ESUR prostate MR guidelines 2012. Eur Radiol 2012;22(4):746–57.

62. Choi YJ, Kim JK, Kim N, et al. Functional MR imaging of prostate cancer. Radiographics 2007;27(1): 63–75.

63. Yacoe ME, Sommer G, Peehl D. In vitro proton spectroscopy of normal and abnormal prostate. Magn Reson Med 1991;19(2):429–38.

64. Kurhanewicz J, Swanson MG, Nelson SJ, et al. Combined magnetic resonance imaging and spectroscopic imaging approach to molecular imaging of prostate cancer. J Magn Reson Imaging 2002; 16(4):451–63.

65. Oliveira Neto JA, Parente DB. Multiparametric magnetic resonance imaging of the prostate. Magn Reson Imaging Clin North Am 2013;21(2): 409–26.

66. Klijn S, De Visschere PJ, De Meerleer GO, et al. Comparison of qualitative and quantitative approach to prostate MR spectroscopy in peripheral zone cancer detection. Eur J Radiol 2012;81(3):411–6.

67. Jung JA, Coakley FV, Vigneron DB, et al. Prostate depiction at endorectal MR spectroscopic imaging: investigation of a standardized evaluation system. Radiology 2004;233(3):701–8.

68. Fütterer JJ, Scheenen TWJ, Heijmink SWTPJ, et al. Standardized threshold approach using three-dimensional proton magnetic resonance spectroscopic imaging in prostate cancer localization of the entire prostate. Invest Radiol 2007;42(2):116–22.

69. Kurhanewicz J, Vigneron DB. Advances in MR spectroscopy of the prostate. Magn Reson Imaging Clin North Am 2008;16(4):697–710.

70. Shukla-Dave A, Hricak H, Eberhardt SC, et al. Chronic prostatitis: MR imaging and 1H MR spectroscopic imaging findings–initial observations. Radiology 2004;231(3):717–24.

71. Scheidler J, Hricak H, Vigneron DB, et al. Prostate cancer: localization with three-dimensional proton MR spectroscopic imaging–clinicopathologic study. Radiology 1999;213(2):473–80.

72. Kumar V, Jagannathan NR, Thulkar S, et al. Prebiopsy magnetic resonance spectroscopy and imaging in the diagnosis of prostate cancer. Int J Urol 2012;19(7):602–13.

73. Reinsberg SA, Payne GS, Riches SF, et al. Combined use of diffusion-weighted MRI and 1H MR spectroscopy to increase accuracy in prostate cancer detection. AJR Am J Roentgenol 2007; 188(1):91–8.

74. Vilanova JC, Comet J, Barceló-Vidal C, et al. Peripheral zone prostate cancer in patients with elevated PSA levels and low free-to-total PSA ratio: detection with MR imaging and MR spectroscopy. Radiology 2009;253(1):135–43.

75. Aydin H, Kizilgöz V, Tatar IG, et al. Detection of prostate cancer with magnetic resonance imaging: optimization of T1-weighted, T2-weighted, dynamic-enhanced T1-weighted, diffusion-weighted imaging apparent diffusion coefficient mapping sequences and MR spectroscopy, correlated with biopsy a. J Comput Assist Tomogr 2012;36(1):30–45.

76. Umbehr M, Bachmann LM, Held U, et al. Combined magnetic resonance imaging and magnetic resonance spectroscopy imaging in the diagnosis of prostate cancer: a systematic review and meta-analysis. Eur Urol 2009;55(3):575–91.

77. Wetter A, Engl TA, Nadjmabadi D, et al. Combined MRI and MR spectroscopy of the prostate before radical prostatectomy. Am J Roentgenol 2006; 187(3):724–30.

78. Claus FG, Hricak H, Hattery RR. Pretreatment evaluation of prostate cancer: role of MR imaging and 1H MR spectroscopy. Radiographics 2004; 24(Suppl 1):S167–80.

79. Kurhanewicz J, McKenna DA, Coakley FV, et al. Role of magnetic resonance imaging and magnetic resonance spectroscopic imaging before and after radiotherapy for prostate cancer. J Endourol 2008; 22(4):789–94.

80. Kobus T, Wright AJ, Scheenen TWJ, et al. Mapping of prostate cancer by 1H MRSI. NMR Biomed 2014;27(1):39–52.

81. Mottet N, Bellmunt J, Briers E, et al. Guidelines on prostate cancer. European Association of Urology; 2015. Available at: http://uroweb.org/wp-content/uploads/09-Prostate-Cancer_LR.pdf.

82. Chatfield M, Weinreb JC, Barentsz JO, et al. PI-RADS version 2. American College of Radiology; 2015. Available at: http://www.acr.org/~/media/ACR/Documents/PDF/QualitySafety/Resources/PIRADS/PIRADS V2.pdf.

83. Partridge SC, Rahbar H, Murthy R, et al. Improved diagnostic accuracy of breast MRI through combined apparent diffusion coefficients and dynamic contrast-enhanced kinetics. Magn Reson Med 2011;65(6):1759–67.

84. Huang W, Fisher PR, Dulaimy K, et al. Detection of breast malignancy: diagnostic MR protocol for improved specificity. Radiology 2004;232(2):585–91.

85. Meisamy S, Bolan PJ, Baker EH, et al. Adding in vivo quantitative 1H MR spectroscopy to improve diagnostic accuracy of breast MR imaging: preliminary results of observer performance study at 4.0 T. Radiology 2005;236(2):465–75.

86. Baltzer PAT, Dietzel M. Breast lesions: diagnosis by using proton MR spectroscopy at 1.5 and 3.0 T–systematic review and meta-analysis. Radiology 2013;267(3):735–46.

87. Bolan PJ. Magnetic resonance spectroscopy of the breast: current status. Magn Reson Imaging Clin North Am 2013;21(3):625–39.

88. Haddadin IS, McIntosh A, Meisamy S, et al. Metabolite quantification and high-field MRS in breast cancer. NMR Biomed 2009;22(1):65–76.

89. Shin HJ, Baek H-M, Cha JH, et al. Evaluation of breast cancer using proton MR spectroscopy: total choline peak integral and signal-to-noise ratio as prognostic indicators. AJR Am J Roentgenol 2012;198(5):W488–97.

90. Bathen TF, Heldahl MG, Sitter B, et al. In vivo MRS of locally advanced breast cancer: characteristics related to negative or positive choline detection and early monitoring of treatment response. MAGMA 2011;24(6):347–57.

91. Jagannathan NR, Kumar M, Seenu V, et al. Evaluation of total choline from in-vivo volume localized proton MR spectroscopy and its response to neoadjuvant chemotherapy in locally advanced breast cancer. Br J Cancer 2001;84(8):1016–22.

92. Cao MD, Sitter B, Bathen TF, et al. Predicting long-term survival and treatment response in breast cancer patients receiving neoadjuvant chemotherapy by MR metabolic profiling. NMR Biomed 2012;25(2):369–78.

93. Hammer S, de Vries APJ, de Heer P, et al. Metabolic imaging of human kidney triglyceride content: reproducibility of proton magnetic resonance spectroscopy. PLoS One 2013;8(4):e62209.

94. Van der Meer RW, Doornbos J, Kozerke S, et al. Metabolic imaging of myocardial triglyceride content: reproducibility of 1H MR spectroscopy with respiratory navigator gating in volunteers. Radiology 2007;245(1):251–7.

95. Lee SS, Park SH. Radiologic evaluation of nonalcoholic fatty liver disease. World J Gastroenterol 2014;20(23):7392–402.

96. ter Voert E. Magnetic resonance spectroscopy of liver tumors and metastases. World J Gastroenterol 2011;17(47):5133.

97. Li CW, Kuo YC, Chen CY, et al. Quantification of choline compounds in human hepatic tumors by proton MR spectroscopy at 3 T. Magn Reson Med 2005;53(4):770–6.

98. Kuo YT, Li CW, Chen CY, et al. In vivo proton magnetic resonance spectroscopy of large focal hepatic lesions and metabolite change of hepatocellular carcinoma before and after transcatheter arterial chemoembolization using 3.0-T MR scanner. J Magn Reson Imaging 2004;19(5):598–604.

99. Wang D, Li Y. 1H magnetic resonance spectroscopy predicts hepatocellular carcinoma in a subset of patients with liver cirrhosis: a randomized trial. Med (Baltimore) 2015;94(27):e1006.

100. Fischbach F, Schirmer T, Thormann M, et al. Quantitative proton magnetic resonance spectroscopy of the normal liver and malignant hepatic lesions at 3.0 Tesla. Eur Radiol 2008;18(11):2549–58.

101. Bian DJ, Xiao EH, Hu DX, et al. Magnetic resonance spectroscopy on hepatocellular carcinoma after transcatheter arterial chemoembolization. Chin J Cancer 2010;29(2):200–1.

102. Ma X, Zhao X, Ouyang H, et al. The metabolic features of normal pancreas and pancreatic adenocarcinoma: preliminary result of in vivo proton magnetic resonance spectroscopy at 3.0 T. J Comput Assist Tomogr 2011;35(5):539–43.

103. Süllentrop F, Hahn J, Moka D. In vitro and in vivo 1 H-MR spectroscopic examination of the renal cell carcinoma. Int J Biomed Sci 2012;8(2):94–108.

104. Han X, Kang J, Zhang J, et al. Can the signal-to-noise ratio of choline in magnetic resonance spectroscopy reflect the aggressiveness of endometrial cancer? Acad Radiol 2015;22(4):453–9.

105. Celik O, Hascalik S, Sarac K, et al. Magnetic resonance spectroscopy of premalignant and malignant endometrial disorders: a feasibility of in vivo study. Eur J Obstet Gynecol Reprod Biol 2005; 118(2):241–5.

106. De Silva SS, Payne GS, Thomas V, et al. Investigation of metabolite changes in the transition from pre-invasive to invasive cervical cancer measured using 1H and 31P magic angle spinning MRS of intact tissue. NMR Biomed 2009;22(2):191–8.

107. Takeuchi M, Matsuzaki K, Harada M. Preliminary observations and clinical value of lipid peak in high-grade uterine sarcomas using in vivo proton MR spectroscopy. Eur Radiol 2013;23(9): 2358–63.

108. Dzik-Jurasz AS, Murphy PS, George M, et al. Human rectal adenocarcinoma: demonstration of 1H-MR spectra in vivo at 1.5 T. Magn Reson Med 2002;47(4):809–11.

109. Kim MJ, Lee SJ, Lee JH, et al. Detection of rectal cancer and response to concurrent chemoradiotherapy by proton magnetic resonance spectroscopy. Magn Reson Imaging 2012;30(6):848–53.

110. Jeon YS, Cho SG, Choi SK, et al. Differentiation of recurrent rectal cancer and postoperative fibrosis: preliminary report by proton MR spectroscopy. J Korean Soc Magn Reson Med 2004;8(1):24–31.

111. Fayad LM, Wang X, Salibi N, et al. A feasibility study of quantitative molecular characterization of musculoskeletal lesions by proton MR spectroscopy at 3 T. AJR Am J Roentgenol 2010;195(1):W69–75.

112. Doganay S, Altinok T, Alkan A, et al. The role of MRS in the differentiation of benign and malignant soft tissue and bone tumors. Eur J Radiol 2011; 79(2):e33–7.

113. Subhawong TK, Wang X, Durand DJ, et al. Proton MR spectroscopy in metabolic assessment of musculoskeletal lesions. Am J Roentgenol 2012; 198(1):162–72.

114. Drapé J-L. Advances in magnetic resonance imaging of musculoskeletal tumours. Orthop Traumatol Surg Res 2013;99(1 Suppl):S115–23.

115. Jensen KE, Jensen M, Grundtvig P, et al. Localized in vivo proton spectroscopy of the bone marrow in patients with leukemia. Magn Reson Imaging 1990; 8(6):779–89.

116. Oriol A, Valverde D, Capellades J, et al. In vivo quantification of response to treatment in patients with multiple myeloma by 1H magnetic resonance spectroscopy of bone marrow. MAGMA 2007; 20(2):93–101.

117. Hsieh TJ, Li CW, Chuang HY, et al. Longitudinally monitoring chemotherapy effect of malignant musculoskeletal tumors with in vivo proton magnetic resonance spectroscopy: an initial experience. J Comput Assist Tomogr 2008; 32(6):987–94.

118. Fayad LM, Barker PB, Jacobs MA, et al. Characterization of musculoskeletal lesions on 3-T proton MR spectroscopy. Am J Roentgenol 2007;188(6): 1513–20.

119. Tse GM, King AD, Yu AMC, et al. Correlation of biomarkers in head and neck squamous cell carcinoma. Otolaryngol Head Neck Surg 2010;143(6): 795–800.

120. Varoquaux A, Le Fur Y, Imperiale A, et al. Magnetic resonance spectroscopy of paragangliomas: new insights into in vivo metabolomics. Endocr Relat Cancer 2015, in press.

Multiparametric MR Imaging in the Assessment of Brain Tumors

Margareth Kimura, MD[a],*, L. Celso Hygino da Cruz Jr, MD, PhD[b]

KEYWORDS

- Perfusion • Permeability • Diffusion-weighted imaging • Spectroscopy • Tractography
- Diffusion tensor imaging • BOLD • Brain tumor

KEY POINTS

- A multiparametric MR imaging approach can better guide lesion biopsy to the place of higher perfusion, lower ADC, and increased levels of choline, representing the most aggressive areas within a neoplasm.
- Multiparametric MRI can also predict the histopathologic diagnosis of the lesion; some specific neoplasms have particular MR imaging characteristics, for example lymphoma, which presents low ADC values, low perfusion, and high choline associated with lipids and lactate peaks on MRS.
- In general, anaplastic neoplasms have higher perfusion and permeability, higher choline levels, and lower ADC values than low-grade gliomas.
- Tumor treatment response can be assessed by changes depicted in the advanced MR imaging sequences in the sequential examinations performed before, during, and after the therapy.
- Overall survival is worse if a tumor presents high choline, lipids and lactate, restricted diffusion, and high perfusion (rCBV >1.75).

INTRODUCTION

Brain tumors represent 1.4% of all new cases of cancer in the United States annually, but underlie 2.4% of all deaths caused by cancer.[1] Most brain tumors diagnosed are metastatic; the annual incidence of new metastatic brain cancer cases in the United States is 150,000 to 200,000.[2,3] Several recently developed physiology-based MR imaging methods, such as diffusion-weighted imaging (DWI), diffusion tensor imaging (DTI), permeability, perfusion imaging, and magnetic resonance spectroscopy (MRS), have become widely used in the assessment of brain lesions. A multiparametric brain tumor diagnostic approach allows for better lesion evaluation, including more accurate tumor grading, surgical biopsy guidance, and enhanced treatment response monitoring. Although advanced imaging techniques are in routine clinical use internationally, and their use is widely accepted in brain oncology treatment settings, they have not been standardized in large clinical trials.

IMAGING BIOMARKERS

Physiology-based MR imaging methods enable dynamic physiologic processes in the brain to be

Disclosure: The authors have nothing to disclose.
[a] Magnetic Resonance Department of Clínica de Diagnóstico por Imagem (CDPI), Centro Médico Barrashopping, Av. das Américas, 4666, grupo 325, Barra da Tijuca, Rio de Janeiro, RJ, CEP: 22649-900, Brazil;
[b] Magnetic Resonance Department of Clínica de Diagnóstico por Imagem (CDPI), IRM Ressonância Magnética, Av. das Américas, 4666, grupo 325, Barra da Tijuca, Rio de Janeiro, RJ, CEP: 22649-900, Brazil
* Corresponding author.
E-mail address: detekimura@hotmail.com

Magn Reson Imaging Clin N Am 24 (2016) 87–122
http://dx.doi.org/10.1016/j.mric.2015.09.001
1064-9689/16/$ – see front matter © 2016 Elsevier Inc. All rights reserved.

mri.theclinics.com

quantified. Quantitative images that index parameters such as cerebral blood flow (CBF), cellularity, water mobility, and biochemical composition can be used as biomarkers. Biomarkers are objectively measured characteristics that can indicate normal and pathogenic biological processes as well as pharmacologic responses to therapeutic intervention.[4] Although histopathology remains the gold standard diagnostic and prognostic tool in clinical practice, imaging biomarkers are used routinely to evaluate patients with brain tumors. Imaging biomarkers that are already widely used in neuro-oncology include cerebral blood volume (CBV), volume transfer constant between plasma and extracellular extravascular space (K^{trans}), CBF, apparent diffusion coefficient (ADC), fractional anisotropy (FA), and metabolites analysis by MRS (Table 1).

PERFUSION MR IMAGING

Perfusion MR imaging or dynamic susceptibility contrast-enhanced (DSC)-MR imaging is performed by means of 2 major methods, namely T1-weighted imaging steady-state dynamic contrast-enhanced (DCE) and perfusion DSC-MR imaging, which encompasses T2*-weighted imaging in the first pass of a contrast effusion. This last approach is particularly sensitive to paramagnetic changes in local magnetic susceptibility between vessels and surrounding tissue and is, therefore, used commonly in daily clinical practice.

DCE data are simple measurements of MR signal change over a specified time course and can be thought of as changes in the shape of the enhancement-time curve.[5,6] Commonly, DSC-MR imaging is performed according to the indicator dilution method with nondiffusible tracers,[7] which enables one to obtain a signal intensity versus time curve after an endovenous contrast injection. The clinical parameter CBV is proportional to the area under the contrast agent concentration × signal intensity-time curve, in the absence of recirculation and contrast leakage. Several methods are used to minimize susceptibility effects, including preacquisition gadolinium dosing, gamma variate fitting, and baseline correction.[8,9]

DCE-MR imaging and DSC-MR imaging sequences can be performed in the same procedure to obtain complementary information regarding the vascular physiology of brain tumors. DCE-MR imaging is less susceptible than DSC-MR imaging to artifacts from blood products, calcium, and metals; and it is sensitive to capillaries and can be used near the skull and at brain-bone-air interfaces (Fig. 1).[8] On the other hand, relative to DCE-MR imaging, DSC-MR imaging involves a simpler postprocessing procedure, has a better signal-to-noise ratio with a standard dose of contrast, and is more sensitive to paramagnetic changes between vessels and tissue, making it a more sensible choice for analysis of capillaries and larger vessels (Table 2).[10,11]

Because of the complexity of angiogenesis processes, some institutions perform both methods when evaluating brain tumor vascularity. Two types of vascular permeability have been described: a very high vascular permeability and a steady-state permeability.[12,13] The former is flow-related and can be characterized by the first pass of endovascular contrast material. The latter is believed to depend on the bidirectional exchange between plasma and extravascular extracellular spaces and should be measured in a steady-state condition. Hence, the main biomarkers obtained by these methods, which are known as K^{trans} and CBV, reflect different vascular parameters. Areas of high CBV do not necessarily correspond to areas of high permeability.[14]

Table 1
Main imaging biomarkers in neuro-oncology

Biomarker	What They Detect	MR Imaging Sequence
rCBV	Neoangiogenesis (flow-related)	DSC-MR imaging
K^{trans}	Neoangiogenesis (permeability)	DCE-MR imaging
ADC	Cellularity	DWI
FA	White matter integrity	DTI
Cho	Cellular turnover	MRS

Abbreviations: ADC, apparent diffusion coefficient; Cho, choline; DCE or vascular permeability, T1-weighted steady-state dynamic contrast-enhanced turbo spin echo sequence; DSC-MR imaging, T2*-weighted first-pass, dynamic susceptibility contrast-enhanced gradient-echo/EPI sequence; DTI, diffusion tensor imaging; DWI, diffusion-weighted imaging; FA, fractional anisotropy; K^{trans}, volume transfer constant or vascular permeability; MRS, proton magnetic resonance spectroscopy; rCBV, relative cerebral blood volume.

IMMUNOHISTOCHEMISTRY CORRELATES OF PERFUSION IMAGING

Angiogenesis, that is, vascular proliferation, is associated with tumoral growth.[15] Vascular endothelial growth factor (VEGF) and vascular permeability factor (VPF) are important mediators of tumor growth and angiogenesis.[16,17] Indirect

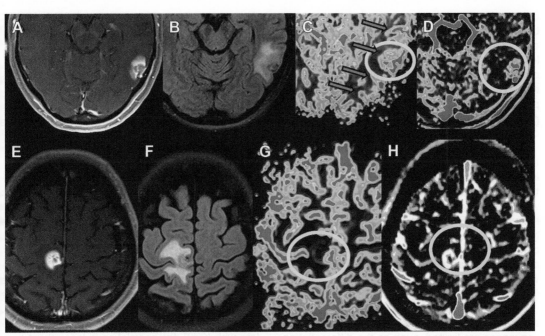

Fig. 1. 56-year-old man with lung metastases treated with radiotherapy. Enhancing lesions surrounded by vasogenic edema (A, E, postcontrast fast spin echo (FSE) T1-weighted image); (B, F, FLAIR) located at the cortico-subcortical junction. DSC-MR imaging derived rCBV maps (C, G) can be difficult to analyze. Cortical veins (C, arrows) may be misdiagnosed as cortical lesion. Also, a cortical lesion with hemorrhagic component may present susceptibility artifact, which may prevent a correct interpretation of the DSC-MR imaging perfusion sequence, as shown in this example, which seems to not have high perfusion (G, rCBV map). In both cases, high permeability can be seen on DCE-MR imaging maps (D, H) related to recurrent/residual lesions.

measurements of angiogenesis can be performed noninvasively by DSC-MR imaging and DCE-MR imaging. Parameters such as CBV and K^{trans}, derived from perfusion and permeability imaging, respectively, correlate with molecular markers of VEGF/VPF and histopathologic changes.[18,19] Furthermore, relative CBV (rCBV) measurements have been reported to correlate with tumor grade and histologic findings of high tumor vascularity.[20–23]

CLINICAL APPLICATIONS
Differential Diagnosis of Solitary Brain Lesions

Perfusion MR imaging is useful for the assessment and differential diagnosis of solitary expansive brain lesions. Determination of the histologic characteristics of a lesion is crucial for guiding treatment plans and determining prognoses. Advanced MR imaging techniques can add previously unavailable physiologic information to the evaluation of brain lesions. Imaging biomarkers

Table 2
Dynamic susceptibility contrast-enhanced MR imaging and dynamic contrast-enhanced MR imaging sequences parameters protocols for 1.5-T and 3.0-T MR scanners

Technical Parameters	DSC-MR Imaging (1.5 T)	DCE-MR Imaging (1.5 T)	DSC-MR Imaging (3.0 T)	DCE-MR Imaging (3.0 T)
Repetition time (ms)	1440	4.16	1600	5.17
Excitation time (ms)	65	1.51	30	1.81
Acquisition time (s)	1.19	4.55	1.25	4.56
Field of view (mm)	230	220	220	200
Slice thickness (mm)	5.0	3.0	4.0	4.0
Contrast volume (mL)	15	5	15	5

Abbreviations: mL, Milliliters; mm, Millimeters; ms, Milliseconds; s, Seconds.

derived from microvascular structural data have been shown to be of enormous usefulness in discriminating between some solitary expansive lesion types that need of different therapeutic approaches. Angiogenic metrics can be used to facilitate differentiation of cerebral tumors and their principal differential diagnosis. Physiopathologic properties underlie angiogenic particularities that can be related to tumor histology (Boxes 1–4).

For example, although lymphoma and glioblastoma multiforme (GBM) tumors have similar imaging features in conventional MR sequences, the 2 tumor types can be distinguished with perfusion-weighted imaging. In particular, GBM tumors have high rCBV values (see Box 3), whereas lymphomas, in general, do not have increased perfusion (Fig. 2). In one series, the rCBV ratio of primary intracranial lymphomas was 1.72 ± 0.59, whereas the rCBV ratio of high-grade gliomas (HGGs) was 4.86 ± 2.18 (P<0.001).[26]

Perfusion imaging can also help in tumor characterization in specific scenarios where other sequences are limited, such as the differentiation between GBM and solitary metastasis (see Box 1; Fig. 3), ependymoma versus medulloblastoma (see Box 2) and hemangioblastoma versus pilocitic astrocytoma (see Box 4; Fig. 4).

Tumor Grading

DSC-MR imaging improves image sensitivity and is of predictive value for glioma grading relative to conventional contrast-enhanced MR imaging.[21] DSC-MR imaging has been demonstrated to be useful for predicting tumor grade in several studies. HGGs exhibit a very high rCBV (3.54–7.32), whereas low-grade gliomas (LGGs) exhibit a relatively lower rCBV (1.11–2.14).[21,23,27] An rCBV threshold of ≥1.75 can be used to differentiate HGGs from LGGs with 95% to 100% sensitivity (Fig. 5). Meanwhile, an rCBV less than 1.5 has

---

Box 1

Glioblastoma multiforme versus solitary metastasis

Metastases have greater permeability than GBM.

Metastases have no blood-brain barrier (BBB) infiltration and GBM has a "damaged" BBB.

High CBV may be demonstrated in the hyperintensity area surrounding the enhancing portion of a GBM, probably related to infiltrative neoplastic cells (see Fig. 3).

The signal intensity recovery curve is greater in patients with GBM compared with metastasis.[24]

Box 2

Ependymomas versus medulloblastomas

Both lesions can demonstrate markedly increased rCBV and K^{trans}.

Ependymoma exhibits a poor return to baseline in the signal intensity recovery curve, attributable to fenestrated blood vessels and an incomplete blood-brain barrier.[25]

---

been associated with LGG tumor identity.[21] Published specificities for rCBV-threshold glioma dissociation have been mediocre, in the range of 57.5% to 69.0%, because of a high number of LGGs with increased rCBVs being misclassified as HGGs.

rCBV has been shown to have a good correlation with tumor grade and is considered to be the most robust standard hemodynamic variable derived from perfusion-weighted MR imaging. Although tumor grade has been reported to correlate with K^{trans}, the correlation is less robust than that with rCBV.[28,29]

LGGs go on to differentiate into a more aggressive malignancy in most LGG cases. The associated dedifferentiation process can be demonstrated in rCBV maps before there are signs of it in conventional MR sequences. The concept of an "angiogenic switch" refers to the moment when an avascular tumor becomes angiogenic and represents a transition point in the malignant transformation of gliomas.[30,31] The angiogenic switch is characterized by an increase in rCBV, which can be detected up to 12 months before contrast enhancement is apparent on T1-weighted images (Fig. 6).[32]

Guiding Stereotactic Biopsy and Radiosurgery

Undergrading of gliomas is a major clinical problem, occurring in about 30% of cases, which can affect the management and outcome of patients. Lesion heterogeneity can put unguided biopsy procedures at risk of sampling errors. Although contrast enhancement is the MR imaging feature commonly used to assess GBMs, it has limited specificity in tumor grading. Recent findings suggest that aggressiveness-related genetic and

---

Box3

Lymphoma versus GBM

rCBV are much lower in lymphomas than in GBM.

GBM has higher permeability than lymphoma.

Box 4
Hemangioblastoma versus pilocitic astrocytoma

High rCBV and permeability are demonstrated in pilocitic astrocytoma, but rCBV is higher in hemangioblastomas (see Fig. 4).

cellular features of GBMs influence MR imaging results, especially rCBV values in areas of angiogenesis and high cellularity.[33] In this context, perfusion imaging techniques can be used to define the most vascularized, and thus the most malignant, regions of tumors to be biopsied or irradiated.

Assessing Tumor Extension

Perfusion and permeability maps of areas of increased rCBV or K^{trans} enable tumor infiltration beyond areas of enhancement on conventional MR imaging to be evaluated (see Fig. 3). Such maps allow for a more accurate assessment of tumor extension to be made (Fig. 7), which may in

turn be helpful in surgery planning.[34] Surgical approach still remains the first line therapy. Greater extension of resection is associated with a survival benefit, specifically improved overall survival, progression-free survival, and malignant progression-free survival. Thus, a more precise identification of tumor borders can indicate more aggressive surgical resection in order to improve median overall survival.

Monitoring Therapeutic Response

Tumor recurrence versus radiation necrosis

Chemoradiotherapy-induced necrosis and tumor recurrence/growth can coexist. Determining the relative predominance of each process is challenging and may be supported by single or serial multiparametric MR imaging examinations. Transient increases in contrast enhancement in conventional MR imaging scans immediately after completion of chemoradiotherapy in patients with HGGs are an important factor in the clinical management of such patients, because they make it difficult to determine whether to continue with standard adjuvant chemotherapy or to switch to a second-line therapy for recurrence. Thus,

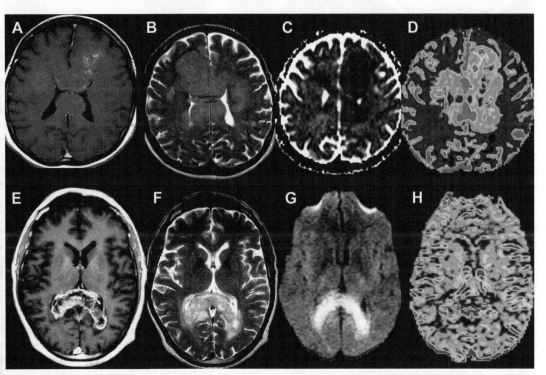

Fig. 2. Glioblastoma (A–D). A not enhancing (A, postcontrast FSE T1-weighted image), infiltrating lesion (B, T2-weighted image), with restricted diffusion (C, ADC map) and high perfusion on DSC-MR imaging map (D, rCBV map) is seen in the frontal lobes, which involves the corpus callosum. Lymphoma (E–H). A contrast-enhancing (E, postcontrast FSE T1-weighted image) heterogeneous lesion, surrounded by edema (F, T2-weighted image), with restricted diffusion (G, high b value DWI image) is seen in the splenium of the corpus callosum. In contrast to GBM, the lesion does not demonstrate high perfusion on DSC-MR imaging sequence (H, rCBV map).

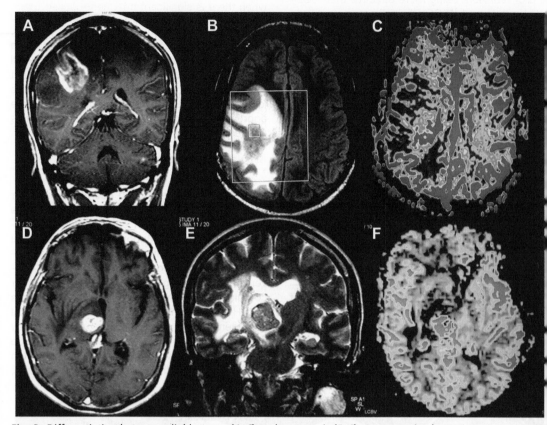

Fig. 3. Differentiation between glioblastoma (*A–C*) and metastasis (*D–F*). An expansive heterogeneous contrast enhancing (*A*, postcontrast FSE T1-weighted image) lesion, associated with a hyperintense area, which corresponds to vasogenic edema and infiltrating tumor (*B*, FLAIR). DSC-MR imaging map shows high perfusion in the nonenhancing, hyperintense surrounding area, suggesting an infiltrating neoplastic lesion (*C*). An enhancing lung metastasis (*D* postcontrast FSE T1-weighted image), surrounded by vasogenic edema in the right thalamus (*E*, FLAIR), shows high perfusion (*F*, DSC-MR imaging map). There is no high perfusion in the hyperintense area surrounding the enhancing portion of the lesion, corresponding to the vasogenic edema.

distinguishing true progression from pseudoprogression is a critically important issue in oncology (Fig. 8).[35]

Delayed radiation necrosis is a histopathological occlusive vasculopathy that results in stroke-like episodes. Endothelial proliferation, which represents pseudoprogression, can be seen in early-phase radionecrosis (Fig. 9). It is associated with some concerns, such as fibrinoid necrosis of small vessels, endothelial thickening, hyalinization, and vascular thrombosis. On the other hand, recurrent tumors are associated with vascular proliferation and angiogenesis, without vascular luminal obliteration.[8]

Many investigators have suggested using CBV and K^{trans} to differentiate radiation necrosis from recurrent tumor.[11,36,37] Hu and colleagues[38] studied 13 patients with HGGs who were treated with multimodality therapy and examined how CBV data correlated with tissue specimen findings. They found that new enhancing lesions with

rCBV values in the range of 0.21 to 0.71 were likely to be radionecrosis, whereas lesions with rCBV values in the range of 0.55 to 4.64 were likely to be recurrent tumors, with an accuracy of 95.9% Consequently, they recommended that an rCBV greater than 0.71 indicates tumor growth, whereas an rCBV less than 0.71 indicates radionecrosis Mangla and colleagues[39] evaluated rCBV values in patients with GBM tumors before and 1 month after radiotherapy concurrent with temozolomide therapy. The patients with pseudoprogression had a 41% mean decrease in rCBV from pretreatment to posttreatment, whereas patients with true tumor progression showed a 12% mean increase in rCBV (Fig. 10). However, to date, no single imaging technique has been validated to recognize and adequately establish a diagnosis of pseudoprogression.[35]

A multiparametric assessment of posttreatment brain tumor changes can enhance diagnostic accuracy.[11] Vascular permeability is reduced in

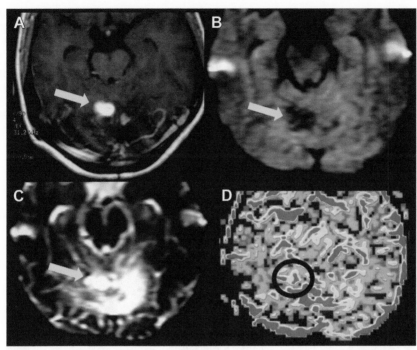

Fig. 4. Hemangioblastoma. The solid-enhancing portions of the lesion on postcontrast turbo spin echo (TSE) T1-weighted image (*A, arrow*), have high diffusibility shown on DWI (*B, arrow*) and confirmed on the ADC map (*C, arrow*). The lesion also presents high perfusion on the rCBV map (*D, circle*).

radiation-induced necrosis because the rate of enhancement is slow. Conversely, steady-state permeability studies have demonstrated a rapid initial increase in the vascular permeability curve, compatible with a vascular phase, in recurrent tumors. Subsequently, a more steady leakage, typical for a highly vascular and highly permeable recurrent tumor, can be observed.[8] Perfusion and vascular permeability seem to be measuring different pathophysiologic changes in the brain. As a result, there are some instances where there are not only spatial differences in the distribution of rCBV versus permeability but also differences in the significance of changes between different metrics for differentiating radiation necrosis from recurrent tumor.[8] It may happen because of the location of the lesion in relation to bone structures and air or the presence of blood products. The spatial resolution of perfusion or permeability maps may vary, and one may show better resolution to depict increased angiogenesis foci in a treated tumor in relation to the other because of the different protocol parameters.

Pseudoresponse

Antiangiogenic agents, such as the anti-VEGF antibody bevacizumab and the VEGF receptor tyrosine kinase inhibitor cediranib, have been tested in recent HGG treatment trials. Although these agents produce a rapid decrease in contrast enhancement with a high response rate and increased 6-month progression-free survival, only modest effects on overall survival have been observed.[40,41]

Malignant gliomas tend to infiltrate surrounding tissues and this property makes them difficult to eradicate surgically. For instance, infiltrated brain parenchyma adjacent to a surgical bed is characterized by areas of enhanced signal on fluid attenuated inversion recovery (FLAIR) and T2-weighted images; their associated nonenhancing contrast areas persist and enlarge with disease progression. As cells in these areas dedifferentiate into more malignant forms, the angiogenic switch occurs, resulting in the development of contrast enhancement. When antiangiogenic agents are introduced in the context of tumor recurrence, they decrease contrast enhancement by changing vascular permeability and pruning of vessels with BBB normalization, rather than by true tumor reduction (see **Fig. 10**). Such results can be observed within hours of therapy commencement.

The visible responses to antiangiogenic therapy may be due, at least in part, to a normalization of abnormally permeable tumor vessels.[41,42] Thus, radiologic changes should be interpreted with caution because an apparent improvement may be a temporary pseudoresponse that lasts only

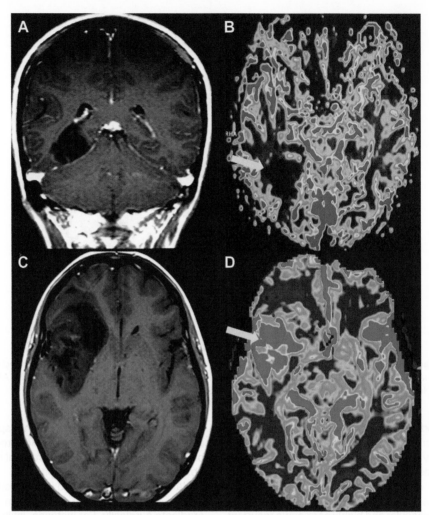

Fig. 5. Glioma grading. A nonenhancing LGG (*A*, postcontrast FSE T1-weighted image) does not show increased perfusion on DSC-MR imaging perfusion (*B*, rCBV map, *arrow*). On the other hand, a nonenhancing right insular HGG (*C*, postcontrast FSE T1-weighted image) demonstrates high perfusion on DSC-MR imaging perfusion (*D*, rCBV map, *arrow*).

days or weeks. Reversibility of this vascular normalization, with rebound enhancement and edema, have been described when patients went off the drugs, mostly for toxicity concerns.[43] Moreover, in glioma cases, antiangiogenic therapy reduces cerebral edema through elimination of VEGF, which may reduce the need for steroid use and be beneficial for neurologic function.[35] In this context, it is recommended that MR perfusion and permeability imaging are used routinely in the initial assessment, as well, in subsequent treatment monitoring evaluations to reveal possible new areas of dedifferentiation and to enable better evaluation of the treatment response to new antiangiogenic agents and chemoradiotherapy.

Prognosis

The usefulness of rCBV in brain tumor patients' prognoses was illustrated well in a previous study[29] examining the value of rCBV measurements in predicting tumor biology, with patient outcome as the gold standard readout. In that study, patients with histopathologic diagnoses of HGG or LGG were stratified into 2 groups based on rCBV. A Kaplan-Meier curve demonstrated significantly longer progression-free survival for the low-perfusion (rCBV <1.75) LGG group than for the high-perfusion (rCBV >1.75) HGG group (*P*<.0001). Similarly, there was a significant difference in the progression of gliomas with a high rCBV versus gliomas with a low rCBV (*P*<.0001). Lesions with low baseline rCBV (<1.75)

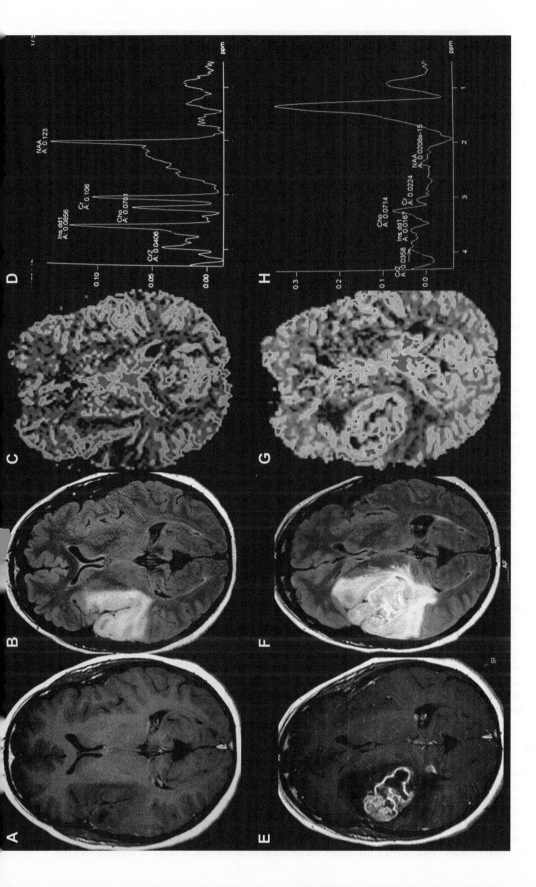

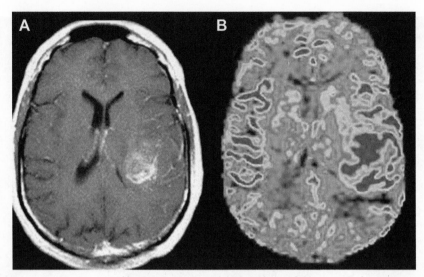

Fig. 7. Anaplastic astrocytoma. An infiltrating, expansive lesion is seen, which presents heterogeneous and irregular contrast enhancement, mostly in the posterior and medial aspects of the lesion (*A*, postcontrast FSE T1-weighted image). DSC-MR imaging perfusion map (*B*) shows a more widespread area of high perfusion, demonstrating areas of higher anaplasia, which do not demonstrate enhancement on the postcontrast T1-weighted sequence.

demonstrated stable tumor volumes when followed over time, and lesions with high baseline rCBV (>1.75) demonstrated progressively increasing tumor volumes over time. These results demonstrate that rCBV measurements from DSC-MR imaging may provide an additional prognostic factor for tumor biology. Thereby, the predictive value of perfusion MR imaging for the prognosis of patients with gliomas has been well documented.[44]

DIFFUSION-WEIGHTED IMAGING AND DIFFUSION TENSOR IMAGING

DWI can detect water movement at a molecular level. It is based on the random or Brownian motion of water molecules, typically in relation to their thermal energy. MR imaging makes it possible to estimate the diffusivity of water molecules. Most diffusion measurements are made using a variant of the diffusion-weighted sequence first described by Stejskal and Tanner.[45] For practical purposes, an echo-planar imaging (EPI) spin echo T2-weighted sequence is used, because of its ability to reduce motion artifacts and its rapid acquisition time. By acquiring an image with little diffusion weighting and another image with substantial diffusion weighting, the ADC can be calculated on a voxel-by-voxel basis (**Table 3**).[45]

DTI is a powerful approach and is widely popular; however, the limitations of this technique have begun to become apparent. Nevertheless, the Gaussian approximation has definite usefulness. In a tensor model, water mobility is described by a 3×3 matrix. To estimate the 9-tensor matrix elements, the diffusion gradients must be applied to at least 6 noncollinear directions. The eigenvalues represent the 3 principal diffusion coefficients measured along the 3 coordinate directions of the ellipsoid. FA measures the fraction of the total magnitude of diffusion anisotropy. DTI has been used to attempt to map the white matter fiber tracts. This is typically done by connecting each voxel eigenvector to its adjacent one in accordance with the direction in which the fibers are pointing.[45]

Fig. 6. "Angiogenic switch." A nonenhancing (*A*, postcontrast FSE T1-weighted image) right insular biopsy-proven low-grade glioma (*B*, FLAIR) does not have high perfusion (*C*, DSC-MR imaging map). MR spectroscopy (*D*) shows a reduction of NAA peak and a high myoinositol peak. After clinical deterioration, a new MR examination demonstrates enlargement of the lesion, which currently presents irregular contrast enhancement (*E*, postcontrast FSE T1-weighted image), with necrotic central areas and surrounding heterogeneous portion consistent with vasogenic edema and neoplastic infiltration (*F*, FLAIR). Increased perfusion can be demonstrated on the DSC-MR imaging map (*G*) and MRS shows a high peak of choline and a very high peak of lactate/lipids. The "angiogenic switch" represents a malignant transformation of gliomas, related to angiogenesis (*H*).

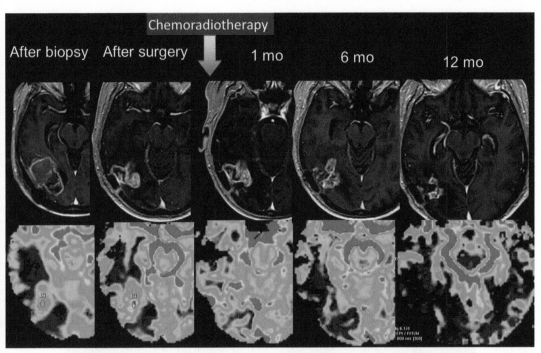

Fig. 8. Pseudoprogression in a treated glioblastoma. Postcontrast FSE T1-weighted images (*top line*) and DSC-MR imaging maps (*bottom line*) pretreatment and posttreatment (surgery and chemoradiotherapy) are shown. MR imaging obtained 1 month after concomitant radiotherapy and temozolomide chemotherapy demonstrate an expansion of the right temporal lesion. Reductions in both the enhancing portion and the corresponding high perfusion area in the DSC-MR imaging are seen in the follow-up MR imaging examinations, which characterize pseudoprogression, a reversible increase in the enhancing portion of the lesion at the end of treatment.

Diffusion kurtosis imaging (DKI) is a clinically feasible extension of DWI and DTI, which enables the assessment of non-Gaussianity properties of water diffusion. Whereas in DTI the water mobility is based on the assumption that the displacement probability function of water diffusion follows a Gaussian distribution, DKI assumes a non-Gaussian probability of water diffusion. DKI has been considered to be a technique that can provide additional information about microstructure in the brain in comparison to DTI.[45]

DWI has been studied extensively in the context of brain tumor evaluation. Several papers have demonstrated its usefulness for grading brain tumors according to tumor cellularity. Low ADC values have been correlated with increasing cellularity, increasing grade, and an increasing Ki-67 cellular proliferation index in cerebral gliomas.[45–49] It has been described as a useful method of assessing tumor treatment response after chemotherapy, radiotherapy, and antiangiogenic therapy owing to its property of being sensitive to macromolecular and microstructural changes occurring before anatomic changes are evident.[50–52]

DTI may enable oncologists to more accurately distinguish tumor tissue from infiltrating tumor cells in peritumoral edema and normal brain parenchyma.[53] It has been used widely because of its apparent ability to illustrate the relationship between a tumor and its nearby main fiber tracts (**Fig. 11**). This information should help surgeons achieve as complete a lesion resection as possible without harming vital brain functions.[54] Accordingly, a preoperative diagnostic tool that maps, even imperfectly, a tumor and its relationship to nearby functional structures has the potential to improve patient outcome.

CLINICAL APPLICATIONS
Differential Diagnosis of Cerebral Neoplasms

ADC is a remarkable quantitative biomarker of cellularity that has been described as a means to help stratify tumor histology.[46] With the wide clinical availability of DWI, ADC measurement is being integrated into conventional imaging analyses with increasing frequency, in particular for tumor characterization (**Boxes 5–10**). In some studies, lymphoma, a highly cellular tumor, has

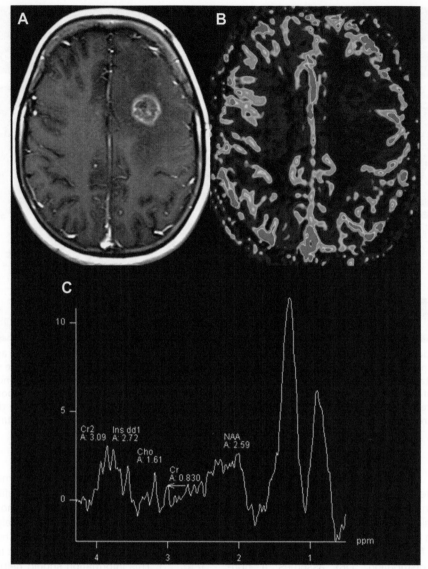

Fig. 9. Radionecrosis. MR imaging was performed in an anaplastic astrocytoma submitted to radiotherapy, which demonstrates a round enhancing lesion in the left frontal lobe (*A*, postcontrast FSE T1-weighted image) that does not have high perfusion (*B*, DSC-MR imaging map). (*C*) MRS also shows a not very high peak of choline and a predominant peak of lipids/lactate because of necrosis.

been found to present a hyperintense DWI signal with reduced ADC values,[55] suggesting that DWI may be helpful in differentiating lymphoma from lesions with higher characteristic ADC values. Some studies have shown statistically significant differences in ADC values between GBM and lymphoma.[56,57] GBM is a heterogeneous neoplasm in which areas of restricted diffusion related to high cellularity may coexist with very-high-ADC areas corresponding to high vascularity and necrosis.[58,59] This mixing can complicate discrimination of lymphomas from some GBMs (see **Fig. 2**).

However, lymphomas have been reported to have lower ADC values than GBMs.[60] Indeed, the 2 tumor types could be distinguished with an accuracy of 100% when an ADC ratio ($ADC_{lesion}/ADC_{normal\ white\ matter}$) cutoff value of 1.06 was used (**Box 7**).

DWI can also be used to differentiate arachnoid cysts from epidermoid tumors (see **Box 5**).[55] Arachnoid cysts tend to have high ADC values, whereas epidermoid lesions tend to present with high DWI signal intensity, due mostly to restricted diffusion (**Fig. 12**).

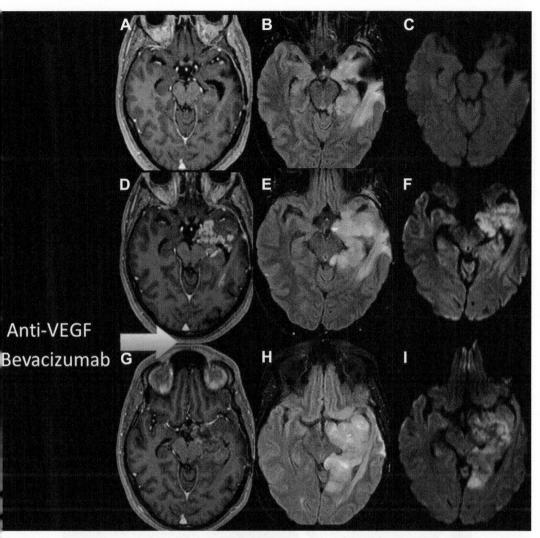

Fig. 10. Pseudoresponse. A patient with anaplastic astrocytoma was submitted to surgical resection and radiotherapy. The first follow-up MR examination (*A–C*) shows an area of hyperintensity in the left temporal lobe in the FLAIR image (*B*), without contrast enhancement (*A*, postcontrast FSE T1-weighted image) or restricted diffusion (*C*, DWI). Two months later, a new MR examination (*D–F*) shows enlargement of the lesion, with new areas of enhancement (*D*, postcontrast FSE T1-weighted image) and areas of restricted diffusion (*F*, DWI), consistent with a recurrent lesion. Antiangiogenic therapy is then initiated, and the following MR examination performed 45 days later shows a marked reduction in the enhancing portion of the lesion (*G*, postcontrast FSE T1-weighted image). However, an enlargement of the nonenhancing hyperintense portion is seen (*H*, FLAIR), associated with restricted diffusion (*I*, DWI).

Preoperative ADC values may predict meningioma malignancy, and therefore may be useful in preoperative planning, particularly regarding the establishment of surgical strategies and the decision on whether adjunctive therapy should be prescribed (**Fig. 13**).

Tumor grading

Tumor grading is a critical component of treatment planning and evaluation of prognosis. Imaging has

the potential to improve tumor grading accuracy, which is complicated by tissue sample heterogeneity, as well as the monitoring of malignant dedifferentiation.[45]

DWI may increase MR imaging sensitivity and specificity in brain tumor evaluation by providing information about tumor cellularity, which may, in turn, improve tumor grading accuracy.[53,64] The mechanism by which DWI may help with tumor grading is based on the restriction of free water

Table 3
Parameters of diffusion-weighted imaging and diffusion tensor imaging sequences for a 1.5-T MR scanner

Technical Parameters	DWI	DTI
Repetition time (ms)	1900	1900
Excitation time (ms)	81	81
Acquisition time (s)	0.57	>1.14
Slice (mm)	5.0	5.0
Number of directions	2	>6
Field of view (mm)	160	160

molecules in areas of high cellularity, high nuclear-cytoplasmic ratios, and reduction of extracellular space (**Fig. 17**).[65,66] Extracellular space reduction and the high nuclear-to-cytoplasmic ratios of some cancer cells produce a relative reduction in ADC values (see **Fig. 12**).[38] Some researchers have reported a correlation between ADC values and tumor cellularity,[66] with lower ADC values being associated with higher-grade lesions.[43] However, ADC values for HGGs and LGGs may overlap somewhat because of the heterogeneity of gliomas within and across grades. Consequently, the range of ADC values within a given glioma classification can vary greatly.

Guiding Stereotactic Biopsy and Radiosurgery

DWI has been useful for guiding operators toward high-cellularity areas during brain tumor biopsy procedures, owing to the relatively low ADC values

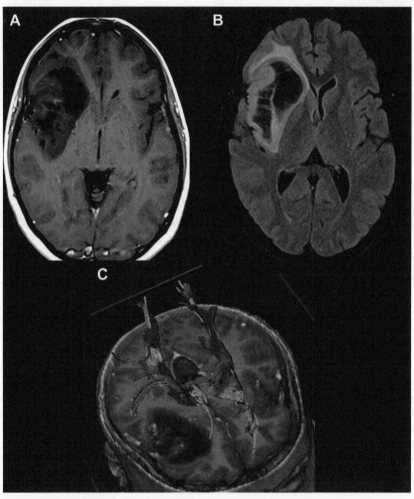

Fig. 11. Same case as in the high-grade glioma (HGG) in Fig. 5C, D. An HGG of the right insula (*A*, postcontrast TSE T1-weighted image and *B*, FLAIR) demonstrating reduction of the anterior fibers and deviation of the medial and posterior main fibers of the right corticospinal tract on tractography (*C*).

Box 5
Arachnoid cyst versus epidermoid tumor

ADC values of epidermoid tumor are similar or slightly lower than those of the brain parenchyma.

The ADC value of an arachnoid cyst is similar to that of CSF.[61]

Box 6
Benign meningioma versus malignant meningioma

Malignant and atypical meningiomas demonstrated low ADC values compared with typical meningiomas[62]

Box 7
GBM versus lymphoma

Lymphomas demonstrate lower ADC values than GBM.

A cutoff value of 1 for the ADC ratio (ADC_{lesion}/$ADC_{normal\ white\ matter}$) can be used to differentiate lymphoma from GBM with an accuracy of 100%.[63]

Box 8
Ependymomas versus medulloblastomas

Medulloblastomas have lower ADC values than all other posterior fossa tumors (Fig. 14).

Classic ependymoma does not show restricted diffusion.

Box 9
Hemangioblastoma versus pilocitic astrocytoma

ADC values are increased in the solid-enhancing portion of hemangioblastoma, because of the large amount of capillaries (see Fig. 4).

ADC values are similar to brain parenchyma within the solid-enhancing portion of pilocitic astrocytoma (Fig. 15).

Box 10
Intra-axial ring-enhancing lesions

Abscess has restricted diffusion within the cavity, related to pus viscosity.

Necrotic and cystic tumors have increased ADC values within the lesions (Fig. 16).

of these areas (Fig. 18). Previous studies[67,68] have shown that minimum-ADC regions within glial tumors correspond to the highest-grade foci of those tumors.

Preoperative planning and evaluation of tumor extension
The precise determination of tumor margins is considered by many investigators to be of the utmost importance to the management of brain tumors. The goal of surgical interventions in patients with brain neoplasms is complete resection of the tumor, coupled with minimal neurologic deficits.[69]

Some have suggested that DWI can provide information about peritumoral neoplastic cell infiltration,[53] and perhaps even be used to help discriminate boundaries between tumor, infiltrating tumor, peritumoral edema, and normal brain parenchyma.[53,70] High-grade tumors tend to spread diffusely across the brain, moving along fiber tracts,[71,72] most likely because of the difficulty associated with finding the borders of some tumors, even histopathologically. Hence, it remains unclear whether DWI and DTI are useful tools for predicting the true extent of a brain tumor. Because of the challenges of obtaining a histologic standard of reference (ie, a gold standard), it is reasonable to question DWI's capacity to distinguish neoplastic cell infiltration beyond the enhancing portion of the lesion in abnormal hyperintense T2-weighted images, which is believed to represent vasogenic edema with or without tumor invasion. DTI findings have suggested that the periphery of an LGG contains preserved fiber tracts, whereas most tracts are disarranged in grade III gliomas. However, the presence of edema can obscure the visibility of fiber tracts. Involvement of white matter tracts in brain tumors can be revealed by anisotropy maps (eg, FA maps), tractography, or a combination of both.

Monitoring Therapeutic Response

Postsurgery evaluation
Postoperative DWI can immediately reveal areas of restricted diffusion adjacent to a low-grade or

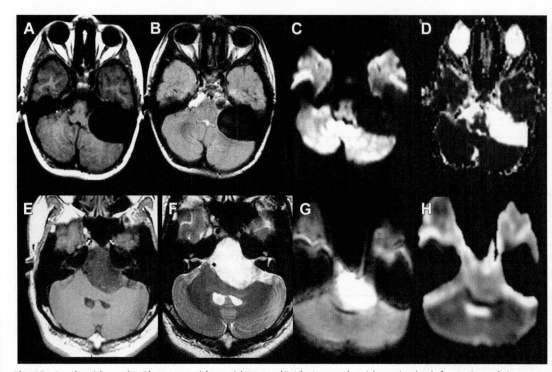

Fig. 12. Arachnoid cyst (*A–D*) versus epidermoid tumor (*E–H*). An arachnoid cyst in the left portion of the posterior fossa (*A*, postcontrast TSE T1-weighted image and *B*, FLAIR) that has high diffusibility on DWI (*C*) and ADC map (*D*). An epidermoid tumor causing a mass effect and dislocation of the brain stem, as well as distortion of the fourth ventricle (*E*, postcontrast TSE T1-weighted image and *F*, TSE T2-weighted image). On DWI (*G*), the lesion has high diffusibility, consistent with restricted diffusion, confirmed by the ADC map (*H*).

high-grade tumor resection cavity. Follow-up MR imaging examinations have shown that these areas of restricted diffusion can persist for up to 2 to 3 months before they are resolved, when contrast enhancement appears in the corresponding location. This enhancement may regress to form an area of encephalomalacia (**Fig. 19**). Images obtained by conventional MR imaging during the enhancement period can suggest tumor recurrence or progression, leading to a false determination of treatment failure and, potentially, the initiation of new, unwarranted adjuvant therapy.[45] Areas of restricted diffusion around the surgery bed may represent areas of infarct, ischemia, or even venous congestion secondary to acute cellular damage, such as surgical trauma, retraction, vascular damage, or tumor devascularization.[38]

Posttreatment Evaluation

DWI can be used to evaluate the extension of surgical resection of epidermoid tumor. As this lesion has similar signal intensity of cerebrospinal fluid (CSF) on conventional MR sequences, to determine whether there is or is not a complete resection is a challenge. As this lesion shows hyperintensity on DWI, this technique is able to differentiate the surgical cavity filled with CSF, which presents hypointensity on DWI, and the residual tumor, which presents hyperintensity (**Fig. 20**).

DWI may be useful for assessment of treatment response because changes in tumor water diffusibility can occur secondarily to reductions in cell density. In this setting, ADC seems to be a sensitive and early predictor of therapeutic efficacy.[73] In a prospective study, investigators compared tumor diffusion values 3 weeks after therapy initiation versus pretreatment values with the aim of documenting therapy-induced ADC changes. The logic behind this methodology is that a successful treatment should result in extensive cell damage, leading to a reduction in cell density[74] (**Fig. 21**). Neoplasm cell loss results in an increase in extracellular space, which can increase free water molecule diffusibility. Long-term follow-up study findings demonstrating that increases in brain tumor ADC values correspond with decreases in tumor volume support the suggestion

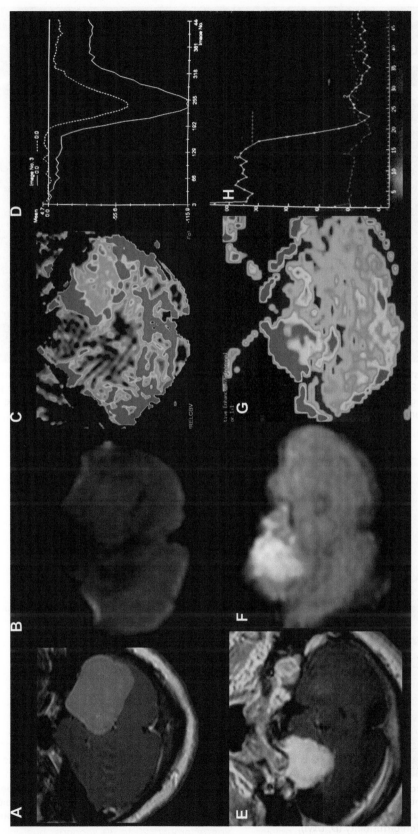

Fig. 13. Grading meningioma. A left posterior fossa low-grade meningioma (*A–D*). An extra-axial enhancing lesion (*A*, postcontrast T1-weighted image), which does not have restricted diffusion (*B*, DWI), demonstrates high perfusion on DSC-MR imaging map (*C*, rCBV map). However, the dynamic curves originated from DSC-MR imaging perfusion (*D*) show that the curve tends to return to the baseline. An enhancing (*E*, postcontrast T1-weighted image) right pontocerebellar cistern anaplastic meningioma (*E–H*), which has restricted diffusion (*F*, DWI) and high perfusion in DSC-MR imaging perfusion sequence (*G*, rCBV map). The dynamic curve originated from DSC-MR imaging perfusion (*H*) does not return to the baseline, secondary to high permeability.

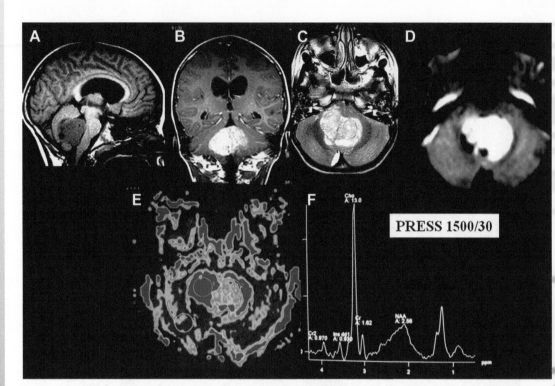

Fig. 14. Medulloblastoma. A fourth ventricle, enhancing expansive lesion (*A–C*, precontrast and postcontrast TSE T1-weighted and TSE T2-weighted images, respectively), which has restricted diffusion (*D*, DWI) and high perfusion in DSC-MR imaging perfusion sequence (*E*, rCBV map). MRS (*F*) demonstrates an important choline peak, reduction of NAA, and a lipids/lactate peak.

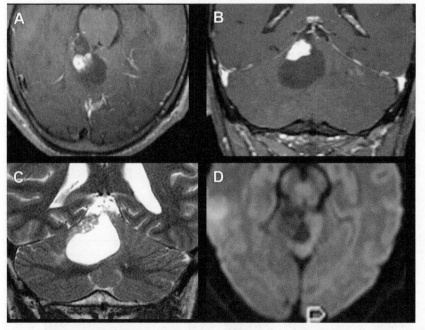

Fig. 15. Pilocitic astrocytoma. A predominant cystic lesion with an enhancing solid mural component in the right cerebellum hemisphere is identified in (*A, B*, postcontrast TSE T1-weighted sequences and *C*, TSE T2-weighted sequence). The diffusibility of the solid component of the lesion is similar to the normal parenchyma, and the cystic portion has high diffusibility (*D*, DWI).

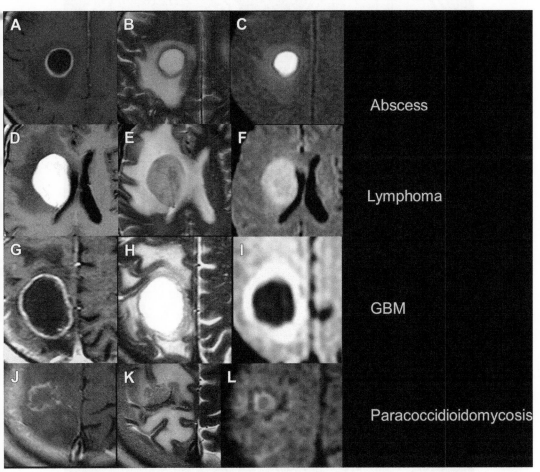

Abscess

Lymphoma

GBM

Paracoccidioidomycosis

Fig. 16. Differential diagnosis of intra-axial enhancing lesions. (*A–C*) Abscess. Ring-enhancing lesion (*A*, postcontrast FSE T1-weighted image) presenting marked surrounding edema on a TSE T2-weighted image (*B*) and restricted diffusion within the cavity (*C*, high *b* value DWI). (*D–F*) Lymphoma. Solid-enhancing lesion (*D*, postcontrast FSE T1-weighted image), with low signal intensity on T2-weighted image (*E*) and restricted diffusion on a high *b* value image (*F*). (*G–I*) Glioblastoma. Expansive ring-enhancing lesion (*G*, postcontrast FSE T1-weighted image), with surrounding edema demonstrated on a TSE T2-weighted image (*H*) and restricted diffusion in the borders and high diffusibility within the lesion cavity, related to necrosis, as shown in a high *b* value image (*I*, DWI). Granulomatous lesion (*J–L*). A case of paracoccidioidomycosis with a ring-enhancing lesion (*J*, postcontrast FSE T1-weighted image), with low signal intensity on T2-weighted image (*K*) and restricted diffusion in the lesion borders as shown on a high *b* value image (*L*, DWI).

that DWI may provide an important surrogate marker for treatment response quantitation. This sequence is important to be performed in follow-up brain tumor treatment.[45,49,74]

Pseudoprogression

Clinically, it is difficult to differentiate tumor progression from pseudoprogression based on ADCs, because of lesion heterogeneity. Currently, there is insufficient evidence to suggest that DWI or DTI should be used make such differentiation judgments.[35]

Pseudoresponse

Antiangiogenesis therapy involving VEGF pathway inhibition in the treatment of HGGs can result in reductions of tumor ADC values that coincide with reductions in contrast enhancement. The principal explanation for this phenomenon seems to be reduction of the lesion's extravascular extracellular space secondary to vascular normalization and a lessening of vascular permeability.[75] However, ADCs may increase if there is significant treatment-induced tumor necrosis. Vascular disrupting agents,

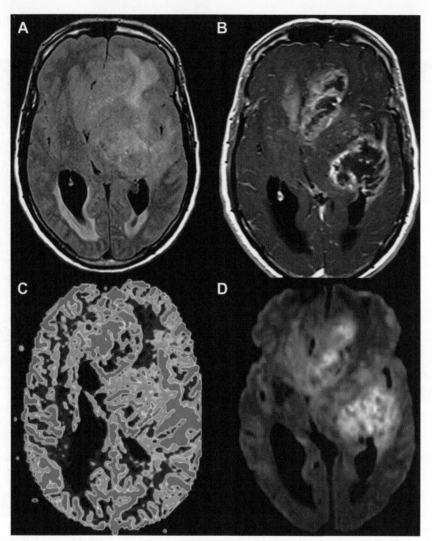

Fig. 17. Multicenter high-grade glioma (*A–D*). An expansive multicenter, infiltrating (*A*, FLAIR) and enhancing (*B*, postcontrast FSE T1-weighted image) lesion, in the frontal and left temporoparietal lobes, involving the insula and thalamus, shows high perfusion in DSC-MR imaging perfusion sequence (*C*, rCBV map). The lesion presents areas of restricted diffusion that may correspond to higher neoplastic cellularity (*D*, DWI).

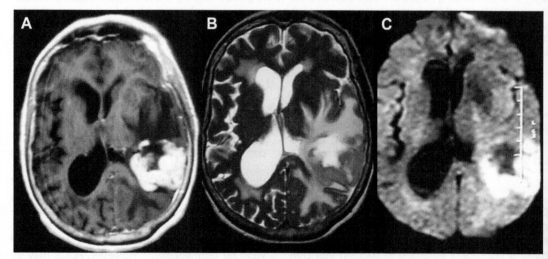

Fig. 18. Glioblastoma (*A–C*). Heterogeneous, irregular contrast-enhancing expansive lesion, with central areas of necrosis (*A*, postcontrast TSE T1-weighted image and *B*, TSE T2-weighted image). Diffusion-weighted image with high *b* value demonstrates an area of restricted diffusion in the posterior aspect of the lesion, related to higher cellularity and central anterior region of necrosis, which has high diffusibility (*C*, DWI).

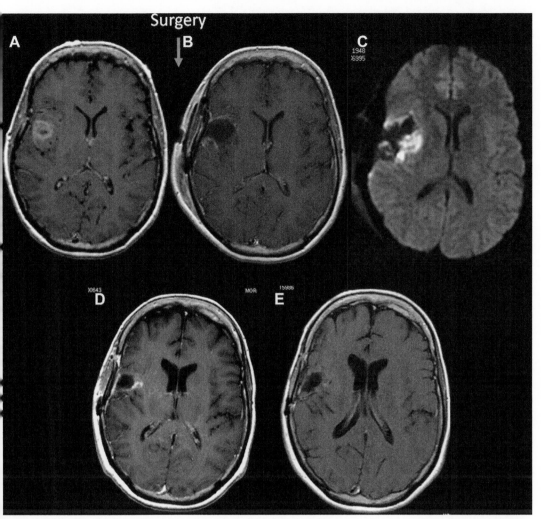

Fig. 19. Enhancing glioblastoma in the right insula (*A*, preoperative postcontrast T1-weighted sequence). Postoperative examination show a surgical cavity with tiny contrast enhancement in its border (*B*, postcontrast T1-weighted sequence) and an area of restricted diffusion mostly in the right posterior aspect, related to the surgery (*C*, DWI). Follow-up MR examination performed 2 months after surgery demonstrates a focal area of contrast enhancement (*D*, postcontrast FSE T1-weighted image), in the same area that demonstrated restricted diffusibility in the previous examination, which is no longer seen in the MR examination performed 1 month later (*E*, postcontrast T1-weighted sequence).

which induce massive necrosis, can also increase ADC values.[76–78] Thus, DWI can reveal drug-induced changes in the microenvironmental architecture, including apoptosis and angiolysis.[75] In other words, any therapy that causes necrosis or cellular lysis would be expected to create increases in ADCs.

Restricted diffusion can also be observed preceding the appearance of tumor enhancement in patients undergoing antiangiogenic therapy. In the absence of abnormal contrast enhancement, areas of low ADC values may correspond to a so-called pseudoresponse (ie, tumor cell infiltration heralding tumor promulgation) (**Fig. 22**).[35] Thus, one must be aware that an area of restricted diffusion could signify an ischemic area secondary to efficacious treatment or tumor spread. The use of other physiologic MR imaging modalities, such as perfusion or spectroscopy, may add information and help physicians to define the nature of the area in question. Nonetheless, it may not always be possible to obtain an accurate answer, in which case serial examinations may be necessary.

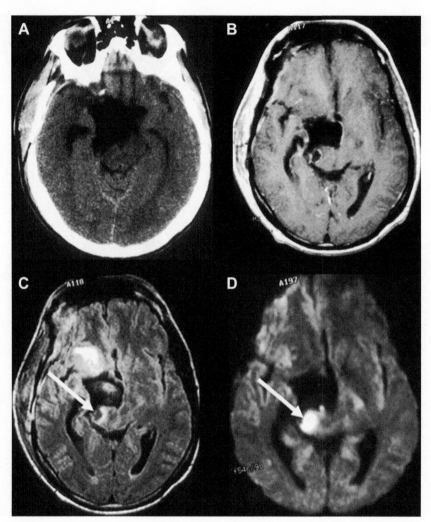

Fig. 20. Postoperative evaluation of epidermoid tumor (*A–D*). Computed tomography (*A*) and postgadolinium T1-weighted image (*B*) are not able to detect residual lesion in the surgical bed. On FLAIR sequence (*C*), there is a slight hyperintense area in the posterior aspect of the surgical bed, laterally to the brainstem (*C*, FLAIR *arrow*), which also presents restricted diffusion (*D*, DWI, *arrow*) and represents residual tumor.

Prognosis

Previous reports have described a close relationship between ADC values and tumor prognosis. Tumors presenting with restricted diffusion have been associated with a dismal prognosis. Patients with malignant supratentorial astrocytomas or brain lymphomas demonstrating lower ADCs have been reported to have worse prognoses than patients whose tumors had higher ADCs.[79]

¹H MAGNETIC RESONANCE SPECTROSCOPY

In general, multivoxel MRS is preferred to single-voxel MRS in the evaluation of brain tumors with metabolic inhomogeneity because the spectrum from a necrotic core of a high-grade tumor is different from that of the actively growing rim and of surrounding tumor-invaded parenchyma. MRS parameters may be optimized by adjusting the echo time (TE) (**Table 4**). Relative to a long TE, a short TE allows for the recognition of more metabolites, which may be important for differential diagnosis of brain masses and tumor grading. Myoinositol (Myo), an LGG marker, is only seen with short TE acquisitions. The brain tumor metabolite signature is characterized by a high level of choline (Cho) and a low N-acetyl-aspartate (NAA) signal, yielding increased Cho/NAA and Cho/creatine (Cr) ratios. Reduced NAA levels in tumors indicate decreased viability and numbers of neurons, whereas increased Cho is

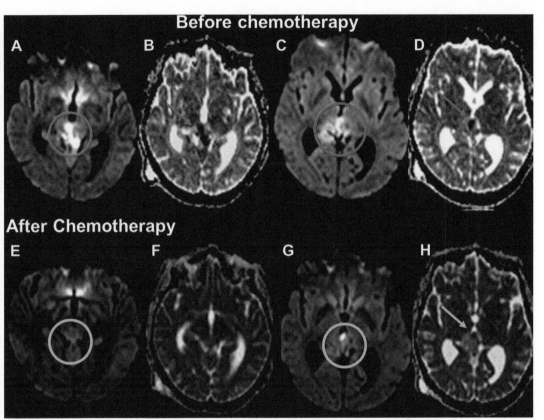

Fig. 21. Pineoblastoma. An expansive lesion in the pineal region with restriction of diffusion (*A, C, circles* in DWI), confirmed in the ADC maps (*B, D, arrows*), is depicted. In the postchemotherapy MR examination (*E–H*), there is a reduction in the lesion size. Also, the area of restricted diffusion decreased substantially (*E, G, circles* in DWI), confirmed by ADC maps (*F, H, arrows*), representing a good treatment response, secondary to reduction on tumor cellularity.

associated with a high cell-membrane turnover and a high cell density produced by tumor cell proliferation.[80] Myo is a glial marker synthesized primarily by astrocytes. Increased lactate levels are likely the result of anaerobic glycolysis, although they can also be consequent to ischemia or necrosis caused by insufficient blood flow.[81] Increased levels of lipids are believed to be secondary to necrosis and membrane breakdown.

CLINICAL APPLICATIONS OF SPECTROSCOPY
Differential Diagnosis of Cerebral Tumors

MRS is used to assess the biochemical composition of brain lesions. It may help with differentiation between neoplastic and non-neoplastic lesions or between types of tumor. Analysis of peri-enhancing tumor regions can be helpful for discriminating solitary metastases from primary brain tumors. Gliomas are often invasive lesions

with increased Cho levels in surrounding tissues, whereas metastatic lesions tend to be encapsulated without high Cho signals or other abnormalities outside the region of enhancement (**Fig. 23**).[82,83]

The role of MRS in the differentiation of brain tumors is reviewed in **Boxes 11–15**.

Tumor grading

MRS can help differentiate between high-grade and low-grade tumors noninvasively. It is important to perform this distinction in order to develop a treatment plan appropriate for the aggressiveness of the target tumor. A higher Cho concentration has been related to a more aggressive neoplasm.[89] The region of interest chosen for analysis has a large influence on the results, and MRS is the preferred approach for this differentiation because it allows metabolic heterogeneity to be evaluated and enables the voxel with the maximum Cho signal to be targeted for analysis.[90]

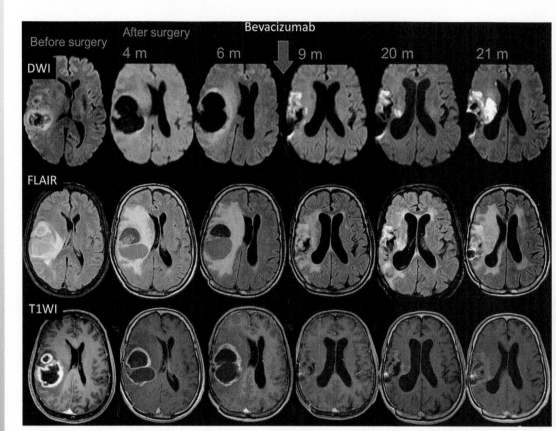

Fig. 22. Pseudoresponse in anaplastic astrocytoma. After surgical resection and radiotherapy and chemotherapy with temozolomide, a recurrent lesion is seen. Thus, antiangiogenic therapy is initiated and a marked decreased in the contrast enhancement of the lesion is demonstrated. However, after several months, the FLAIR sequence shows a clear expansion of the lesion and the area of restricted diffusion progressively enlarges, although without significant contrast enhancement increase.

MRS accuracy has been reported to be 96% accurate for differentiation between LGG and HGG, where HGGs have higher Cho/Cr and Cho/NAA ratios than LGGs[91,92]; the former is the most frequently used ratio for LGG-HGG differentiation.

The suggested cutoff value for this differentiation varies between studies, ranging from 2.0 to 2.5.[21]

Lipids and lactate can also be used to grade astrocytomas. High lipid and lactate peaks are associated with necrosis and indicate a high-grade

Table 4
Magnetic resonance spectroscopy sequences parameters protocols for 1.5-T MR scanners

Technical Parameters	Single-Voxel Excitation Time 30 ms	Single-Voxel Excitation Time 135 ms	Multivoxel Excitation Time 30 ms
Repetition time (ms)	1500	1500	1500
Excitation time (ms)	30	135	30
Acquisition time (ms)	3.18	6.05	7.12
Field of view (mm)	160	160	160
Voxel size (mm)	20 × 20 × 20	10 × 10 × 12.5	10 × 10 × 15
Slice thickness (mm)	15	15	15

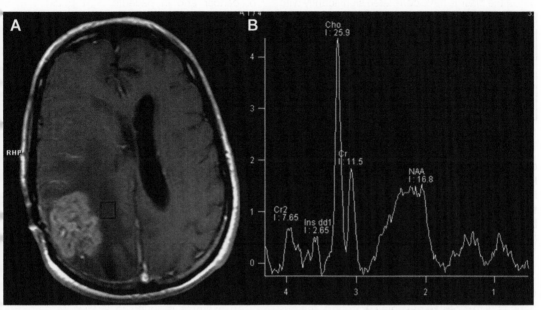

Fig. 23. Postsurgical and radiotherapy evaluation of a glioblastoma (*A*, postcontrast T1-weighted sequence). MRS TE = 30ms shows an increased choline peak at the nonenhancing area of the lesion (*Blue box*), secondary to neoplastic cell infiltration (*B*).

Box 11
Primary brain tumor versus solitary metastasis

High-grade glioma has high Cho signals in surrounding tissue in the nonenhancing portion of the lesion, whereas metastasis does not.

Box 12
GBM versus lymphoma

Both demonstrate lipids/lactate peak.

GBM demonstrates a high choline peak; low levels of all other metabolites may characterize GBM with a major necrotic component.

Lymphoma also has increased choline and reduction in Myo (**Fig. 24**). The choline peak in lymphoma is usually lower compared with GBM.

Box 13
Medulloblastoma versus ependymoma

Ependymomas have low NAA, high Myo, moderately increased Cho and Cr.[84,85]

Significant increase in Cho peak with a reduction in NAA and Myo peaks and taurine at 3.3 ppm characterize medulloblastomas (see **Fig. 14**).[86,87]

---

tumor.[91] High Myo levels indicate low-grade astrocytomas, in which the Cho/Cr ratio is usually not altered (**Fig. 25**).[81]

Assess tumor extension
Similar to DSC-MR imaging and DWI, MRS can be used to detect areas of metabolic abnormality, which may not correspond to areas of enhancement in conventional MR imaging or may even exceed the area of an abnormal T2-weighted signal.[93,94] MRS may be more useful for delineating tumor extension than conventional MR imaging.[95] NAA/Cho ratio data can be used to distinguish the likely center of the lesion and low-infiltration borders. NAA concentration is considered to be a particularly useful parameter for detection of low levels of tumor

---

Box 14
Hemangioblastomas versus pilocytic astrocytoma

Pilocytic astrocytoma demonstrates a prominent peak of choline, and reduction of NAA peak and the presence of lipids/lactate, simulating HGG.

Hemangioblastoma may have lipids peak related to the presence of cysts.

cell infiltration, whereas Cho levels may be too low to be detected by spectroscopy.[96] Accordingly, there may be too few neoplastic cells in the border regions of the lesion to be detected by MRS; thus infiltration cannot be ruled out (see **Fig. 23**).

Guiding Stereotactic Biopsy and Radiosurgery

MRS is useful for identifying regions of high metabolic activity for stereotactic biopsy guidance toward the area of a tumor that is most representative for grading. Likewise, MRS data can be useful in guiding deliverance of radiotherapy, maximizing the dose delivered to areas of active tumor growth and minimizing the dose delivered to surrounding normal tissues. Elevated Cho levels and low NAA levels indicate viable tumor tissue.[97,98] Meanwhile, low Cho and low NAA levels can correspond to areas of radiation necrosis, astrogliosis, macrophage infiltration, or mixed tissue.[99]

Monitoring Therapeutic Response

Posttreatment evaluation

MRS can be used to differentiate radiation induced tissue injury and tumor recurrence after radiation therapy, gamma knife radiosurgery, or brachytherapy. A high Cho/Cr or Cho/NAA ratio suggests the presence of a recurrent tumor.[10] Conversely, marked reductions in Cho and Cr levels suggest radiation necrosis.[97,98,10] Although MRS cannot differentiate mixed tumor radiation necrosis tissue from either tumor or radiation necrosis in a consistent manner, it can provide good separation between pure necrosis and pure tumor tissues.[98] In addition, MRS can be used to monitor the clinical response to temozolamide in LGG cases[102] and to detect tumor recurrence at sites remote from irradiated areas. Metabolic alterations can be detected by MRS several months before changes in tumor volume are evident.[101,102] Radiation necrosis can yield a slight increase in Cho levels, perhaps because of cell damage and astrogliosis; care should be taken to avoid misclassification of such sites of necrosis as tumors.[103] If the metabolic findings are indeterminate, there may be both residual tumor and radiation-related changes. Therefore, in such cases, another MRI evaluation must be performed 6 to 8 weeks later.[104,105] A discrete isolated increase in Cho levels should not be considered as evidence of tumor recurrence. Only when a Cho level increase exceeds 45% and is associated with increased blood volume and permeability should the finding be considered

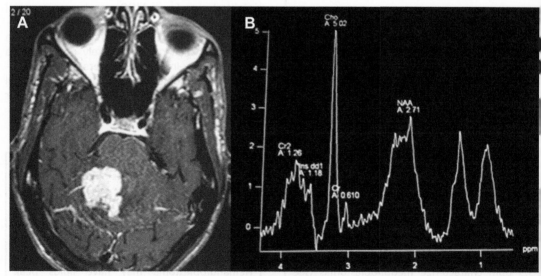

Fig. 24. Lymphoma in the right cerebellum hemisphere (*A*, postcontrast T1-weighted sequence). The MRS with TE = 30ms analysis (*B*) shows a high peak of choline, reduction of NAA, and peak of lipids/lactate.

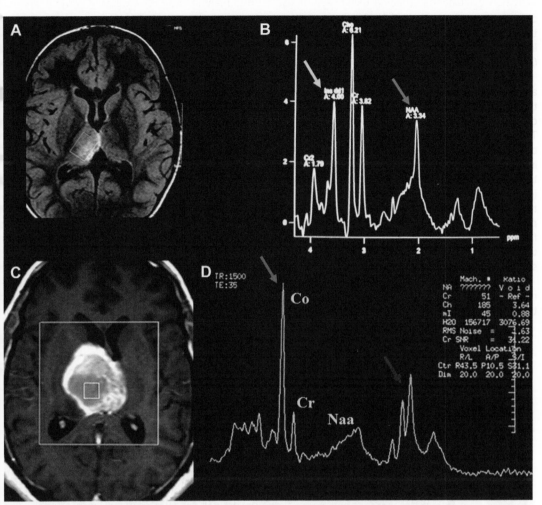

Fig. 25. Tumor grading. Low-grade glioma (*A, B*). Right thalamus low-grade glioma with hyperintense signal on FLAIR image (*A*) that presents on MRS with TE = 30ms (*B*) a high peak of myoinositol (*yellow arrow*) and a slight reduction of NAA (*green arrow*). HGG (*C, D*). Expansive and contrast-enhancing lesion (*C*, postcontrast T1-weighted sequence), of which MRS (*D*) analysis demonstrates a very high peak of choline (*red arrow*), reduction of NAA, and a double peak of lipids/lactate (*blue arrow*).

to indicate probable malignancy progression/tumor recurrence.

Prognosis

MRS findings have been related to overall survival. High lactate and lipid levels together with a high Cho/NAA index have been reported to correlate inversely with survival time.[99] Particular spectral resonances (ie, Cho-containing compounds, NAA, Cr, lipids, and lactate) have been found to be useful for predicting outcomes in patients with gliomas.[106] MRS, diffusion-weighted MR imaging, and perfusion-weighted MR imaging can provide oncologists a greater insight into tumor functionality, allowing better prognostic stratification of brain tumors than histopathology.[106]

PREOPERATIVE PLANNING

Precise determination of a lesion's relationship with surrounding functionally important tissue is of the utmost importance for optimizing surgical outcomes. Among the various advanced MR imaging techniques used to assess brain lesions, some techniques, such as DTI and blood oxygen level-dependent (BOLD)-contrast functional MR (fMR) imaging, provide particularly important information for neurosurgical planning (**Fig. 26**).

In BOLD-contrast fMR imaging, a specific brain area is stimulated causing a transient increase in the blood flow in that area and a consequent increase in the associated oxyhemoglobin supply. The diamagnetic effect of this transient increase of oxyhemoglobin causes an increase in the signal intensity of that area. This technique can be used to establish the involvement of particular cortical (gray matter) areas in particular tasks and functions, and thus enables surgeons to distinguish particular areas of brain tissue for which sparing from resection should be prioritized, such as motor, visual, and auditory cortices and language-specialized areas (**Fig. 27**).[107–111]

DTI can provide information about how a neoplastic lesion is interacting with nearby fibers tracts, perhaps even helping to discriminate boundaries between primary tumor, infiltrating tumor, peritumoral edema, and normal brain parenchyma. It is unclear how useful DTI is for evaluating tumor extensions and their relationships with nearby fibers around them, most likely because of the difficulty of establishing tumor borders. Because tumor borders are even difficult to establish histopathologically with certainty, there is not yet a reliable histologic standard with which to compare imaging data.

Although the specific biophysics of perilesional edema remains unclear, and ADC alone may not differentiate peritumoral edema with infiltration from peritumoral edema without infiltration, several investigators have reported that DTI can detect variations in FA values around lesions.

This has in turn led some to speculate that these variations may be caused by the presence of infiltrative tumor. However, it is not clear if infiltrating tumor will destroy fibers, and therefore results in

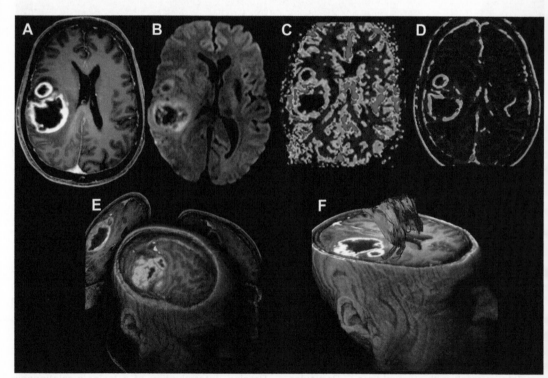

Fig. 26. Multiparametric approach (same case as in **Fig. 23**) in an anaplastic astrocytoma. An expansive, heterogeneous contrast-enhancing lesion, with central areas of necrosis (*A*, postcontrast T1-weighted sequence) shows restricted diffusion at the periphery (*B*, DWI), which also demonstrates high perfusion on DSC-MR imaging perfusion (*C*, rCBV map) and DCE-MR imaging permeability (*D*). The motor cortical area is displaced but not infiltrated posteriorly on a BOLD sequence image (*E*). Tractography also shows a dislocation of the main corticospinal fiber tracts (*F*).

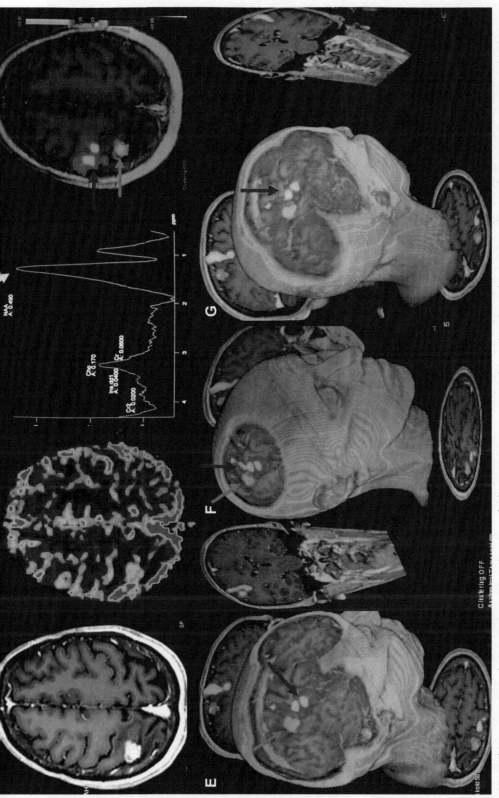

Fig. 27. Multiparametric analysis in preoperative planning of a breast cancer metastasis located in the right postcentral gyrus (A, postcontrast T1-weighted sequence) that has high perfusion on DSC-MR imaging perfusion (B, rCBV). MRS (C) shows a high peak of choline, reduction of NAA, and a very high peak of lipids/lactate (arrow). BOLD sequence (D) reveals a close relationship of the metastasis (red arrows) with the cortical activation of the sensitive motor region (blue arrows) on the 3D reconstruction images, with fusion of BOLD and postgadolinium T1-weighted sequences (E–G).

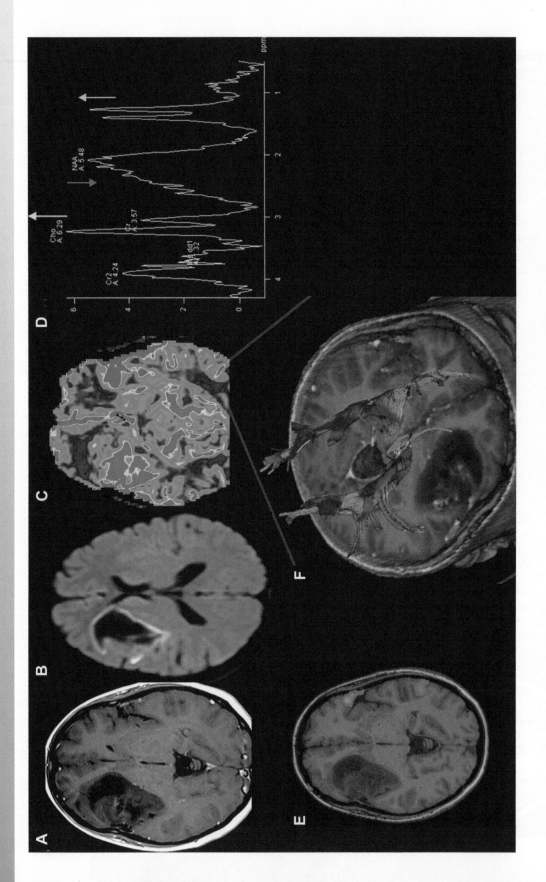

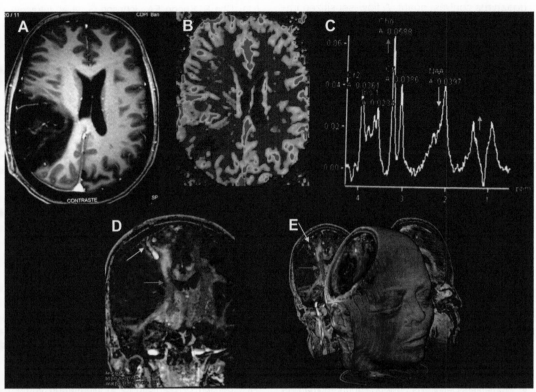

Fig. 29. Multiparametric analysis of an anaplastic oligodendroglioma. An infiltrating, expansive lesion that does not show significant contrast enhancement (*A*, postcontrast T1-weighted image), with foci of high perfusion in DSC-MR imaging perfusion (*B*, rCBV map) is depicted. MRS (*C*) reveals high peak of choline (*red arrow*), reduction of NAA (*yellow arrow*), and peak of lipids/lactate (*blue arrow*). DTI and BOLD sequences fusion images (*D*, *E*) demonstrate motor cortical activation (*yellow arrow*) closely related to the superior and medial margin of the lesion and a dislocation of the corticospinal tract (*red arrow*).

lower FA, or if the tumor infiltrating along the fibers actually increases FA by having more ultrastructure aligned with the fibers.[45]

Previous reports have suggested that DTI may reveal patterns of white matter involvement in tumor extensions. The following 4 categories of white matter involvement have been suggested based on FA maps: displaced, infiltrated, disrupted, and edematous. The displaced category includes cases where a lesion has displaced the main fibers of a tract, while FA remains normal or only slightly reduced. The infiltrated category includes cases where FA values have been clearly reduced by lesion incursion but the affected tracts are still identifiable. The disrupted category includes cases where tract fibers can no longer be identified anatomically and FA values are markedly reduced.[60,112] A marked reduction in FA values for tracts in the peritumoral region also occurs with edematous white matter involvement, with or without tumor infiltration[45] (**Figs. 28** and **29**).

Fig. 28. Multiparametric approach (same case as in **Figs. 5** and **12**) of an HGG of the right insula (*A–F*). An infiltrative expansive lesion with irregular and subtle contrast enhancement (*A*, postcontrast T1-weighted sequence) demonstrates restricted diffusion at the peripheral border (*B*, DWI) and high perfusion in the DSC-MR imaging sequence (*D*, rCBV map). MRS (*C*) shows a high peak of choline (*yellow arrow*), reduction of NAA (*red arrow*), and a double peak of lipids/lactate (*blue arrow*). The BOLD sequence reveals cortical activation in the left frontal orpercular region and posterior superior temporal aspect related to the language activation areas (*E*). A fusion reconstruction map with postcontrast T1-weighted and tractography images (*F*) also demonstrates a reduction of the anterior fibers and deviation of the medial and posterior main fibers of the right corticospinal tract in the tractography. Note that with this imaging approach, one may suggest that there is no tumor infiltration of the language area.

SUMMARY

Advanced MR imaging techniques can be useful in the assessment of brain neoplasms by allowing correct diagnosis and differentiation with other nontumoral brain lesions. These techniques also allow for the pretreatment and posttreatment evaluation of these tumors and help in their surgical planning. Advanced MR imaging techniques have been proving to be of upmost importance in clinical daily decisions enabling physiologic evaluation of brain tumors in relation to diagnosis and treatment.

REFERENCES

1. Ostrom QT, Gittleman H, Farah P, et al. CBTRUS statistical report: primary brain and central nervous system tumors diagnosed in the United States in 2006-2010. Neuro Oncol 2013;15(2):1–56.

2. Gavrilovic IT, Posner JB. Brain metastases: epidemiology and pathophysiology. J Neurooncol 2005; 75:5–14.

3. Sul J, Posner JB. Brain metastases: epidemiology and pathophysiology. Cancer Treat Res 2007;136: 1–21.

4. Biomarkers Definitions Working Group. Biomarkers and surrogate endpoints: preferred definitions and conceptual framework. Clin Pharmacol Ther 2001; 69(3):89–95.

5. Stack J, Redmond O, Codd M, et al. Breast disease: tissue characterization with Gd-DTPA enhancement profiles. Radiology 1990;174:491–4.

6. Flickinger F, Allison J, Sherry R, et al. Differentiation of benign from malignant breast masses by time intensity evaluation of contrast enhanced MRI. Magn Reson Imaging 1993;11:617–20.

7. Zierler KL. Circulation times and the theory of indicator-dilution methods for determining blood flow and volume. In: Hamilton VF, editor. Handbook of physiology. Baltimore (MD): Williams & Wilkins; 1962. p. 585–615.

8. Lacerda S, Law M. Magnetic resonance perfusion and permeability imaging in brain tumors. Neuroimaging Clin N Am 2009;19:527–57.

9. Hu LS, Baxter LC, Pinnaduwage DS, et al. Optimized preload leakage correction methods to improve the diagnostic accuracy of dynamic susceptibility-weighted contrast-enhanced perfusion MR imaging in posttreatment gliomas. AJNR Am J Neuroradiol 2010;31(1):40–8.

10. Roberts HC, Roberts TPL, Brasch RC, et al. Quantitative measurement of microvascular permeability in human brain tumors achieved using dynamic contrast-enhanced MR imaging: correlation with histologic grade. AJNR Am J Neuroradiol 2000; 21(5):891–9.

11. Cha S, Knopp EA, Johnson G, et al. Intracranial mass lesions: dynamic contrast-enhanced susceptibility-weighted echo-planar perfusion MR imaging. Radiology 2002;223(1):11–29.

12. Padhani AR, Dzik-Jurasz A. Perfusion MR imaging of extracranial tumor angiogenesis. Top Magn Reson Imaging 2004;15(1):41–57.

13. Cha S, Yang L, Johnson G, et al. Comparison of microvascular permeability measurements, Ktrans, determined with conventional steady-state T1-weighted and first-pass T2*-weighted MR imaging methods in gliomas and meningiomas. AJNR Am J Neuroradiol 2006;27(2):409–17.

14. Provenzale JM, York G, Moya MG, et al. Correlation of relative permeability and relative cerebral blood volume in high-grade cerebral neoplasms. AJR Am J Roentgenol 2006;187:1036–42.

15. Folkman J. Tumor angiogenesis: therapeutic implications. N Engl J Med 1971;285:1182–6.

16. Vajkoczy P, Menger MD. Vascular microenvironment in gliomas. J Neurooncol 2000;50(1–2):99–108.

17. Dvorak HF, Brown LF, Detmar M, et al. Vascular permeability factor/vascular endothelial growth factor, microvascular hyperpermeability, and angiogenesis. Am J Pathol 1995;146(5):1029–39.

18. Provenzale JM, Wang GR, Brenner T, et al. Comparison of permeability in high-grade and low-grade brain tumors using dynamic susceptibility contrast MR imaging. AJR Am J Roentgenol 2002;178(3):711–6.

19. Maia ACM Jr, Malheiros SMF, da Rocha AJ, et al. MR cerebral blood volume maps correlated with vascular endothelial growth factor expression and tumor grade in nonenhancing gliomas. AJNR Am J Neuroradiol 2005;26(4):777–83.

20. Cha S. Perfusion MR imaging: basic principles and clinical applications. Magn Reson Imaging Clin N Am 2003;11(3):403–13.

21. Law M, Yang S, Wang H, et al. Glioma grading: sensitivity, specificity, and predictive values of perfusion MR imaging and proton MR spectroscopic imaging compared with conventional MR imaging. AJNR Am J Neuroradiol 2003;24(10):1989–98.

22. Petrella JR, Provenzale JM. MR perfusion imaging of the brain: techniques and applications. Am J Roentgenol 2000;175(1):207–19.

23. Sugahara T, Korogi Y, Kochi M, et al. Correlation of MR imaging-determined cerebral blood volume maps with histologic and angiographic determination of vascularity of gliomas. AJR Am J Roentgenol 1998;171(6):1479–86.

24. Cha S, Lupo JM, Chen MH. Differentiation of glioblastoma multiforme and single brain metastasis by peak height and percentage of signal intensity recovery derived from dynamic susceptibility weighted contrast-enhanced perfusion MR imaging. AJNR Am J Neuroradiol 2007;28:1078–84.

25. Yuh EL, Barkovich AJ, Gupta N. Imaging of ependymomas: MRI and CT. Childs Nerv Syst 2009; 25:1203–13, 100.

26. Liao W, Liu Y, Wang X, et al. Differentiation of primary central nervous system lymphoma and high-grade glioma with dynamic susceptibility contrast-enhanced perfusion magnetic resonance imaging. Acta Radiol 2009;50(2):217–25.

27. Yang D, Korogi Y, Sugahara T, et al. Cerebral gliomas: prospective comparison of multivoxel 2D chemical-shift imaging proton MR spectroscopy, echoplanar perfusion and diffusion-weighted MRI. Neuroradiology 2002;44(8):656–66.

28. Patankar TF, Haroon HA, Mills SJ, et al. Is volume transfer coefficient (Ktrans) related to histologic grade in human gliomas? AJNR Am J Neuroradiol 2005;26:2455–65.

29. Law M, Yang S, Babb JS, et al. Comparison of cerebral blood volume and vascular permeability from dynamic susceptibility contrast-enhanced perfusion MR imaging with glioma grade. AJNR Am J Neuroradiol 2004;25:746–55.

30. Kerbel RS. Tumor angiogenesis. N Engl J Med 2008;358(19):2039–49.

31. Jain RK, di Tomaso E, Duda DG, et al. Angiogenesis in brain tumours. Nat Rev Neurosci 2007; 8(8):610–22.

32. Danchaivijitr N, Waldman AD, Tozer DJ, et al. Low grade gliomas: do changes in rCBV measurements at longitudinal perfusion-weighted MR imaging predict malignant transformation? Radiology 2008;247(1):170–8.

33. Barajas RF, Hodgson JG, Chang JS, et al. Glioblastoma multiform regional genetic and cellular expression patterns: influence on anatomic and physiologic MR imaging. Radiology 2010;254(2):564–76.

34. Provenzale JM, Schmainda K. Perfusion imaging for brain tumor characterization and assessment of treatment response. In: Newton HB, Jolesz FA, editors. Handbook of neuro-oncology neuroimaging. New York: Elsevier; 2008. p. 264–77.

35. Hygino da Cruz LC Jr, Rodriguez I, Domingues RC, et al. Pseudoprogression and pseudoresponse: imaging challenges in the assessment of post treatment glioma. AJNR Am J Neuroradiol 2011; 32(11):1978–85.

36. Sugahara T, Korogi Y, Tomiguchi S, et al. Post therapeutic intra axial brain tumor: the value of perfusion sensitive contrast-enhanced MR imaging for differentiating tumor recurrence from non neoplastic contrast-enhancing tissue. AJNR Am J Neuroradiol 2000;21(5):901–9.

37. Cha S. Update on brain tumor imaging: from anatomy to physiology. AJNR Am J Neuroradiol 2006; 27:475–87.

38. Hu LS, Baxter LC, Smith KA, et al. Relative cerebral blood volume values to differentiate high-grade glioma recurrence from posttreatment radiation effect: direct correlation between image-guided tissue histopathology and localized dynamic susceptibility-weighted contrast-enhanced perfusion MR imaging measurements. AJNR Am J Neuroradiol 2009;30(3):552–8.

39. Mangla R, Singh G, Ziegelitz D, et al. Changes in relative cerebral blood volume 1 month after radiation-temozolomide therapy can help predict overall survival in patients with glioblastoma. Radiology 2010;256:575–84.

40. Batchelor TT, Sorensen AG, di Tomaso E, et al. AZD2171, a pan-VEGF receptor tyrosine kinase inhibitor, normalizes tumor vasculature and alleviates edema in glioblastoma patients. Cancer Cell 2007; 11:83–95.

41. Gerstner ER, Duda DG, di Tomaso E, et al. VEGF inhibitors in the treatment of cerebral edema in patients with brain cancer. Nat Rev Clin Oncol 2009;6: 229–36.

42. de Groot JF, Yung WK. Bevacizumab and irinotecan in the treatment of recurrent malignant gliomas. Cancer J 2008;14(5):279–85.

43. Noguchi K, Watanabe N, Nagayoshi T, et al. Role of diffusion-weighted echo-planar MRI in distinguishing between brain abscess and tumor: a preliminary report. Neuroradiology 1999; 41:171–4.

44. Mills SJ, Patankar TA, Haroon HA, et al. Do cerebral blood volume and contrast transfer coefficient predict prognosis in human glioma? AJNR Am J Neuroradiol 2006;27:853–8.

45. Cruz LC, Kimura M. Diffusion magnetic resonance imaging in brain tumors. In: Newton HB, Jolesz FA, editors. Handbook of neuro-oncology neuroimaging. 2nd edition.

46. Rumboldt A, Camacho DL, Lake CT, et al. Apparent diffusion coefficients for differentiation of cerebellar tumors in children. AJNR Am J Neuroradiol 2006;27:1362–9, 21.

47. Mills SJ, Soh C, Rose CJ, et al. Candidate biomarkers of extravascular extracellular space: a direct comparison of apparent diffusion coefficient and dynamic contrast-enhanced MR imaging derived measurement of the volume of the extravascular extracellular space in glioblastoma multiforme. AJNR Am J Neuroradiol 2010;31: 549–53, 32.

48. Gupta A, Young RJ, Karimi A, et al. Isolated diffusion restriction precedes the development of enhancing tumor in a subset of patients with glioblastoma. AJNR Am J Neuroradiol 2011;32: 1301–6, 33.

49. Cruz LC, Vieira IG, Domingues R. Diffusion MR imaging: an important tool in the assessment of brain tumors. Neuroimaging Clin N Am 2011; 21(1):27–49.

50. Pope WB, Qiao XJ, Kim HJ, et al. Apparent diffusion coefficient histogram analysis stratifies progression-free and overall survival in patients with recurrent GBM treated with bevacizumab: a multi-center study. J Neurooncol 2012;108:491–8.

51. Hwang EJ, Cha Y, Leum Lee A, et al. Early response evaluation for recurrent high grade gliomas treated with bevacizumab: a volumetric analysis using diffusion-weighted imaging. J Neurooncol 2013;112:427–35.

52. Chapman CH, Nazem-Zadeh M, Lee OE, et al. Regional variation in brain white matter diffusion index changes following chemoradiotherapy: a prospective study using tract-based spatial statistics. PLoS ONE 2013;8(3):e57768.

53. Brunberg JA, Chenevert TL, McKeever PE, et al. In vivo MR determination of water diffusion coefficients and diffusion anisotropy: Correlation with structural alteration in gliomas of the cerebral hemispheres. AJNR Am J Neuroradiol 1995;16:361–71.

54. Schulder M, Maldjian JA, Liu WC, et al. Functional image-guided surgery of intracranial tumors located in or near the sensorimotor cortex. J Neurosurg 1998;89:412–8.

55. Toh CH, Castillo M, Wong AM-C, et al. Primary cerebral lymphoma and glioblastoma multiforme: differences in diffusion characteristics evaluated with diffusion tensor imaging. AJNR Am J Neuroradiol 2008;29:471–5.

56. Guo AC, Cummings TJ, Dash RC, et al. Lymphomas and high-grade astrocytomas: comparison of water diffusibility and histologic characteristics. Radiology 2002;224(1):177–83, 49.

57. Yamasaki F, Kurisu K, Satoh K, et al. Apparent diffusion coefficient of human brain tumors at MR imaging. Radiology 2005;235:985–91.

58. Toh CH, Chen YL, Hsieh TC, et al. Glioblastoma multiforme with diffusion-weighted magnetic resonance imaging characteristics mimicking primary brain lymphoma. Case report. J Neurosurg 2006; 105:132–5, 68.

59. Baehring JM, Bi WL, Bannykh S, et al. Diffusion MRI in the early diagnosis of malignant glioma. J Neurooncol 2007;82:221–5.

60. Goebell E, Paustenbach S, Vaeterlein O, et al. Low-grade and anaplastic gliomas: differences in architecture evaluated with diffusion-tensor MR imaging. Radiology 2006;239:217–22.

61. Chen S, Ikawa F, Kurisu K, et al. Quantitative MR evaluation of intracranial epidermoid tumors by fast fluid-attenuated inversion recovery imaging and echo-planar diffusion-weighted imaging. AJNR Am J Neuroradiol 2001;22(6):1089–96.

62. Filippi CG, Edgar MA, Ulug AM, et al. Appearance of meningiomas on diffusion-weighted images: correlation diffusion constants with histopathologic findings. AJNR Am J Neuroradiol 2001;22:65–72.

63. Melhem ER, Mori S, Mukundan G, et al. Diffusion tensor MR imaging of the brain and white matter tractography. AJR Am J Roentgenol 2002;178(1): 3–16.

64. Cruz LCH Jr, Sorensen GS. Diffusion tensor magnetic resonance imaging of brain tumors. Neurosurg Clin N Am 2005;16:115–34.

65. Pierpaoli C, Jezzard P, Basser P, et al. Diffusion tensor MR imaging of the human brain. Radiology 1996;201:637–48.

66. Sugahara T, Korogi Y, Kochi M, et al. Usefulness of diffusion-weighted MRI with echo-planar technique in the evaluation of cellularity in gliomas. J Magn Reson Imaging 1999;9:53–60.

67. Murakami R, Hirai T, Sugahara T, et al. Grading astrocytic tumors by using apparent diffusion coefficient parameters: superiority of a one- versus two-parameter pilot method. Radiology 2009;251: 838–45, 108.

68. Lee EJ, Lee SK, Agid R, et al. Preoperative grading of presumptive low-grade astrocytomas on MR imaging: diagnostic value of minimum apparent diffusion coefficient. AJNR Am J Neuroradiol 2008;29: 1872–7.

69. Jellinson BJ, Field AS, Medow J, et al. Diffusion tensor imaging of cerebral white matter: a pictorial review of physics, fiber tract anatomy, and tumor imaging patterns. AJNR Am J Neuroradiol 2004; 23:356–69.

70. Yoshiura T, Wu O, Zaheer A, et al. Highly diffusion-sensitized MRI of brain: dissociation of gray and white matter. Magn Reson Med 2001;45:734–40.

71. Johnson PC, Hunt SJ, Drayer BP. Human cerebral gliomas: correlation of postmortem MR imaging and neuropathologic findings. Radiology 1989; 170:211–7.

72. Castillo M, Smith JK, Kwock L, et al. Apparent diffusion coefficients in the evaluation of high-grade cerebral gliomas. AJNR Am J Neuroradiol 2001; 22(1):60–4.

73. Ross BD, Chenevert TL, Kim B, et al. Magnetic resonance imaging and spectroscopy: application to experimental neuro-oncology. Q Magn Reson Biol Med 1994;1:89–106.

74. Moffat BA, Chenevert TL, Lawrence TS, et al. Functional diffusion map: a noninvasive MRI biomarker for early stratification of clinical brain tumor response. Proc Natl Acad Sci U S A 2005; 102(15):5524–9.

75. Figueiras RG, Padhani AR, Goh VJ, et al. Novel oncologic drugs: what they do and how they affect images. RadioGraphics 2011;31:2059–91.

76. Sorensen AG, Batchelor TT, Wen PY, et al. Response criteria for glioma. Nat Clin Pract Oncol 2008;5(11):634–44.

77. Rieger J, Bähr O, Ronellenfitsch MW, et al. Bevacizumab-induced diffusion restriction in patients with

glioma: tumor progression or surrogate marker of hypoxia? J Clin Oncol 2010;28(27):e477.

78. Higano S, Yun X, Kumabe T, et al. Malignant astrocytic tumors: clinical importance of apparent diffusion coefficient in prediction of grade and prognosis. Radiology 2006;241:839–46, 151.

79. Murakami R, Sugahara T, Nakamura H, et al. Malignant supratentorial astrocytoma treated with postoperative radiation therapy: prognostic value of pretreatment quantitative diffusion-weighted MR imaging. Radiology 2007;243:493–9, 2011;196: 71–6.

80. Michaelis T, Merboldt KD, Bruhn H, et al. Absolute concentrations of metabolites in the adult human brain in vivo: quantification of localized proton MR spectra. Neuroradiology 1993;187:219–27.

81. Castillo M, Smith JK, Kwock L. Correlation of myo-inositol levels and grading of cerebral astrocytomas. AJNR Am J Neuroradiol 2000;21: 1645–9.

82. Fan G, Sun B, Wu Z, et al. In vivo single-voxel proton MR spectroscopy in the differentiation of high-grade gliomas and solitary metastases. Clin Radiol 2004;59(1):77–85, 35.

83. Chiang IC, Kuo YT, Lu CY, et al. Distinction between high-grade gliomas and solitary metastases using peritumoral 3-T magnetic resonance spectroscopy, diffusion, and perfusion imagings. Neuroradiology 2004;46(8):619–27.

84. Raybaud C, Barkovich AJ. Intracranial, orbital and neck masses of childhood. In: Barkovich AJ, Raybaud C, editors. Pediatric neuroimaging. 5th edition. Philadelphia: Lippincott Williams & Wilkins; 2012. p. 637–711, 63.

85. Harris L, Davies N, MacPherson L, et al. The use of short-echo time 1H MRS for childhood cerebellar tumors prior to histopathological diagnosis. Pediatr Radiol 2007;37:1101–9.

86. Majós C, Aguilera C, Cos M, et al. In vivo proton magnetic resonance spectroscopy of intraventricular tumors of the brain. Eur Radiol 2009;19: 2049–59.

87. Jouanneau E, Tovar RA, Desuzinges C. Very late frontal relapse of medulloblastoma mimicking a meningioma in an adult. Usefulness of 1H magnetic resonance spectroscopy and diffusion-perfusion magnetic resonance imaging for preoperative diagnosis: case report. Neurosurgery 2006;58(4):E789, 55.

88. Demir MK, Iplikcioglu AC, Dincer A, et al. Single voxel proton MR spectroscopy findings of typical and atypical intracranial meningiomas. Eur J Radiol 2006;60:48–55, 37.

89. Gill SS, Thomas DG, Van Bruggen N, et al. Proton MR spectroscopy of intracranial tumours: in vivo and in vitro studies. J Comput Assist Tomogr 1990;14:497–504.

90. Senft C, Hattingen E, Pilatus U, et al. Diagnostic value of proton magnetic resonance spectroscopy in the noninvasive grading of solid gliomas: comparison of maximum and mean choline values. Neurosurgery 2009;65(5):908–13.

91. Howe FA, Barton SJ, Cudlip SA, et al. Metabolic profiles of human brain tumors using quantitative in vivo 1H magnetic resonance spectroscopy. Magn Reson Med 2003;49:223–32.

92. Di Costanzo A, Scarabino T, Trojsi F, et al. Multiparametric 3T MR approach to the assessment of cerebral gliomas: tumor extent and malignancy. Neuroradiology 2006;48:622–31.

93. Ganslandt O, Stadlbauer A, Fahlbusch R, et al. Proton magnetic resonance spectroscopic imaging integrated into image-guided surgery: correlation to standard magnetic resonance imaging and tumor cell density. Neurosurgery 2005;56: 291–8, 90.

94. McKnight TR, Von Dem Bussche MH, Vigneron DB, et al. Histopathological validation of a three dimensional magnetic resonance spectroscopy index as a predictor of tumor presence. J Neurosurg 2002; 97:794–802.

95. Poussaint TY. Pediatric brain tumors. In: Newton HB, Jolesz FA, editors. Handbook of neuro-oncology neuroimaging. New York: Academic Press; 2008. p. 469–84.

96. Stadlbauer A, Nimsky C, Buslei R, et al. Proton magnetic resonance spectroscopic imaging in the border zone of gliomas: correlation of metabolic and histological changes at low tumor infiltration—initial results. Invest Radiol 2007;42(4):218–30.

97. Dowling C, Bollen AW, Noworolski SM, et al. Preoperative proton MR spectroscopic imaging of brain tumors: correlation with histopathologic analysis of resection specimens. AJNR Am J Neuroradiol 2001;22(4):604–12.

98. Hall WA, Galicich W, Bergman T, et al. 3-Tesla intraoperative MR imaging for neurosurgery. J Neurooncol 2006;77(3):297–303.

99. Saraswathy S, Crawford FW, Lamborn KR, et al. Evaluation of MR markers that predict survival in patients with newly diagnosed GBM prior to adjuvant therapy. J Neurooncol 2009;91(1): 69–81.

100. Smith EA, Carlos RC, Junck LR, et al. Developing a clinical decision model: MR spectroscopy to differentiate between recurrent tumor and radiation change in patients with new contrast-enhancing lesions. AJR Am J Roentgenol 2009; 192:W45–52, 119.

101. Chernov MF, Hayashi M, Izawa M, et al. Multivoxel proton MRS for differentiation of radiation-induced necrosis and tumor recurrence after gamma knife radiosurgery for brain metastases. Brain Tumor Pathol 2006;23:19–27.

102. Murphy PS, Viviers L, Abson C, et al. Monitoring te-mozolomide treatment of low-grade glioma with proton magnetic resonance spectroscopy. Br J Cancer 2004;90:781–6.

103. Hourani R, Brant LJ, Rizk T, et al. Can proton MR spectroscopic and perfusion imaging differentiate between neoplastic and non-neoplastic brain lesions in adults? AJNR Am J Neuroradiol 2008; 29(2):366–72.

104. Law M. MR spectroscopy of brain tumors. Top Magn Reson Imaging 2004;15:291–313.

105. Li X, Jin H, Lu Y, et al. Identification of MRI and 1H MRSI parameters that may predict survival for patients with malignant gliomas. NMR Biomed 2004; 17:10–20.

106. Majós C, Bruna J, Julià-Sapé M, et al. Proton MR spectroscopy provides relevant prognostic information in high-grade astrocytomas. AJNR Am J Neuroradiol 2011;32:74–80.

107. Ramsey NF, Sommer IE, Rutten GJ, et al. Combined analysis of language tasks in fMRI improves assessment of hemispheric dominance for language functions in individual subjects. Neuroimage 2001;13(4):719–33.

108. Abou-Khalil B. Methods for determination of language dominance: the Wada test and proposed noninvasive alternatives. Curr Neurol Neurosci Rep 2007;7(6):483–90.

109. Roux FE, Boulanouar K, Lotterie JA, et al. Language functional magnetic resonance imaging in preoperative assessment of language areas: correlation with direct cortical stimulation. Neurosurgery 2003;52(6):1335–45 [discussion 1345–7].

110. Rutten GJ, Ramsey NF, van Rijen PC, et al. Development of a functional magnetic resonance imaging protocol for intraoperative localization of critical temporoparietal language areas. Ann Neurol 2002;51(3):350–60.

111. Bizzi A, Blasi V, Falini A, et al. Presurgical functional MR imaging of language and motor functions: validation with intraoperative electrocortical mapping. Radiology 2008;248(2): 579–89.

112. Tsuchiya K, Fujikawa A, Nakajima M, et al. Differentiation between solitary metastasis and high-grade gliomas by diffusion tensor imaging. Br J Radiol 2005;78:533–7.

Evaluation of Head and Neck Tumors with Functional MR Imaging

Jacobus F.A. Jansen, PhD[a],*, Carlos Parra, PhD[b],
Yonggang Lu, PhD[c], Amita Shukla-Dave, PhD[b,d]

KEYWORDS

• Head and neck cancer • MR imaging • Diffusion • Perfusion • Data processing

KEY POINTS

• Functional MR imaging techniques (diffusion and perfusion MR imaging) allow for quantifying tumor characteristics related to tumor physiology and biology.
• Compared with anatomic imaging techniques, functional MR imaging techniques have shown their added value in head and neck tumor detection, characterization, staging, treatment response monitoring, and prediction.
• Dedicated MR imaging hardware and software and knowledgeable personnel are essential to obtain reliable data and to translate to the head and neck clinic.

DISCUSSION OF PROBLEM/CLINICAL PRESENTATION

Head and neck (HN) cancer is one of the major types of cancer, affecting 50,000 new patients in the United States every year.[1] HN cancers typically originate from the mucosal epithelia of the oral cavity, pharynx, and larynx and can be linked to alcohol consumption and tobacco smoking.[2] For early HN cancers, encouraging locoregional control can be reached through radiation or surgery treatment. However, for advanced HN cancer, the odds are less favorable, as with standard therapy, only 60% of patients will survive 5 years.[1] HN cancers frequently metastasize to (cervical) lymph nodes before they penetrate distant organs such as the lungs. In spite of recent advances in surgical and oncologic treatments, the overall survival rate of patients with HN cancer has unfortunately not improved much over recent years.[1] Important causes for unfavorable outcome in advanced HN cancer can be a delayed diagnosis (followed by loco regional failure) and a tardy salvage treatment at the recurrence of the disease. A priori predictors of outcome and predictive biomarkers of treatment response are desperately needed to advance patient care and individualized treatment. For example, noninvasive imaging biomarkers could have an important role in the clinical decision-making process, thereby allowing oncologists to use interventions with alternative therapy strategies. Imaging has several benefits as a method for improving the tumor treatment evaluation, as it can sample the entire tumor noninvasively and can be repeated longitudinally to monitor changes at regular intervals.

The authors are supported by the National Cancer Institute/National Institutes of Health (grant number 1 R21CA176660-01A1).
[a] Department of Radiology, Maastricht University Medical Center, PO Box 5800, Maastricht 6202 AZ, The Netherlands; [b] Department of Medical Physics, Memorial Sloan-Kettering Cancer Center, 1275 York Avenue, New York, NY 10065, USA; [c] Department of Radiation Oncology, University of Washington, 4921 Parkview Pl, St Louis, MO 63110, USA; [d] Department of Radiology, Memorial Sloan-Kettering Cancer Center, 1275 York Avenue, New York, NY 10065, USA
* Corresponding author.
E-mail address: jacobus.jansen@mumc.nl

Magn Reson Imaging Clin N Am 24 (2016) 123–133
http://dx.doi.org/10.1016/j.mric.2015.08.011
1064-9689/16/$ – see front matter © 2016 Elsevier Inc. All rights reserved.

Functional MR imaging might provide the ideal tools yielding such noninvasive markers.[3,4] This review focuses on the promises of diffusion- and perfusion-weighted MR imaging techniques in HN cancer. Diffusion-weighted (DW) MR imaging can quantify and map the diffusion of molecules (typically water), in biological tissues,[5] whereas perfusion-weighted MR imaging can assess the passage of blood through vessels through tissue.[6,7] Both MR imaging techniques have a rich history that extends decades, and the MR imaging tools available to assess the associated processes are currently very mature, providing excellent opportunities to study both diffusion and perfusion in HN cancer. Although some might consider magnetic resonance (MR) spectroscopy also to be a functional MR imaging technique, it falls beyond the scope of this review, and we refer the reader to an excellent review by Razek and Poptani.[8]

Diffusion

DW imaging (DWI) is an MR technique that allows the measurement of water self-diffusivity.[5] Because freedom of motion of water molecules is hindered by interactions with other molecules and cellular barriers, water molecule diffusion abnormalities can reflect changes of tissue organization at the cellular level (eg, increase of extracellular space owing to cell death). These microstructural changes affect the (hindered) motion of water molecules and consequently alter the water diffusion properties and thus the MR signal. Apart from deriving a measure for the average extent of molecular motion that is affected by cellular organization and integrity (apparent diffusion coefficient [ADC]), it is also possible using diffusion tensor imaging (in which diffusion is measured in several directions) to measure the preferred direction of molecular motion, which provides information on the degree of alignment of cellular structures and their structural integrity (fractional anisotropy). Recently, also DWI techniques have entered the HN cancer clinic, in which images are acquired with multiple b values, yielding techniques such as intravoxel incoherent imaging (IVIM)[9] or diffusion kurtosis imaging,[10] techniques that aim to provide information that extends diffusion of water, such as perfusion (for IVIM) or non-Gaussian diffusion behavior (for diffusion kurtosis imaging).

Perfusion

Perfusion is physiologically defined as the steady-state delivery of blood to tissue.[6,7] Two major approaches exist to assess perfusion with MR imaging. The first is the application of an exogenous contrast agent (usually gadolinium based), exploiting the susceptibility effects or relaxivity effects of the contrast agents on the signal, respectively, dynamic susceptibility contrast–enhanced MR perfusion or dynamic contrast–enhanced (DCE) MR perfusion. The second application involves the use of an endogenous contrast agent, namely, magnetically labeled arterial blood water, as a diffusible flow tracer in arterial spin labeling (ASL) MR perfusion. DCE and, to a lesser extend ASL, are currently being used to study HN cancer.

Outline

This review summarizes recent literature and provides an overview of the various studies in which diffusion- or perfusion-based MR imaging studies are applied to HN cancer. This review provides an overview of commonly used acquisition protocols and postprocessing methods, advanced data analysis, imaging findings regarding tumor characterization and differentiation, tumor risk stratification and staging, monitoring, and prediction of treatment response. Subsequently, limitations are highlighted followed by a conclusion with recommendations for future research.

IMAGING PROTOCOLS
Diffusion-Weighted MR Imaging

Data acquisition

- *MR imaging scanner and coil:* DW MR imaging studies for HN cancers are commonly carried out on 1.5-T or 3-T MR imaging scanners using dedicated neurovascular phase array coils.[10–12]
- *Pulse sequence:* Clinical DW MR imaging is most commonly performed using single-shot spin-echo echo planar imaging (EPI), axial free breathing.
- *Acquisition parameters* (Table 1): Protocol optimization is a prerequisite for obtaining optimum signal-to-noise ratio in DW images. The number of b values for mono exponential modeling of the data are 2 to 3 and the b values are greater than 100 s/mm²; (usually between 500 and 1200 s/mm²), whereas the number of b values increases up to 10 or more (usually between 0 to 1500 s/mm²) including both the high and low b values for biexponential modeling of the data[9,10,13]; slice thickness, 5 to 8 mm, gap thickness, 0 mm, field of view, 200 to 380 mm[14]; acquired matrix, 128 x 128 or higher[5]; number of averages, 2 to 4; parallel imaging (SENSE or ASSET), factor, 2; echo time (TE, ideal/target), minimum TE; acceptable

Table 1
Typical acquisition parameters

Contrast	Sequence	TE/TR (ms)	Slice Thickness (mm)	FOV (mm)	Matrix	Extras
DW MR imaging	Single-shot spin-echo EPI	<110/2000–4000	5–8	200–380	≥128x128	>2 b values, 0–1500 s/mm^2
DCE MR imaging	3-D spoiled gradient echo	~1.4/5.3	5–8	~220	≥128x128	Gd-DTPA bolus 0.1 mmol/kg at 2 ml/s, followed by a 20-mL saline flush Temporal resolution: 3–6 s; ~50 phases
ASL	Multishot spin-echo echo-planar, pCASL	~20/4000	5	~230	~80x80	Labeling duration: 1650 ms; postlabel delay: 1280 ms; 2 shots; labeling just under the bifurcation

less than 110 milliseconds; repetition time (TR), 2 to 4 seconds; receiver bandwidth, greater than 1000 Hz/voxel.

Diffusion-weighted MR imaging data processing

- *Region of interest analysis:* The regions of interest (ROIs) are usually drawn on the DW MR images by an experienced neuroradiologist based on the radiologic and clinical information. The ROI encompasses the entire tumor and node of interest.
- *Quantitative methods:* Mono- and biexponential models[9,10,13,15] are usually used for quantifying diffusion either based on voxel by voxel or the ROI. For monoexponential models, ADC value can be quantified using S/S0 = exp(-b × ADC), where S and S0 are the signal intensities with and without diffusion weighting, respectively, and b is the gradient factor (b value, seconds per millimeter squared).[11,15] For biexponential models,[9,16] metrics related to intravoxel incoherent motions can be calculated using

$$S = S_0((1-f)\exp(-bD) + f\exp(-bD^*))$$

or

$$S = S_0\left((1-f)\exp\left(-bD + \frac{1}{6}b^2D^2K\right) + f\exp(-bD^*)\right)$$

where f is the vascular volume fraction or perfusion factor, D is the pure diffusion coefficient (millimeter squared per second), D* is the pseudodiffusion coefficient (millimeter squared per second) associated with blood velocity and capillary geometry, and K is the diffusion kurtosis coefficient. Noise floor rectification schemes are commonly used in the above diffusion quantifications.[17]

Dynamic Contrast–Enhanced MR Imaging Data Acquisition

- *MR imaging scanner and coil:* DCE MR imaging studies for HN cancers are commonly being carried out on 1.5-T or 3-T MR imaging scanners using dedicated neurovascular phase array coils.
- *Contrast agent:* The most commonly used contrast agent is paramagnetic gadolinium chelates, such as Gd-DTPA (gadopentetic diethylenetriamine pentaacetic acid) (Magnevist; Berlex Laboratories, Wayne, NJ).[18–20] The bolus of contrast agent is typically delivered at 0.1 mmol/kg body weight at 2 mL/s followed by a 20-mL saline flush with a flow rate of 2 mL/s using an MR-compatible, programmable power injector (eg, Spectris; Medrad, Indianola, PA).[20–22]
- *Pulse sequence:* Most of the DCE MR imaging data acquisition is performed using a fast 2-dimensional (D) or 3-D gradient-echo sequence because of its high T1 sensitivity and rapid image acquisition.[18–20] A 3-D spoiled gradient-echo sequence is more widely applied than 2-D spoiled gradient-echo because of its ability to achieve higher spatial resolution and signal-to-noise ratio.

- *Acquisition parameters* (see **Table 1**): The acquisition parameters can be tailored depending on whether the study design needs higher spatial resolution or higher temporal resolution. Approximate typical parameters on gradient-echo MR scanners are field of view (FOV), 22 cm; TR, 5.3 milliseconds; TE, 1.4 milliseconds; temporal resolution, 4 seconds; phases, 50; number of excitations (NEX), 1. Temporal resolution ranges from 3 to 6 seconds and acquisition time is generally in the range of 2 to 10 minutes.[18,20,23]

Dynamic contrast–enhanced MR imaging data processing

- *Radiofrequency (RF) field inhomogeneity correction:* RF field nonuniformities often cause inhomogeneity in image profile. Image correction methods, such as an edge-completed low pass filter algorithm, can be used to correct this kind of image artifacts.[19] Additionally, this inhomogeneity can result in deviation of the flip angles from nominal values when using gradient-echo sequences for data acquisition. This flip angle deviation has a great impact on the calculation of native T1 relaxation time values, further influencing the accuracies of the estimated pharmacokinetic parameters. A double-echo method can be used to correct this artifact.[24,25]
- *Motion artifact correction:* DCE MR images in the HN region suffer from motion artifacts caused by the voluntary and involuntary motions of patients. The motions can cause in-plane and through-plane image artifacts. Image registration methods are commonly used to correct the through-plane image artifacts by realigning the DCE MR imaging time series image itself or coregistering DCE MR images with other image modalities, such as T1- or T2-weighted images.[18,19,26] Rigid body alignments are more readily performed than nonrigid deformations.[19]

Dynamic contrast–enhanced MR imaging data quantification

- *Semiquantitative methods:* Semiquantitative methods classify the signal intensity time curve of DCE MR imaging into different patterns or provide some simple summary descriptors about the curve. For curve pattern classification, the initial enhancement (1–2 min) of the curve is usually described as fast, medium, and slow uptake. The late enhancement (>2 min) of the curve is often classified as persistent, plateau, and washout.[27] Normal tissues and tumor tissues with different degrees of malignancy could show different curve patterns. This feature can be used for tumor detection and tumor differentiation.[28,29] For curve summary description, several summary parameters, such as maximum *contrast index* (CI), time to reach maximum CI, maximum slope, washout slope, area under the curve (AUC) at a specific time (eg, AUC90 means the area under the curve 90 seconds after contrast injection), are used.[6,19]

- *Pharmacokinetic modeling methods:* Pharmacokinetic modeling methods provide characteristics of tumor microvasculature (related to endothelial permeability, the size of extracellular extravascular space [EES], and the size of intravascular space) by modeling tumor contrast kinetics into separate compartments and establishing the transport equation of the contrast agent. Commonly used models are the Tofts model, extended T model, shutter speed model, and the 2-compartment exchange model.[18,20,26,30,31] Among these models, the Tofts model is used the most. From the Tofts model, kinetic parameters such as K^{trans} (volume transfer rate between vascular space and EES min^{-1}) and v_e (volume fraction of the EES) can be characterized on a basis of tumor ROI or voxel by voxel.[18–20] For these models accurate estimation of the arterial input function (AIF) is required, and when this is not possible in individual cases, also averaged population-based AIF functions can be used.[23]

Arterial Spin Labeling MR Imaging Data Acquisition

- *MR imaging scanner and coil:* ASL MR imaging studies for HN cancers[32,33] have been reported using 3-T MR imaging scanners using dedicated neurovascular phase array coils.
- *Pulse sequence:* ASL can be acquired with a sequence using echo-planar MR imaging signal targeted by alternating RF pulses (EPISTAR).[32] Magnetic labeling of in-flowing arterial blood can be achieved using section-selective 180° RF pulses in labeling slab. After the labeling, a Look-Locker readout of gradient-echo EPI with an excitation pulse of 30° can be used for image acquisition. Additionally, control images without labeling need to be acquired. Also, pCASL (Pseudocontinuous arterial spin labeling) techniques have

been reported.[34] The acquisition of pCASL can be performed by using multishot spin-echo echo-planar imaging to obtain control and labeled images. The labeling slab can be placed just under the bifurcation of the internal and external carotid arteries.

- *Acquisition parameters* (see **Table 1**): Typical parameters on 3-T Philips MR scanners for EPI STAR are TR, 3000 milliseconds; TE, 24 milliseconds; FOV, 230 × 230 mm; matrix, 80 x 80; slice thickness, 10 mm; interslice gap, 30%; NEX 30. Label slab is 58.5 mm thick located 20 mm proximal to the imaging section. For pCASL, parameters are labeling duration, 1650 milliseconds; postlabel delay, 1280 milliseconds; TR, 3619 milliseconds; TE, 18 milliseconds; flip angle, 90°; number of shots, 2; FOV, 230 × 230 mm; matrix, 80 x 80; slice thickness, 5 mm; number of slices, 15; acceleration factor for parallel imaging, 2.

Arterial spin labeling data quantification

- Tumor blood flow (TBF) can be calculated using image processing software such as MatLab (MathWorks, Natick, MA). TBF can be calculated from analysis of magnetization difference obtained by subtracting the labeled images from the ASL control images.[32,34] TBF maps can be created on a pixel-by-pixel basis.

Advanced data analysis

In addition to using perfusion- or diffusion-based MR imaging contrasts for a better evaluation of HN cancer, on the data analysis side, improvements in the applicability of MR images in HN cancer are developing. Most of these techniques do not need specific MR imaging contrasts as input, because, in principle, they work on any quantitative map. For example, the parametric response map approach[35] is a voxel-based approach that allows segmentation of a tumor volume based on regional intratumoral changes in the MR signal. It is ideally suited to accurately follow treatment-induced changes in tumors on a voxel-by-voxel basis. Another analysis method allows for accurate assessment of tumor heterogeneity. HN cancer can be very heterogeneous in nature, as the tumor vascular system is typically chaotic and poorly organized, and tumor heterogeneity itself is a well-recognized feature that is associated with tumor malignancy.[36] In particular, tumor heterogeneity in the blood supply may prevent therapeutic efficacy and result in treatment resistance. Therefore, tumor heterogeneity may play an important role in assessing tumor malignancy and predicting treatment response. Most studies typically use summarizing characteristics, such as mean, median, or standard deviation of voxel-wise measures, to describe the nature of the whole tumor volume. However, these commonly used measures do not necessarily reflect the marked morphologic heterogeneity in nodal metastases of HN cancer. Image texture analysis may be an ideal candidate to assess tumor tissue heterogeneity in a reliable manner.[37–39] In texture analysis, an algorithm that assesses spatial intensity coherence is applied to an image yielding several textural features (reflecting heterogeneity), independent of the image's mean and variance. The gray-level co-occurrence matrix, or gray-level spatial dependence matrix, is one of the most important algorithms used for texture analysis.[40]

IMAGING FINDINGS
Tumor Characterization and Differentiation

Studies have found that DW MR imaging and DCE MR imaging can be used to differentiate tumor types. Sumi and Nakamura[41] combined use of IVIM and time-signal intensity curve (TIC) analyses to diagnose HN tumors. IVIM parameters (f and D values) and TIC profiles in combination were distinct among the different types of HN tumors, including squamous cell carcinomas (SCCs), lymphomas, malignant salivary gland tumors, Warthin's tumors, pleomorphic adenomas, and schwannomas; a multiparametric approach using both measures differentiated between benign and malignant tumors with 97% accuracy and diagnosed different tumor types with 89% accuracy. A combined use of IVIM parameters and TIC profiles may have high efficacy in diagnosing HN tumors.

Lee and colleagues[6] used DCE MR imaging–derived parameters to differentiate SCC, undifferentiated carcinoma (UD), and lymphoma; they showed that K^{trans}, AUC60, and AUC90 were significantly different between UD and SCC and UD and lymphoma but not between SCC and lymphoma.

Similarly, Asaumi and colleagues[42] attempted to differentiate malignant lymphomas from SCCs using DCE MR imaging with 17 lesions of malignant lymphoma and 30 cases of SCC. The results showed that there was a significant difference between SCC and malignant lymphoma in the time to reach the maximum CI.

Fong and colleagues[43] found that DW MR imaging was successful in 45 of 65 with nasopharynx cancer (NPC), 5 of 7 with lymphoma, and 26 of 28 with SCC, and the mean ADCs (± standard deviation [SD]) of NPC, lymphoma, and SCC were 0.98 ± 0.161, 0.75 ± 0.190, and 1.14 ± 0.196 (×10[−3] mm[2]/s), respectively, which were significantly different (P<.001–.003).

Srinivasan and colleagues[44] in their DWI study found that HN squamous cell cancer (HNSCC) patients had a significantly lower mean ADC value (1.101 [±0.214] × 10[−3] mm[2]/s) than paraspinal muscles, pterygoid muscle, masseter muscle, thyroid gland, and base of the tongue (P = .0006, .0002, .0001, .001, and .002, respectively). The tumor ADC values were not significantly different from ADC values of parotid and submandibular glands (P = .057 and .14, respectively).[14] In their other study with 33 patients at 3-T MR scanner, they found that there was a statistically significant difference (P = .004) between the mean ADC values (10[−3] mm[2]/s) in the benign and malignant lesions (1.505 ± 0.487; 95% confidence interval, 1.305–1.706, and 1.071 ± 0.293; 95% confidence interval, 0.864–1.277, respectively), and suggested that a 3-T ADC value of 1.3 × 10−3 mm2/s may be the threshold value for differentiation between benign and malignant HN lesions.

Tumor Risk Stratification and Staging

In a recent study by Lu and colleagues,[15] the utility of DW MR imaging as a novel preoperative tool for risk stratification in thyroid cancer was evaluated. The study concluded that ADC values of papillary thyroid cancers (PTCs) with extrathyroidal extension (ETE; 1.53 ± 0.25 × 10−3 mm2/s) were significantly lower than corresponding values from PTCs without ETE (2.37 ± 0.67 × 10−3 mm2/s; P<.005), and the cutoff ADC was determined at 1.85 × 10−3 mm2/s with a sensitivity of 85%, specificity of 85%, and receiving operating characteristic curve area of 0.85 that had ETE from those patients that did not have ETE. ETE was assessed at pathology, making DW MR imaging a tool of choice for preoperative clinical workup.

Vandecaveye and colleagues,[45] investigated the role of DWI in nodal staging in HNSCC patients. In their study, DWI led to a correct change in nodal stage for 12 (36%) of 33 patients. The nodal stage of 2 patients was downgraded from N1 to N0 in one patient and from N2b to N0 in the other. In 4 patients, a contralateral metastasis that was initially undetected at preoperative MR imaging was diagnosed at DWI. The nodal stage of the lymph node in the neck of 6 patients was upgraded from N0 to N1 or N2b in 3 patients with laryngeal cancer, to N2b in 2 patients with tongue cancer, and to ipsilateral metastasis in 1 patient with mouth floor cancer. In the patient with mouth floor cancer, a contralateral lymph node at neck

level 2 that was considered suspicious at turbo spin-echo imaging was correctly diagnosed as benign at DWI, and the extent of the contralateral neck dissection was consequently reduced. Compared with turbo spin-echo imaging, DW imaging performed with ADC b 0 to 1000 values had higher accuracy than MR imaging in nodal staging, providing added value in the detection of subcentimeter nodal metastases.

Monitoring of Treatment Response

To evaluate DWI for assessment of early treatment response in HNSCC after the end of chemoradio therapy, Vandecaveye and colleagues[12] found that the ADC change between pretreatment and after treatment (ΔADC) of lesions with later tumor recurrence was significantly lower than that in lesions with complete remission for both primary lesions (-2.3% ± 0.3% vs 80% ± 41%; P<.0001 and adenopathies (19.9% ± 32% vs 63% ± 36%; P = .003). The ΔADC showed a PPV of 89% and an NPV of 100% for primary lesions and a PPV of 70% and an NPV of 96% for adenopathies per neck side. DWI improved positive predictive value and negative predictive value compared with anatomic imaging.

Kim and colleagues[11] investigated the ADC change in 40 newly diagnosed HNSCC, before, during, and after the end of chemoradiation therapy and found that pretreatment ADC value of complete responders (1.04 ± 0.19 × 10−3 mm2/s) was significantly lower (P<.05) than that from partial responders (1.35 ± 0.30 × 10−3 mm2/s). A significant increase in ADC was observed in complete responders within 1 week of treatment (P<.01), which remained high until the end of the treatment. The complete responders also showed significantly higher increase in ADC than the partial responders by the first week of chemoradiation (P<.01). These results suggest that ADC can be used as a marker for early detection of response to concurrent chemoradiation therapy in HNSCC (Fig. 1).

Prediction of Treatment Response

Shukla-Dave and colleagues[20] showed in a DCE MR imaging study performed on 74 HNSCC patients that in a stepwise Cox regression, skewness of K[trans] (volume transfer constant) was the strongest predictor for stage IV patients (progression-free survival and overall survival, P<.001). This study suggests an important role for pretreatment DCE MR imaging in prediction of outcome in these patients.

Baer and colleagues[35] reported the utility of DCE MR imaging in assessment of treatment response. They showed in 10 patients with locoregionally HNSCC who underwent definitive

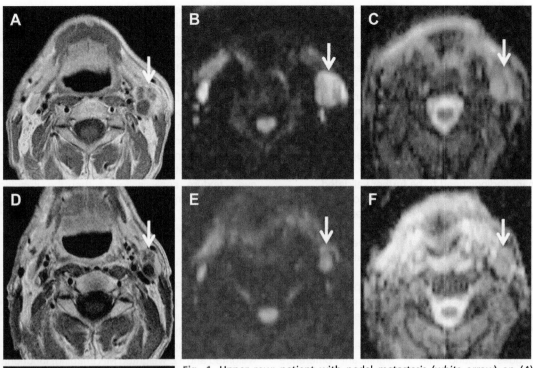

Fig. 1. Upper row: patient with nodal metastasis (*white arrow*) on (*A*) contrast-enhanced T1-weighted image, (*B*) b1000 DWI, and (*C*) ADC map prior to chemorediotherapy. Middle row: (*D*) contrast-enhanced T1-weighted image 3 weeks post-chemorediotherapy shows persistent adenopathy >1.5 cm with intranodal heterogeneity. (*E*) The lymphadenopathy is hyperintense on the b1000 DWI. Bottom row: CT-scan, 2 years post- chemorediotherapy, shows completely calcified, small remnant lymphadenopathy, without evidence of tumor recurrence. (*From* Vandecaveye V, Dirix P, De Keyzer F, et al. Diffusion-weighted magnetic resonance imaging early after chemoradiotherapy to monitor treatment response in head-and-neck squamous cell carcinoma. Int J Radiat Oncol Biol Phys 2012;82:1098–107.)

concurrent chemoradiation therapy that the volume transfer constant and normalized area under the contrast-enhancement time curve at 60 seconds were predictive of survival in parametric response map analysis (volume transfer constant, $P = .002$; normalized area under the contrast-enhancement time curve at 60 seconds, $P = .02$) and in the percentage change analysis (volume transfer constant, $P = .04$; normalized area under the contrast-enhancement time curve at 60 seconds, $P = .02$). After appropriate validation, this method may find use in potentially guide treatment modification in patients with predicted treatment failure.

Bernstein and colleagues[46] performed a study on 37 HNSCC patients undergoing induction chemotherapy (IC), and the median baseline tumor plasma flow (F_p) was 53.2 mL/100 mL/min in 25 responders and 23.9 in 12 nonresponders ($P = .027$). Median baseline F_p in lymph nodes was 25.8 mL/100 mL/min for 37 nodes in 25 responders and 17.1 for 15 nodes in 12 nonresponders ($P = .066$), and frequency of IC response in 37 patients was 68% overall, 83% for tumor F_p greater than the median (40.6 mL/100 mL/min) and 45% less than the median, thereby concluding that pretreatment tumor F_p determined by DCE MR imaging predicts IC response in HNSCC.

In a recent study, Fujima and colleagues[32] used ASL in 22 patients with HN cancer and evaluated perfusion measures before and after nonsurgical treatment. The study found that the TBF reduction rate was significantly lower in patients with residual tumors (0.54 ± 0.12) than in those without

(0.85 ± 0.06); therefore, ASL technique could accurately determine the effect of nonsurgical treatment (Fig. 2).

In a feasibility IVIM study on neck nodal metastases, Hauser and colleagues[47] studied 15 HNSCC patients who received radiotherapy in combination with chemotherapy and/or immunotherapy. They found that the initial perfusion fraction (f) value was significantly higher ($P = .01$) in patients with loco-regional failure (LRF) compared to patients with locoregional control. LRF was present in 3 patients only. These preliminary findings need to be further validated.

Noij and colleagues[48] performed pretreatment MR imaging on 78 HNSCC patients. ADC and contrast-enhanced T1-weighted images were evaluated, and the results showed that tumor volume (sensitivity, 73%; specificity, 57%) and lymph node ADC_{1000} (sensitivity, 71% to 79%; specificity, 77% to 79%) were independent significant predictors of disease-free survival without and with contrast-enhanced T1-weighted images ($P<.05$).

In their HNSCC study, Srinivasan and colleagues[44] found that a significant difference ($P = .03$) in mean ADC between patients showing positive and negative outcomes (1.18 and 1.43 * 10–3 mm²/s, respectively) and patients with lower pretreatment ADC and with greater than 45% of volume less than ADC threshold of 1.15×10 to 3 mm²/s may have better outcomes to chemoradiation at 2 years.

Lu and colleagues[49] assessed the merits of texture analysis on parametric maps derived from pharmacokinetic modeling with DCE MR imaging for the prediction of treatment response in patients with HNSCC. In this retrospective study, 19 HNSCC patients underwent pre- and intratreatment DCE MR imaging scans at a 1.5-T MR imaging scanner. Image texture analysis was then used on maps of K^{trans} and v_e, generating 2 texture measures: energy and homogeneity. No significant changes were found for the mean and standard deviation for K^{trans} and v_e ($P>.09$); however, texture analysis found that the imaging biomarker energy of v_e was significantly higher in intratreatment scans relative to pretreatment scans ($P<.04$; Fig. 3).

PEARLS, PITFALLS, AND VARIANTS

Functional MR imaging techniques such as diffusion and perfusion MR imaging allow for quantifying tumor characteristics related to tumor cellularity and vascularity. Compared with anatomic imaging techniques such as T1-weighted and T2-weighted MR imaging, functional MR imaging techniques have shown their added values in tumor detection, characterization, staging, treatment response monitoring, and prediction. However, there are several limitations for these techniques. In DCE MR imaging, patient voluntary and involuntary motion is a major source of error in the derived metrics of tumor tissues.

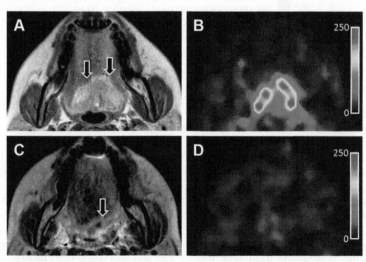

Fig. 2. T2-weighted and ASL-derived TBF maps of a patient (41-year-old woman) with tongue cancer before (A, B) and after (C, D) treatment. (B) Pretreatment TBF map shows high blood flow corresponding to the primary lesion. (D) The posttreatment TBF map shows that higher blood flow is not observed in the PTC area compared with the surrounding soft tissue. The 12-month follow-up confirmed that this lesion was not a residual tumor. Arrows in (A, C) indicate the primary lesion at the root of the tongue. (From Fujima N, Kudo K, Yoshida D, et al. Arterial spin labeling to determine tumor viability in head and neck cancer before and after treatment. J Magn Reson Imaging 2014;40:925; with permission.)

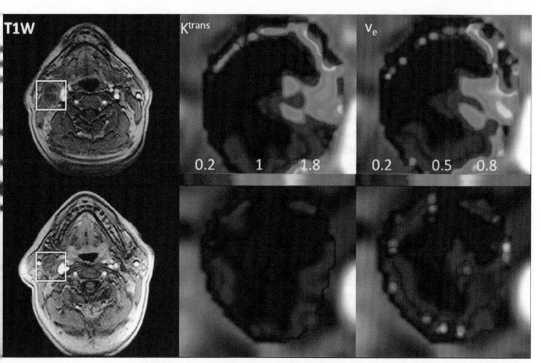

ig. 3. Pretreatment and intratreatment DCE MR images of a patient with locoregional control (63-year-old man). The top row shows pretreatment images, and the bottom row shows images from the intratreatment tage. From left to right, the columns show a T1-weighted image, K^{trans} (min^{-1}) map, and v_e map. The white rectngles delineate the ROIs at the metastatic nodes (outlined in *red*). K^{trans} and v_e maps are zoomed at the locations f ROIs. (*Data from* the authors' clinic.)

nerefore, images should be motion corrected efore further analysis. The nonspecific nature of essel leakage can lead to high false-negative nd false-positive results, which require other naging modalities to correctly interpret tumor haracteristics. Lack of standardized protocols is nother issue that needs consideration to compare the results in different studies. Moreover, he use of individual and population AIF is another source of variability among different studies. In)WI, images suffer from patient motions and susceptibility difference in HN cancers. The selection f b value is crucial to the ADC quantification, as oo low and too high b values can lead to inaccuate estimation of ADC values. For IVIM and its ariant modeling fitting, perfusion metrics are ighly sensitive to image noise thereby limiting he benefits of such techniques. Therefore, to nable clinical applications of DW MR imaging nd DCE MR imaging in HN cancers, the experinents of DW MR imaging and DCE MR imaging hould be carefully designed, standardized, implenented, and interpreted. For most of the discussed techniques, state-of-the-art dedicated MR imaging hardware and software and knowldgeable personnel are needed to obtain reliable lata that can be used in the clinic.

SUMMARY

Considering the diversity of applications and demonstrated potential of diffusion and perfusion imaging methods, the importance of these techniques in assessing HN cancer is expected to grow. Until now, most studies reporting on MR imaging diffusion and perfusion in HN cancer included relatively small populations (ie, n <100), but this number is likely to increase in the future. To obtain reliable biomarkers that extend beyond standard structural scans, however, one has to consider potential complicating factors with respect to both the data acquisition and processing. Yet most problems have been critically addressed and can be taken into account in a satisfying manner. Also, further progress in the development of (eg, automated) analysis methods has to be stimulated to make diffusion and perfusion imaging procedures more easily (ie, push button) applicable in clinical routine.

REFERENCES

1. Jemal A, Siegel R, Xu J, et al. Cancer statistics, 2010. CA Cancer J Clin 2010;60:277–300.

2. Vokes EE, Weichselbaum RR, Lippman SM, et al. Head and neck cancer. N Engl J Med 1993;328:184–94.

3. Jansen JF, Koutcher JA, Shukla-Dave A. Non-invasive imaging of angiogenesis in head and neck squamous cell carcinoma. Angiogenesis 2010;13:149–60.

4. Stephen RM, Gillies RJ. Promise and progress for functional and molecular imaging of response to targeted therapies. Pharm Res 2007;24:1172–85.

5. Chawla S, Kim S, Wang S, et al. Diffusion-weighted imaging in head and neck cancers. Future Oncol 2009;5:959–75.

6. Lee FK, King AD, Ma BB, et al. Dynamic contrast enhancement magnetic resonance imaging (DCE-MRI) for differential diagnosis in head and neck cancers. Eur J Radiol 2012;81(4):784–8.

7. Noij DP, de Jong MC, Mulders LG, et al. Contrast-enhanced perfusion magnetic resonance imaging for head and neck squamous cell carcinoma: a systematic review. Oral Oncol 2015;51:124–38.

8. Abdel Razek AA, Poptani H. MR spectroscopy of head and neck cancer. Eur J Radiol 2013;82: 982–9.

9. Lu Y, Jansen JF, Mazaheri Y, et al. Extension of the intravoxel incoherent motion model to non-gaussian diffusion in head and neck cancer. J Magn Reson Imaging 2012;36:1088–96.

10. Jansen JF, Stambuk HE, Koutcher JA, et al. Non-gaussian analysis of diffusion-weighted MR imaging in head and neck squamous cell carcinoma: a feasibility study. AJNR Am J Neuroradiol 2010; 31:741–8.

11. Kim S, Loevner L, Quon H, et al. Diffusion-weighted magnetic resonance imaging for predicting and detecting early response to chemoradiation therapy of squamous cell carcinomas of the head and neck. Clin Cancer Res 2009;15:986–94.

12. Vandecaveye V, Dirix P, De Keyzer F, et al. Diffusion-weighted magnetic resonance imaging early after chemoradiotherapy to monitor treatment response in head-and-neck squamous cell carcinoma. Int J Radiat Oncol Biol Phys 2012;82:1098–107.

13. Yuan J, Yeung DK, Mok GS, et al. Non-Gaussian analysis of diffusion weighted imaging in head and neck at 3T: a pilot study in patients with nasopharyngeal carcinoma. PLoS One 2014;9:e87024.

14. Lambrecht M, Vandecaveye V, De Keyzer F, et al. Value of diffusion-weighted magnetic resonance imaging for prediction and early assessment of response to neoadjuvant radiochemotherapy in rectal cancer: preliminary results. Int J Radiat Oncol Biol Phys 2012;82:863–70.

15. Lu Y, Moreira AL, Hatzoglou V, et al. Using diffusion-weighted MRI to predict aggressive histological features in papillary thyroid carcinoma: a novel tool for pre-operative risk stratification in thyroid cancer. Thyroid 2015;25(6):672–80.

16. Lu Y, Jansen JF, Stambuk HE, et al. Comparing primary tumors and metastatic nodes in head and neck cancer using intravoxel incoherent motion imaging: a preliminary experience. J Comput Assist Tomog 2013;37:346–52.

17. Prah DE, Paulson ES, Nencka AS, et al. A simple method for rectified noise floor suppression phase-corrected real data reconstruction with application to diffusion-weighted imaging. Magn Reson Med 2010;64:418–29.

18. Kim S, Loevner LA, Quon H, et al. Prediction of response to chemoradiation therapy in squamous cell carcinomas of the head and neck using dynamic contrast-enhanced MR imaging. AJNR Am J Neuroradiol 2010;31:262–8.

19. Noworolski SM, Fischbein NJ, Kaplan MJ, et al. Challenges in dynamic contrast-enhanced MR imaging of cervical lymph nodes to detect metastatic disease. J Magn Reson Imaging 2003;17:455–62.

20. Shukla-Dave A, Lee NY, Jansen JF, et al. Dynamic contrast-enhanced magnetic resonance imaging as a predictor of outcome in head and neck squamous cell carcinoma patients with nodal metastases. Int J Radiat Oncol Biol Phys 2012; 82(5):1837–44.

21. Chawla S, Kim S, Loevner LA, et al. Prediction of disease-free survival in patients with squamous cell carcinomas of the head and neck using dynamic contrast-enhanced MR imaging. AJNR Am J Neuroradiol 2011;32:778–84.

22. Jansen JF, Schoder H, Lee NY, et al. Tumor metabolism and perfusion in head and neck squamous cell carcinoma: pretreatment multimodality imaging with (1)H magnetic resonance spectroscopy, dynamic contrast-enhanced MRI, and [(18)F]FDG PET. Int J Radiat Oncol Biol Phys 2012;82:299–307.

23. Shukla-Dave A, Lee N, Stambuk H, et al. Average arterial input function for quantitative dynamic contrast enhanced magnetic resonance imaging of neck nodal metastases. BMC Med Phys 2009;9:4.

24. Stollberger R, Wach P. Imaging of the active B1 field in vivo. Magn Reson Med 1996;35:246–51.

25. Wang J, Qiu M, Yang QX, et al. Measurement and correction of transmitter and receiver induced non uniformities in vivo. Magn Reson Med 2005;53: 408–17.

26. Kim S, Quon H, Loevner LA, et al. Transcytolemmal water exchange in pharmacokinetic analysis of dynamic contrast-enhanced MRI data in squamous cell carcinoma of the head and neck. J Magn Reson Imaging 2007;26:1607–17.

27. Schnall MD, Ikeda DM. Lesion diagnosis working group report. J Magn Reson Imaging 1999;10: 982–90.

28. Kusunoki T, Murata K, Nishida S, et al. Histopathological findings of human thyroid tumors and dynamic MRI. Auris Nasus Larynx 2002;29:357–60.

29. Tunca F, Giles Y, Salmaslioglu A, et al. The preoperative exclusion of thyroid carcinoma in multinodular goiter: dynamic contrast-enhanced magnetic resonance imaging versus ultrasonography-guided fine-needle aspiration biopsy. Surgery 2007;142: 992–1002 [discussion: e1–2].

30. Donaldson SB, Betts G, Bonington SC, et al. Perfusion estimated with rapid dynamic contrast-enhanced magnetic resonance imaging correlates inversely with vascular endothelial growth factor expression and pimonidazole staining in head-and-neck cancer: a pilot study. Int J Radiat Oncol Biol Phys 2011;81:1176–83.

31. Machiels JP, Henry S, Zanetta S, et al. Phase II study of sunitinib in recurrent or metastatic squamous cell carcinoma of the head and neck: GORTEC 2006-01. J Clin Oncol 2010;28:21–8.

32. Fujima N, Kudo K, Yoshida D, et al. Arterial spin labeling to determine tumor viability in head and neck cancer before and after treatment. J Magn Reson Imaging 2014;40:920–8.

33. Fujima N, Nakamaru Y, Sakashita T, et al. Differentiation of squamous cell carcinoma and inverted papilloma using non-invasive MR perfusion imaging. Dentomaxillofac Radiol 2015;44(9):20150074.

34. Fujima N, Kudo K, Tsukahara A, et al. Measurement of tumor blood flow in head and neck squamous cell carcinoma by pseudo-continuous arterial spin labeling: comparison with dynamic contrast-enhanced MRI. J Magn Reson Imaging 2015;41:983–91.

35. Baer AH, Hoff BA, Srinivasan A, et al. Feasibility analysis of the parametric response map as an early predictor of treatment efficacy in head and neck cancer. AJNR Am J Neuroradiol 2015;36:757–62.

36. Jackson A, O'Connor JP, Parker GJ, et al. Imaging tumor vascular heterogeneity and angiogenesis using dynamic contrast-enhanced magnetic resonance imaging. Clin Cancer Res 2007;13:3449–59.

37. Alic L, van Vliet M, van Dijke CF, et al. Heterogeneity in DCE-MRI parametric maps: a biomarker for treatment response? Phys Med Biol 2011;56:1601–16.

38. Alic L, van Vliet M, Wielopolski PA, et al. Regional heterogeneity changes in DCE-MRI as response to isolated limb perfusion in experimental soft-tissue sarcomas. Contrast Media Mol Imaging 2013;8: 340–9.

39. Davnall F, Yip CS, Ljungqvist G, et al. Assessment of tumor heterogeneity: an emerging imaging tool for clinical practice? Insights Imaging 2012;3:573–89.

40. McNitt-Gray MF, Wyckoff N, Sayre JW, et al. The effects of co-occurrence matrix based texture parameters on the classification of solitary pulmonary nodules imaged on computed tomography. Comput Med Imaging Graph 1999;23:339–48.

41. Sumi M, Nakamura T. Head and neck tumours: combined MRI assessment based on IVIM and TIC analyses for the differentiation of tumors of different histological types. Eur Radiol 2014;24:223–31.

42. Asaumi J, Yanagi Y, Konouchi H, et al. Application of dynamic contrast-enhanced MRI to differentiate malignant lymphoma from squamous cell carcinoma in the head and neck. Oral Oncol 2004;40:579–84.

43. Fong D, Bhatia KS, Yeung D, et al. Diagnostic accuracy of diffusion-weighted MR imaging for nasopharyngeal carcinoma, head and neck lymphoma and squamous cell carcinoma at the primary site. Oral Oncol 2010;46:603–6.

44. Srinivasan A, Chenevert TL, Dwamena BA, et al. Utility of pretreatment mean apparent diffusion coefficient and apparent diffusion coefficient histograms in prediction of outcome to chemoradiation in head and neck squamous cell carcinoma. J Comput Assist Tomogr 2012;36:131–7.

45. Vandecaveye V, De Keyzer F, Vander Poorten V, et al. Head and neck squamous cell carcinoma: value of diffusion-weighted MR imaging for nodal staging. Radiology 2009;251:134–46.

46. Bernstein JM, Kershaw LE, Withey SB, et al. Tumor plasma flow determined by dynamic contrast-enhanced MRI predicts response to induction chemotherapy in head and neck cancer. Oral Oncol 2015;51:508–13.

47. Hauser T, Essig M, Jensen A, et al. Prediction of treatment response in head and neck carcinomas using IVIM-DWI: evaluation of lymph node metastasis. Eur J Radiol 2014;83:783–7.

48. Noij DP, Pouwels PJ, Ljumanovic R, et al. Predictive value of diffusion-weighted imaging without and with including contrast-enhanced magnetic resonance imaging in image analysis of head and neck squamous cell carcinoma. Eur J Radiol 2015;84: 108–16.

49. Lu Y, Jansen JF, Gupta G, et al. Prediction of treatment response using texture analysis on pharmacokinetic maps of dynamic contrast enhanced MRI in patients with head and neck cance. Joint annual meeting ISMRM-ESMRMB 2014. Milan (Italy) May 10-16, 2014., 2014. p. 4076.

Functional MR Imaging in Chest Malignancies

Jordi Broncano, MD[a],*, Antonio Luna, MD[b,c], Javier Sánchez-González, PhD[d], Antonio Alvarez-Kindelan, MD, PhD[e], Sanjeev Bhalla, MD[f]

KEYWORDS

• Functional MR imaging • DWI • DCE–MR imaging • Lung cancer • [18]FDG-PET/CT

KEY POINTS

• Functional MR imaging is an emerging technique in the thorax providing an integral assessment of several characteristics of chest neoplasms by means of prognostic and reproducible quantitative parameters.
• Functional MR imaging represents an alternative to fludeoxyglucose F 18 ([18]FDG)-PET/CT in the differentiation of benign and malignant entities, allowing the accurate staging and treatment response monitoring.
• Although there is only initial experience, the performance of functional MR imaging in the heart and chest wall can enhance its utility in the thorax.

INTRODUCTION

Several tumor characteristics may be assessed using functional imaging techniques (**Table 1**). Currently, the most widely accepted tumor metabolism imaging is performed with [18]FDG-PET/CT.[1]

Although the application of thoracic MR imaging is technically demanding, its great advantage is the possibility of integrating several morphologic and functional techniques in the evaluation of different tumor characteristics. From these techniques, several quantitative and reproducible parameters can be calculated, some of which serve as widely accepted prognostic biomarkers.[2,3] This article reviews currently available techniques and some of the more promising potential applications of thoracic functional MR imaging.

FUNCTIONAL MR IMAGING IN THE CHEST: TECHNICAL CONSIDERATIONS
Diffusion-Weighted Imaging

Diffusion-weighted imaging (DWI) focuses on the evaluation of brownian motion of water motion in biologic tissues, which has been related to tissue cellularity and architecture (see **Table 1**; **Table 2**).[2,4,5] Thoracic application is technically demanding, requiring the application of echo planar imaging (EPI) readout and parallel acquisition strategy. The main hurdle is the presence of motion artifacts and geometric distortion secondary to B0 inhomogeneities and accumulation of phase error during echo train length.[6]

Motion compensation techniques are often necessary to improve image quality. Respiratory

Disclosure Statement: Dr J. Sánchez-González is an employee of Philips Healthcare. Drs J. Broncano, A. Luna, S. Bhalla, and A. Alvarez-Kindelan have nothing to disclose.
[a] Cardiothoracic imaging section, Hospital de la Cruz Roja, RESSALTA, Health-Time Group, Avenida Paseo de la Victoria s/n, Córdoba CP 14014, Spain; [b] Department of Radiology, Health Time, Carmelo Torres 2, Jaén 23006, Spain; [c] Department of Radiology, University Hospitals of Cleveland, Case Western Reserve University, 11100 Euclid Ave, 44106 Cleveland, Ohio, USA; [d] Philips Healthcare Iberia, Maria de Portugal 1, Madrid 28050, Spain; [e] Thoracic Surgery Department, Hospital Universitario Reina Sofía, Av. Menendez Pidal, s/n, Córdoba 14004, Spain; [f] Mallinckrodt Institute of Radiology, Washington University School of Medicine, 510 South Kingshighway, St Louis, MO 63110, USA
* Corresponding author.
E-mail address: j.broncano.c@htime.org

Magn Reson Imaging Clin N Am 24 (2016) 135–155
http://dx.doi.org/10.1016/j.mric.2015.08.004
1064-9689/16/$ – see front matter © 2016 Elsevier Inc. All rights reserved.

mri.theclinics.com

Table 1
Tumor characteristics and functional imaging techniques

Technique	Biophysical Basis	Quantitative Parameters
DWI–MR imaging	Cellularity and tortuosity of interstitial space	ADC
DKI	Tissue microstructure	D_{app}; K_{app}
IVIM	Blood flow and tissue diffusivity	f, D, D*
DCE–MR imaging	Blood flow and permeability	K^{trans}, V_e, V_p, K_{ep}, AUC
BOLD	Hypoxia	Tissue R2* relaxivity
ASL	Blood flow	Flow quantification
Spectroscopy	Metabolism	Ratio of choline to other metabolites

Abbreviations: ASL, arterial spin labeling; AUC, area under the curve; D*, perfusion contribution to signal decay; D_{app}, estimation of diffusion coefficient using nongaussian model; f, perfusion fraction; K_{app}, apparent diffusional kurtosis; K_{ep}, elimination rate; K^{trans}, transfer rate; V_e, extracellular volume; V_p, vascular space volume.

Modified from Luna A, Cunha GM, Sanchez-Sanchez R, et al. Overview of functional Imaging techniques for liver malignancies in current clinical practice or in a very near future. In: Luna A, Vilanova JC, Da Cruz LC, et al, editors. Functional imaging in oncology: clinical applications. vol. 2. Berlin: Springer-Verlag; 2014. p. 953.

triggering is usually preferred to a single breath hold. For avoiding pulsation artifacts, cardiac triggering (which increases acquisition time) may be useful, especially for the assessment of small lesions located near the heart (Table 3).[7]

Apparent diffusion coefficient (ADC) represents the exponential signal decay of water molecules on a voxel by voxel basis.[5] Although ADC may be calculated using only 2 b values, the more b values included in its measurement, the more accurate it is.[5]

Recently, advanced models of DWI have been proposed to better understand the behavior of water motion in the different tissues. The intravoxel incoherent motion (IVIM) model of diffusion signal decay has been shown to better fit than monoexponential analysis, especially in the evaluation of well vascularized organs.[5,7] First, diffusion decay signal shows a rapid attenuation at low b values (b<100–150 s/mm^2) secondary to bulk motion of water molecules in capillaries (perfusion effects on diffusion). With higher b values (more than 100 s/mm^2), a slower decay of signal occurs due to the real diffusion of water molecules (Fig. 1). IVIM-derived parameters are, theoretically, more reliable markers of tissue diffusivity than ADC and can separate both compartments of diffusion signal decay (Box 1). In addition, ADC assumes a gaussian diffusion behavior, which does not always exactly fit to the real signal decay of diffusion signal. Diffusional kurtosis imaging (DKI) quantifies the deviation of tissue diffusion from a gaussian pattern by measuring diffusion with ultrahigh b values greater than 1500 s/mm^2 (see Fig. 1).[8] IVIM and DKI models have been recently explored in the evaluation of chest malignancies and show some promise over conventional ADC measurements.[9–11]

Table 2
Combination of finding in diffusion-weighted imaging and related differential diagnosis

Signal Intensity High b Value	Signal Intensity ADC Map	Interpretation
	■	Hypercellular tumors. Rarely, liquid or viscous abscess or blood products
		T2 shine-through; liquefactive necrosis
■		Fluid, necrosis, low cellularity lesions, well-differentiated adenocarcinomas
■	■	Fibromuscular tissues, fat, susceptibility artifacts (T2 dark-through effect)
	▦	Mature fibrosis with lower water content

White, black and *gray* cells correspond to hyperintense, hypointense and isointense - mild hypointense behaviour for both high b value and ADC map.

Adapted from Padhani AR, Koh DM, Collins DJ. Whole-body diffusion-weighted MR imaging in cancer: current status and research directions. Radiology 2011;261(3):708.

Table 3
Diffusion-weighted imaging sequences performed at our centers at 1.5T and 3T MR imaging

Techniques	Sequence Type/ Parallel Accelerating Factor	B Values (s/mm²)	TR/TE (ms)	Resolution (mm³)	Synchronization	Fat Suppression Technique	Image Evaluation	Quantitative Parameter	Acquisition Time
DWI – 3T (IVIM + DKI)	SS EPI/ factor 2	0, 50, 100, 500, 1000, 1500	5000/55	2.5 × 2.5 × 7	Respiratory triggered	Spectral fat suppression	Monoexponential, IVIM, and DKI model	ADC D, D*, f D_{app}; K_{app}	4 min 41 s
DWI – 1.5T (IVIM + DKI)	SS EPI/ factor 2	0, 50, 100, 500, 1000, 1500	1400/100	3 × 3 × 7	Respiratory triggered	Spectral fat suppression	Monoexponential, IVIM and DKI model	ADC D, D*, f D_{app}; K_{app}	5 min 48 s
DWI cardiac – 3T	SS EPI/ factor 2	0, 50, 150, 300	1000/44	2.58 × 2.54 × 10	Breath hold; ECG based in diastole	Spectral fat suppression	Qualitative/ semiquantitative	ADC ADC ratio SI ratio	1 min 45 s
DWI cardiac – 1.5T	SS EPI/ factor 2	0, 50, 300	2250/96	2.6 × 2.54 × 8	Breath hold; ECG based in diastole	Spectral fat suppression	Qualitative/ semiquantitative	ADC ADC ratio SI ratio	2 min 25 s

Abbreviations: D*, perfusion contribution to diffusion signal decay; D_{app}, estimation of diffusion coefficient using nongaussian model; K_{app}, apparent diffusional kurtosis; SS EPI, single-shot echo planar imaging; TE, echo time; TR, repetition time.

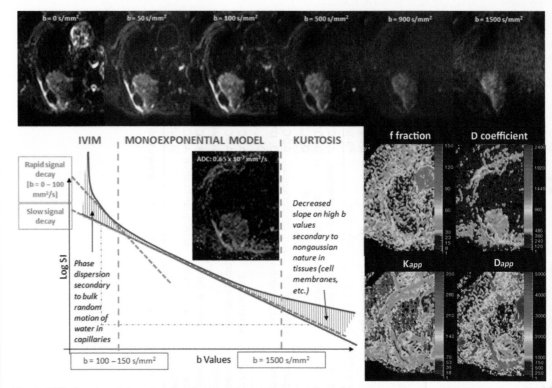

Fig. 1. Diffusion signal decay analyzed using a bicompartmental model and nongaussian diffusion fitting of DWI signal decay on a patient with lung cancer. Graphic represents the differences between the diffusion signal decay using a monoexponential model (ADC measurement) and the better fit to the real behavior of diffusion signal decay using IVIM and DKI models. (*Right*) Color parametric maps are derived from IVIM (f and D) and DKI (K_{app} and D_{app}), which can be calculated with a sequence, including only 6 b values (*top*).

Box 1

Bicompartmental and nongaussian diffusion-weighted imaging–derived parameters

IVIM-derived parameters

True diffusion of tissue H_2O molecules (D): not influenced by movement of water molecules within the capillaries

Perfusion contribution to diffusion signal (f): fractional volume of flowing water molecules within the capillaries.

Perfusion contribution to signal decay (D*): amount of nondiffusional random movements of water molecules

DKI-derived parameters

D_{app} estimation of the diffusion coefficient in the direction parallel to the orientation of diffusion sensitizing gradients.

Apparent diffusional kurtosis (K_{app}): measures the deviation of the true diffusion from a gaussian pattern

---

Dynamic Contrast-Enhanced–MR Imaging

Dynamic contrast-enhanced (DCE)–MR imaging provides information of tumor physiology, including blood flow, vascular volume, and permeability. DCE–MR imaging also provides imaging insight pertinent to tumor angiogenesis.[12]

Free breathing, high temporal resolution, 3-D gradient-echo sequences are usually acquired during a 5-minute period of time. They have limited coverage and require the use of parallel imaging techniques.[13] Motion and respiratory artifacts are common problems that require correction software during postprocessing.[14]

Different strategies for analysis and quantification of DCE–MR imaging have been reported. The easiest and most used approach is to evaluate the variation of contrast enhancement during multiple time points of the lesion, obtaining time intensity curves (TICs). In the graphic representation of contrast dynamics, the first half is correlated with tumor angiogenesis and the second half with tumor interstitium.[15] This approach does not separate perfusion and permeability.[3] There are several TIC-derived descriptors that can be used for assessing perfusion (**Box 2**).

Once the contrast concentration is derived from each dynamic time point acquisition, the tissue status can be quantitatively assessed by calculating the contrast concentrations in the tissue and feeding artery. After applying a contrast kinetic model, quantitative hemodynamic parameters may be obtained. These are based on the use of compartments, defined as spaces where the contrast is evenly distributed. Two well-differentiated models are commonly used, *monocompartmental* and *bicompartmental*, according to if only the vascular volume (P) or also the extracellular compartment (E) is considered (see **Box 2**).[12,16]

The bicompartmental model assumes that: P and E are compartments; E does not exchange tracer with the environment; the clearances for the outlets connecting P and E are equal and the clearance for the outlet of P to the environment equals the plasma flow. In some situations, a tissue with this configuration is reduced to a monocompartmental model:

1. When one of the spaces has a negligible volume

2. When the tracer extravasates with a slow rate (very low concentration at E)
3. When the tracer extravasates with a high rate (single well-mixed space)

Compartmental models are more technically demanding and more time consuming but have demonstrated usefulness in monitoring treatment response and recurrence, because they provide reproducible measurements.[16] Depending on which parametric approximation is used, derived parameters differ in their interpretation (see **Box 2**). Depending on whether or not the delivery of the contrast medium to the tissue is sufficient, K^{trans} approximates the permeability surface area product or blood flow, respectively.[3] Lack of standardization of different models and sequence designs have prevented them from being introduced in the clinical setting.

FUNCTIONAL MR IMAGING OF THE LUNG

Worldwide, lung cancer is the leading cause of cancer-related deaths.[17] CT usually constitutes the first modality in evaluation and staging. It is often complemented with [18]FDG-PET/CT. Other functional modalities have emerged to increase the accuracy of detection, staging, and treatment monitoring. Morphologic MR was classically set as a second-line diagnostic procedure in the evaluation of patients with lung cancer. Recent improvements in hardware and functional techniques, however, have positioned chest MR as an alternative to [18]FDG-PET/CT.[7]

Pulmonary Nodule Detection and Characterization

Functional MR imaging and pulmonary nodule detection
One of the most common challenges in pulmonary medicine is the detection and characterization of pulmonary nodules (PNs).[7] CT is considered the best imaging technique for PN detection.

DWI has been shown useful in the management of PNs. DWI may detect 86.5% of nodules between 6 mm and 9 mm and 97% of PNs greater than 10 mm. In lesions less than 5 mm, the accuracy of DWI falls to only 43.8%,[18] below the sensitivities of other MR imaging sequences, such as short-tau inversion recovery (STIR) (81.5% for lesions >3 mm).[19]

Diffusion-weighted imaging and pulmonary nodule characterization
DWI has shown great usefulness in differentiating benign from malignant PNs (**Table 4**).[20] With an accuracy cited at 91%, it is comparable to other

Table 4
Apparent diffusion coefficient threshold value parameters and reported results

Region/Lesion Evaluation	MR Field Strength	B Values	Threshold	Sensitivity/Specificity/Accuracy	
PN characterization (ADC)[20,26]	1.5T and 3T	0, 500, b1000 s/mm²	$1.1–1.4 \times 10^{-3}$ mm²/s	Pooled 83%/81%/91%	Sensitivity (70%–90%)/specificity (74%–100%)
LN characterization (ADC)[46–49]	1.5T	0, 300, 600 s/mm²	1.85×10^{-3} mm²/s	96.4%/71.4%/83.9%	Pooled sensitivity, specificity, and accuracy: 77.4%–80%, 89%–95%, and 84.4%–97%, respectively. Described PPV and NPV: 95.2% and 77.1%, respectively
Pleural lesion (ADC)[71]	3T	0, 50, 100, 500, 750, 1000 s/mm²	1.52×10^{-3} mm²/s	71.4%/100%/87.1%	Differentiation of benign versus malignant
Mediastinal mass (ADC)[81]	1.5T	0, 300, 600 s/mm²	1.56×10^{-3} mm²/s	95%/96%/94%	Exclusion of cystic mediastinal masses PPV and NPV: 94% and 96%, respectively
Cystic mediastinal mass (ADC)[82]	3T	0, 100, 900 s/mm²	2.5×10^{-3} mm²/s	100%/100%/84%	With this cut-off, the ADCs of all cystic benign lesions were higher and the ADCs of malignant ones lower.

Abbreviations: NPV, negative predictive value; PPV, positive predictive value.

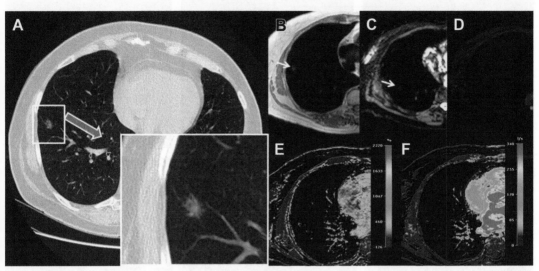

Fig. 2. (*A*) Multidetector CT with focused zoomed image (*inset*) reveals a partially solid millimetric nodule in keeping with minimal invasive adenocarcinoma. (*B*) Proton-density turbo spin-echo (TSE) axial image and (*C*) low b value DWI (b = 0 s/mm²) confirm the solid part of the nodule (*white arrows*). (*D*) DWI confirms absence of high SI on high b value image (b = 1000 s/mm²). (*E*) DCE–MR imaging maximum RSE and (*F*) area under the curve parametric maps show a low enhancement lesion (*gray arrows*). In this case, functional MR imaging rules out biological aggressiveness of this nodule.

functional techniques for this differentiation (93%, 94%, and 94% for DCE-CT, ¹⁸FDG-PET/CT, and DCE–MR imaging, respectively).[21] DWI has similar limitations compared with PET in lesion characterization but with lower false-positive results (**Fig. 2**; **Table 5**).[22]

Varying results among quantitative characterization of PNs with DWI between series may be explained by the lack of standardization of

acquisition and postprocess evaluation (**Figs. 3** and **4**). Koyama and colleagues[23] reported significant differences in minimum and mean ADC in the evaluation of lung tumors, reflecting the inherent heterogeneity of these lesions. Usuda and colleagues[24] applied a DWI signal intensity (SI)-based analysis revealing that DWI SI was an indicator of the amount of tumor cells and its distribution. Tumor SI of the lesion-to–spinal cord ratio (LSR) of

Table 5
False-positive results and false-negative results of diffusion-weighted imaging and fludeoxyglucose F 18–PET/CT in chest lesions

Diagnostic Modality		False-Positive Results	False-Negative Results
¹⁸FDG-PET/CT	PNs	Inflammatory nodules	Well-differentiated adenocarcinoma Small PNs and metastasis
	LNs	Inflammatory LNs	Small intranodal tumor deposits
	Pleural lesions	Inflammatory pleuritis Talc pleurodesis Tuberculous plaques Parapneumonic effusion	Well-differentiated tumors
DWI	PNs	Intranodular inflammation	Mucinous content (T2 shine through) Intranodular necrosis Nonsolid; part-solid lesions (high b value) Low-grade adenocarcinoma Small PNs and metastasis
	LNs	Tuberculous and nontuberculous granulomatous inflammation	Small intranodal tumor deposits
	Pleural lesions	Fibrous plaques (T2 dark-through)	Intratumor necrosis and inflammation

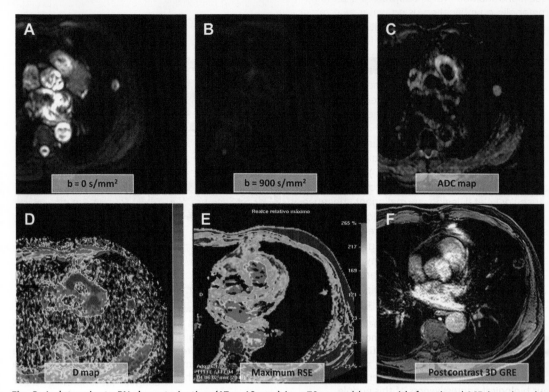

Fig. 3. Indeterminate PN characterization (17 × 19 mm) in a 70-year-old man with functional MR imaging. (A–C) DWI with b values of 0 and 900 s/mm² reveal a nonrestrictive lesion, as confirmed in ADC map (ADC mean = 2.23 × 10⁻³ mm²/s; *white arrows*) (C). (D) IVIM-derived diffusion coefficient map confirming the absence of restriction (1.92 × 10⁻³ mm²/s; *white arrow*). (E) DCE–MR imaging maximum RSE map shows a low enhancing lesion (*white arrow*). (F) Postgadolinium 3-D–GRE sequence shows rim enhancement of this lesion corresponding to an old healed tuberculoma (*white arrow*).

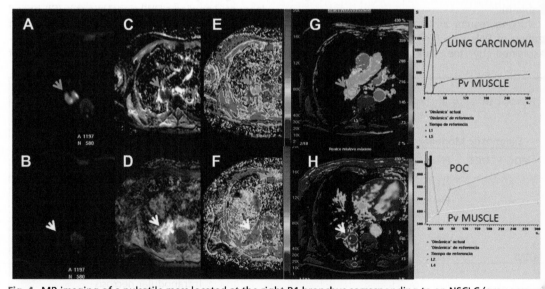

Fig. 4. MR imaging of a pulsatile mass located at the right B1 bronchus corresponding to an NSCLC (*gray arrows*, surrounded by postobstructive consolidation (*POC; white arrows*). There are 2 series of images at different levels (*top and bottom images*, respectively). (A) DWI with high b value shows high SI and low signal of ADC map (C) of the right central mass (*gray arrows*; ADC = 0.594 × 10⁻³ mm²/s). (B–D) However, note the absence, of restriction on DWI and ADC map of distal consolidation (*white arrows*; ADC = 2.77 × 10⁻³ mm²/s). IVIM-derived D map confirms the different behavior of the central mass and the postobstructive consolidation (E, F). (G, H) Maximum RSE maps and (I, J) TICs reflecting (I) a rapid slope with posterior washout for the central mass and (J) a steeper slope with more pronounced WO for the postobstructive consolidation. Both TICs are compared with the TIC of normal paravertebral muscles (*Pv muscle*).

malignant lesions was found higher compared with that of benign ones.[25] Contrarily, Liu and colleagues[26] did not obtain any significant differences of the LSR between malignant and benign nodules. Koyama and coworkers,[27] however, found significantly higher specificity and accuracy of LSR compared with ADC and IVIM-derived parameters in the differentiation of benign and malignant pulmonary nodules. They did not find significant differences in ADC, diffusion coefficient (D), and perfusion fraction (f) between malignant and benign PNs (see **Figs. 3** and **4**).[27]

Dynamic contrast-enhanced–MR imaging and pulmonary nodule characterization

DCE–MR imaging has been used to assess tumor vascularity and interstitium with excellent performance in differentiation of benign and malignant lesions.[28] DCE–MR imaging is used as a problem-solving modality, especially in those cases where multidetector CT and [18]FDG-PET/CT are inconclusive.[7] Also the possibility of combining the same protocol morphologic and functional sequences makes chest MR imaging a powerful tool for assessment of lung cancer and PNs (see **Figs. 3** and **4**). Although the experience reported in the literature is limited, with some difficulties reported in the differentiation of active inflammatory and neoplastic lesions, the application of a multiparametric approach can overcome the limitations of each technique alone.

The patterns of enhancement and morphology of TICs have shown value in characterizing PNs, although some overlap is present (**Fig. 5**).[29–31] Gradual and slow increases in relative signal enhancement (RSE), included in types C and D curves, have been related to benign origin.[28,29,32,33] Donmez and colleagues[29] described a type C curve in atelectasis and postinflammatory lesions, although on some occasions this type of curve can occur in NSCLC. A rapid RSE with washout (WO) or plateau (type A and B curves) has been related to a malignant origin.[28,29,32–34] On the contrary, some investigators have pointed out that active inflammatory lesions had higher RSE with steeper slope compared with malignant ones (**Table 6**).[28]

For Ohno and colleagues,[34] the slope of enhancement showed a more accurate separation of PNs that require further intervention and treatment from benign PNs than did maximum standardized uptake value (SUV$_{max}$) in [18]FDG-PET/CT (see **Table 6**). DWI can improve specificity in lesions displaying a type B curve, due to improvement in diagnosis of lesions with an inflammatory or necrotic component (see **Table 6**).[33]

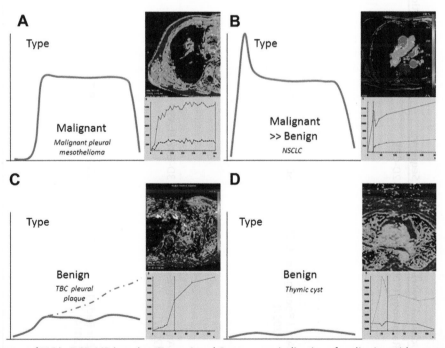

Fig. 5. Patterns of TIC in DCE–MR imaging. Types *A* and *B* curves are indicative of malignity, with some overlap in type *B* curves. Malignant >> bening in type *B* curve means that this profile is more frequently present in malignant lesions compared to benign ones. Types *C* and *D* are indicative of a benign process. (*Adapted from* Coolen J, Vansteenkiste J, De Keyzer F, et al. Characterisation of solitary pulmonary lesions combining visual perfusion and quantitative diffusion MR imaging. Eur Radiol 2014;24(2):531–41; with permission.)

Table 6
Time intensity curves of dynamic contrast-enhanced–MR imaging and pathologic correlation in the characterization of pulmonary nodules—evidence from the literature

Author	Journal (Year)	MR imaging	Sequence	Temporal Resolution	Curve Types	Pathologic Correlation
Schaefer et al[32]	Radiology (2004)	1T	2D-GRE	10 s	A: fast SI increase + obvious WO B: fast SI increase + second moderate increase or plateau C: continuous SI increase + plateau D: no SI increase (mean enhancement <10%)	A: malignant neoplasms only B: overlap malignant/benign lesions C: benign >>> malignant D: benign lesions only
Kono et al[28]	Am J Roentgenol (2007)	0.5T	SE	16 s	A: early peak enhancement (maximum RSE <4 min) A1: WO >10% A2: WO <10% B: late peak enhancement (maximum RSE >4 min) C: gradual increase (maximum RSE 8 min; no WO)	A: focal OP and lung cancer The steeper the slope the higher rate of focal OP B: tuberculoma, hamartoma C: tuberculoma, hamartoma
Donmez et al[29]	Am J Roentgenol (2007)	1.5T	3D-GRE FLASH	12–16 s	A: early RSE + rapid WO B: early RSE + early plateau (<2nd min) C: early RSE + late plateau (4th min) D: gradually RSE	A: malignant (95% sensitivity) B: benign (100% sensitivity/specificity) C: benign (100% sensitivity/specificity) D: benign >>> malignant
Coolen et al[33]	Eur Radiol (2014)	3T	3D-FFE	9.7 s	A: peak RSE without obvious WO B: sharp RSE + obvious WO C: relative contrast uptake >120% RSI D: relative contrast uptake <120% RSI	A: malignant lesions B: overlap malignant >> benign lesions C: benign D: benign

Abbreviations: 2D-GRE, 2-D-gradient echo sequence; 3D-FFE, 3-D-fast field echo sequence; 3D-GRE, 3-D-gradient echo sequence; FLASH, fast low-angle shot; OP, organizing pneumonia; RSI, relative SI; SE, spin-echo sequence. >> in type B curve of coolen et al means that is more frequently present in malignant than benign lesions. >>> seen in type D curves in Donmez et al and type C curves in Schaefer et al means that is a condition much more frequently present in benign than in malignant lesions.

In the authors' experience, the observation of a rapid SI increase after contrast administration with or without obvious WO is highly suspicious of malignant origin, especially in the absence of a plateau.

Lung Cancer Staging and Assessment of Resectability

In lung cancer, differentiation between small cell lung cancer (SCLC) and non-SCLC (NSCLC) is important in clinical practice because of differences in staging, treatment, and prognosis.[23] SCLC is known for its rapid doubling time, rapid growth rate, and early development of metastatic disease.[35] DWI has been shown useful because more aggressive lesions are prone to be more cellular. In this sense, Liu and coworkers[26] obtained significant lower ADC values in SCLC than NSCLC. They also demonstrated that the ADC of NSCLC was significantly lower compared with benign lesions.[23,26]

The differentiation and grading of different types of NSCLC, especially in adenocarcinomas, is of great importance because of the impact shown on progression-free survival (PFS) and overall survival (OS) in patients with stage I adenocarcinoma (AC).[36] Matoba and colleagues[37] demonstrated correlation between ADC values and tumor cellularity. Well-differentiated adenocarcinomas (ACs) usually demonstrated higher ADC values than more aggressive ACs and squamous cell carcinomas (Fig. 6). Negative linear correlation was obtained between tumor cellularity and mean ADC value, which has been confirmed in other studies, including PET/MR imaging.[10,38] The higher cell density seen in tightly packed cells of squamous cells compared with larger cells of AC can lead to lower ADC values and increased SUV.[39]

Tanaka and colleagues,[40] using LSR for evaluating different subtypes of AC, were able to differentiate more invasive lesions based on higher SI. DWI SI may be related to biological cell cancer proliferation, including increased cellularity and larger nuclei.[40] In addition, ADC can differentiate between intermediate versus low-grade tumors (see Fig. 6).[36]

The pattern of SI in DWI is also important in addition to the magnitude. Nomori and colleagues[41] observed that all faint homogeneous SI tumors on DWI were well-differentiated ACs without lymphatic, vascular, pleural invasion, whereas dark homogenous and heterogeneous SI lesions were more aggressive lesions with higher SUV on FDG-PET.

The combination of ADC value and DWI signal has the potential to be a useful biomarker in the

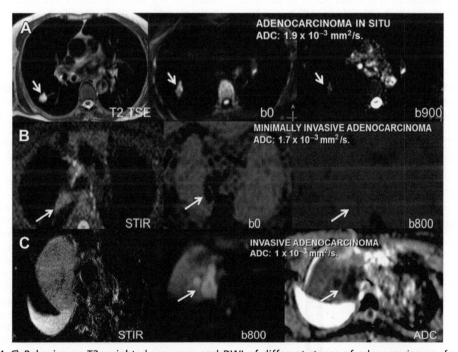

Fig. 6. (A–C) Behavior on T2-weighted sequence and DWI of different stages of adenocarcinoma, from more indolent (adenocarcinoma in situ) to more aggressive (invasive adenocarcinoma). *White arrows* point to primary malignant lung neoplasms in each case.

preoperative assessment of lung cancer.[42] Furthermore, in a recent series by Lee and co-workers,[36] its combined use with SUV_{max} has led to a more useful stratification of patients into different prognostic subsets than the use of each technique alone.

T staging of non–small cell lung cancer

Local staging of NSCLC has not been extensively studied with MR imaging. DWI has shown great utility, however, in evaluating superior sulcus tumors and differentiating central neoplasms from postobstructive consolidation (Fig. 7).[43] Hypercellularity of lung neoplasms contrasts with the composition of the collapsed lung, bronchial impaction, and pneumonia of various types (see Fig. 4).[44] This differentiation is vital not only for cancer staging but also for radiotherapy treatment.

IVIM-derived parameters have shown some promise in this respect, although ADC outperforms IVIM-derived parameters with current experience.[11] DCE–MR imaging also reported utility in this respect by correctly separating tumor lesions from POC (see Fig. 4), showing significantly higher AUC_{60} (initial area under the curve within 60 s) in the former.[11]

Whole-body (WB)-DWI may also show certain advantages over [18]FDG-PET/CT in the T staging of lung cancer. Plathow and colleagues[45] reported that WB-DWI was accurately T staged all cases whereas [18]FDG-PET/CT failed in the evaluation of chest wall infiltration in 4 cases out of 52 patients with NSCLC (sensitivity 92.3%; specificity 100%).

N staging of non–small cell lung cancer

[18]FDG-PET/CT is considered the main imaging modality in the N staging of NSCLC. DWI, using visual assessment or ADC quantification, has demonstrated similar sensitivity and accuracy with higher specificity in N staging of NSCLC versus [18]FDG-PET or [18]FDG-PET/CT. This is due to less overstaging, with a detectable size of metastatic lymph nodes (LNs) for both methods of 4 mm (see Table 5; Fig. 8).[24,46]

[18]FDG-PET/CT false-positive results are related to reactive inflammatory LNs, showing absence of restriction in DWI, whereas false-positive results on DWI were secondary to granulomatous tissue inside LNs.[47] False-negative results for both are due to microscopic cancer deposits in LNs (see Table 5).[47] Better results have been achieved using DWI sequence with selective spectral fat saturation compared with those using DWI with background signal suppression, which showed less accuracy than [18]FDG-PET/CT.[7] A recent meta-analysis proposed DWI as a reliable alternative to [18]FDG-PET/CT for the preoperative N staging of NSCLC.[48] Ohno and coworkers[49] obtained a more sensitive and accurate assessment of N stage of NSCLC with STIR compared with DWI and [18]FDG-PET/CT

In certain situations, such as in LNs from esophageal carcinoma, the ADC of metastatic LNs may be higher than the ADC of benign LNs, secondary to intratumoral microscopic necrosis, with overlap between the 2 groups.[50]

M staging of non–small cell lung cancer

WB–MR imaging with DWI has been reported as a promising tool for M-stage assessment of NSCLC with results similar to [18]FDG-PET/CT.[7,22] Specifically, in the case of bone metastasis, WB-DWI has reported higher specificity and accuracy compared with scintigraphy or [18]FDG-PET/CT.[5] Care must be taken to interpret WB-DWI along with other WB–MR imaging sequences to improve diagnostic accuracy and specificity.[22]

When comparing 3T WB–MR imaging and [18]FDG-PET/CT, similar results were published in the overall distant metastasis detection, although

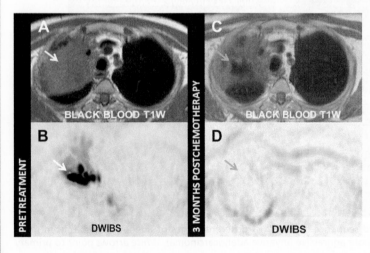

Fig. 7. Follow-up of a superior sulcus (Pancoast) tumor. (A) Pretreatment black blood turbo spin-echo T1-weighted (T1W) sequence shows a large mass involving the right apex. (B) DWI with background signal suppression (DWIBS) differentiates solid tumor from POC because only solid areas demonstrate severe restriction of diffusion (white arrows). (C) In follow-up morphologic MR imaging after 3 months of chemotherapy, the tumor has decreased its size, although residual areas of pleural thickening and atelectasis are depicted. (D) The absence of areas with restricted diffusion rules out the presence of viable tumor (gray arrows).

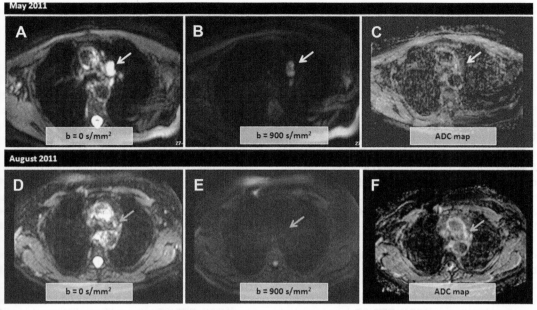

Fig. 8. (*A–C*) LN metastasis of NSCLC located at the aortopulmonary window shows restriction of DWI (*white arrows*; ADC = 0.621 × 10^{-3} mm^2/s). (*D–F*) Post-treatment surveillance demonstrated a reduction in size and SI on high b value image and increase of the ADC = 2.96 × 10^{-3} mm^2/s (*gray arrows*), indicating good response.

each method has its inherent advantages. WB–MR imaging displays higher performance for detection of liver and brain metastasis as well as in other organs, where there is physiologic radiotracer uptake, such as in kidneys. [18]FDG-PET/CT, however, shows better accuracy in the detection of LN and soft tissue metastasis.[22,52]

Recently, hybrid PET/MR imaging systems have been tested with accuracy similar to [18]FDG-PET/CT in the TNM staging of the tumor. Coregistered PET/MR imaging with SI assessment, however, without DWI has demonstrated superior to [18]FDG-PET/CT in the identification of TNM factor, clinical stage, and resectability of NSCLC.[53,54]

Treatment Monitoring and Follow-up

DWI has also been shown great usefulness in treatment monitoring and detection of recurrence in several malignancies.[2] An increase in ADC in NSCLC (advance stage) has been related to good response during and after chemotherapy and/or radiation, being more effective than DCE–MR imaging and [18]FDG-PET/CT parameters.[55–57] DWI may also discriminate between responders and nonresponders even after only 1 cycle of chemotherapy or after CT-guided radiofrequency (see **Figs. 7** and **8**).[58,59] An increase of ADC has also been related to higher PFS and OS compared with those nonresponders.[58,60] Furthermore, initial data suggest a role for DWI in prediction of treatment response to therapy for NSCLC with better results than[18] FDG-PET/CT.[56]

DCE–MR imaging also has shown good performance in treatment monitoring of patients with NSCLC treated with chemotherapy. Monocompartmental-derived parameters, such as maximum RSE ratio and slope of enhancement, were lower in the local control group compared with the local failure group.[60]

Low pretreatment ADC values in the primary tumor are predictive for good response to standard chemotherapy, shown as increase in ADC values compared with pretreatment evaluation.[55] This is due to cell death, necrosis, apoptosis, and cell lysis, which lead to an increase in water mobility in the extracellular space.[61] The differences in the way that novel treatments affect tumor microenvironment architecture are reflected by DWI. Vascular disrupting agents are more effective in tumors with higher pretreatment ADC values, in contrast to general treatments.[62,63] After antiangiogenic therapy, a decrease in ADC values have been reported, comparable to reduction in DCE–MR imaging–derived parameters.[61] In contrast, when there is significant treatment-derived tumor necrosis, the ADC may increase.[63]

With new targeted therapies, such as antiangiogenic drugs, DCE–MR imaging utility has been investigated for detecting early tumor response. Parameters obtained from a bicompartmental analysis have been shown better biomarkers of neoangiogenesis than monocompartmental-derived ones. K_{ep} has been reported a predictor for PFS and OS in stage IV NSCLC treated with sorafenib (**Fig. 9**).[64]

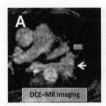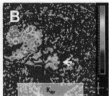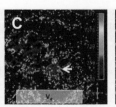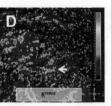

Fig. 9. Angiogenic phenotype of left hilar NSCLC using (*A*) DCE–MR imaging, which shows (*B*) increased permeability (K_{ep}), (*C*) diminished extravascular extracellular volume (V_e), and (*D*) heterogeneous perfusion (K^{trans}). These features favor good response to antivascular agents.

A significant decrease in K_{ep} and K^{trans} was seen in patients with early response to combined bevacizumab, cisplatin, and gemcitabine.[65] Large K_{ep} values and smaller SDs in V_e before treatment were predictors of good response.[65]

The role of functional imaging in early treatment monitoring and prediction of response need to be validated.[60] In some studies, [18]FDG-PET/CT usually showed no changes after antiangiogenic therapy (sorafenib or bevacizumab) in solid malignancies. In others, [18]FDG-PET/CT has reported better predictive performance than DCE–MR imaging for detecting early response in IIIB/IV stage of NSCLC treated with bevacizumab and erlotinib.

Hypoxia in tumor cells leads to chemotherapy and radiotherapy resistance, promoting tumor metabolism, and progression. This trait constitutes an interesting future treatment target and may allow a role for blood oxygen level–dependent (BOLD) MR imaging to depict hypoxic tumor areas by detecting the paramagnetic effects (elevation of transverse magnetization rate: R2*) of endogenous deoxyhemoglobin on surrounding water molecules.[66,67]

FUNCTIONAL IMAGING OF THE PLEURA

Malignant pleural mesothelioma (MPM) is a rare, locally aggressive, and potentially lethal neoplasm originating from the mesothelial cells of pleura, pericardium, or peritoneum.[68] Three types have been described: epithelioid, sarcomatoid, and biphasic (Box 3). Due to its asymmetric morphology, nonspherical, and noncompact growth, it is difficult to stage and follow-up (Box 4).[68]

Metastatic pleural disease (usually from lung cancer) is the most common cause of malignant pleural thickening (Box 5).[69] Lymphoma usually presents as a recurrent disease of contiguous extension whereas sarcomas rarely metastatize to the pleura.[69]

Differentiation of Benign Versus Malignant Pleural Lesions

Although CT is the primary technique for diagnosis and staging MPM, frequently chest MR imaging is used as a problem-solving modality with better differentiation of benign versus malignant disease. MR imaging, with its better contrast resolution than CT, allows for better depiction of pleural thickening and spread to surrounding organs, diaphragm, and chest wall. Infiltration of adjacent structures favors malignancy, although some infections (actynomycosis, nocardiosis, and tuberculosis) are well known to spread to the chest wall (empyema necessitatis).[70]

DWI has shown similar sensitivity and specificity to [18]FDG-PET/CT for differentiating benign versus malignant pleural diseases.[71] It also reduces the number of false-positive results seen with [18]FDG-PET/CT.[71,72] DWI shows diffuse hyperintense focal spots at high b values with low ADC, indicating restrictive tissue diffusivity in malignant lesions (Fig. 10; see Table 4).[7] Significant differences have been described in the ADC between different MPM subtypes (ADC = $1.31 \pm 0.15 \times 10^{-3}$ mm²/s vs ADC = $0.99 \pm 0.07 \times 10^{-3}$ mm²/s for epithelial and sarcomatoid subtypes, respectively) due to different cellular configuration (see Box 3).[73]

Box 3

Malignant pleural mesothelioma hystologic subtypes

Prevalence: 2000 to 3000 new cases/y

Asbestos exposures (40%–80%; 10% incidence)

Epithelioid (55%–65%)

Cuboidal cells

Eosinophilic cytoplasm

Central nuclei

Distinct nucleoli

Sarcomatoid (10%–15%)

Sheets/fascicles of spindle cells

Nuclear atypia

Desmoplasic (collagenous matrix)

Biphasic or mixed type (25%–35%)

10% or more of both types

Pleural effusion

Focal/diffuse pleural thickening

Pleural masses (coalescence)

Shrinking lung sign

Local and diaphragmatic invasion

Multifocal chest wall invasion

Caudocranial gradient growth

Interlobar fissure involvement

Lymphadenopathy (50%)

Metastasis to

   Male: lung, skin, and kidneys

   Female: breast, genitals, bones, and kidneys

MR imaging features

   T1WI: isohyperintense

   T2WI: moderately hyperintense

   DWI: pleural pointillism sign

Adding DCE–MR imaging derived parameters, differentiation of benign versus malignant pleural lesions reduces the number of false-negative results of DWI alone (see **Tables 4** and **5**).[71] It is also useful in the assessment of mediastinal, transdiaphragmatic, chest wall invasion, and fissural extension of MPM.[71,72]

Metastatic pleural disease manifests as multiple nodules or plaques with significant gadolinium uptake and restriction in DWI sequences.

Malignant Pleural Conditions: Staging and Treatment Monitoring

Malignant pleural mesothelioma staging

Because of a direct relationship between the tumor extension assessed by TNM system, treatment, and survival rate, it is critical to differentiate

Lung cancer (40%)

Breast cancer (20%)

Lymphoproliferative disorders (recurrent disease; 10%)

Gastric and ovarian tumors (5%)

Sarcomas (seeding metastasis)

Thymoma and thymic carcinoma (drop metastasis)

resectable (T3) versus nonresectable (T4) disease.[74] Sugarbaker and colleagues[74] pointed out the importance of tumor histology, reporting extended survival rates in treated patients with epithelial histology, negative resection margins, and positive LN.

Because of the characteristic growth pattern of MPM, the staging and measurement of treatment response remain difficult, especially for CT, which underestimates not only local invasion but also N stage.[75]

Treatment monitoring and prognostic factors

Bicompartmental analysis of DCE–MR imaging has been tested in therapy monitoring of MPM and, as a consequence, K_{ep} and K^{trans} have shown a role in the prediction of therapeutic response. Giesel and colleagues[76] monitored treatment response in patients with MPM and found that nonresponders had higher K_{ep} than clinical responders and shorter OS.

Benign Pleural Conditions: Potential Pitfalls

Both solitary fibrous tumor of the pleura and pleural plaques are potential pitfalls for MPM in [18]FDG-PET/CT because they may demonstrate significant radiotracer uptake.[77–79] DWI also potentially detects malignant transformation of solitary fibrous tumor of the pleura (seen in 20% of cases) by showing a decrease in ADC value.[78] A nonrestrictive pleural plaque in DWI or a nonenhancing lesion or showing a slow RSE on DCE–MR imaging is consistent with a pleural plaque of benign origin (**Fig. 11**).[69,80]

Functional MR Imaging and Mediastinal Masses

DWI has great utility in characterizing benign and malignant mediastinal masses without cystic components and in distinguishing between well and poorly differentiated masses (**Fig. 12;** see **Table 4**).[81] Non-neoplastic cysts showed significant higher ADC values compared with tumor lesions (see **Fig. 12**). Therefore, DWI may be useful for characterization of those lesions with questionable findings on CT.[82]

WB-DWI has also been demonstrated as a feasible technique in the initial staging of lymphoma, including mediastinal involvement, with results similar to CT or [18]FDG-PET/CT.[83,84] DWI is a promising tool for treatment monitoring of mediastinal lesions and early prediction of treatment outcome, especially in the evaluation of pediatric and pregnant patients.[7]

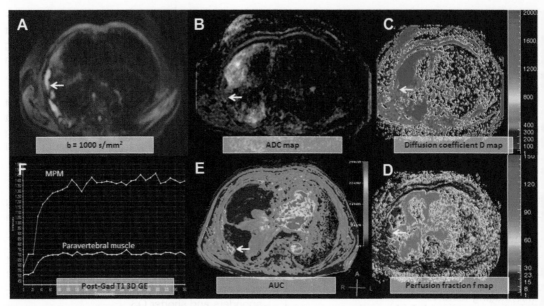

Fig. 10. MPM. (*A, B*) High b value DWI and corresponding ADC map revealing multiple hyperintense and restrictive pleural nodules and plaques (pointillism sign; ADC = 1.44 × 10^{-3} mm^2/s). (*C, D*) IVIM-derived parameters; true diffusion map confirms restriction of water motion (D = 1.03 × 10^{-3} mm^2/s) and high perfusion fraction (f = 22%; *white arrows*) of the pleural thickening is also shown. (*E, F*) Area under the curve (AUC) map shows intense enhancement. TIC of pleural nodule demonstrates a rapid initial slope of enhancement with delayed plateau and absence of significant WO (type A TIC).

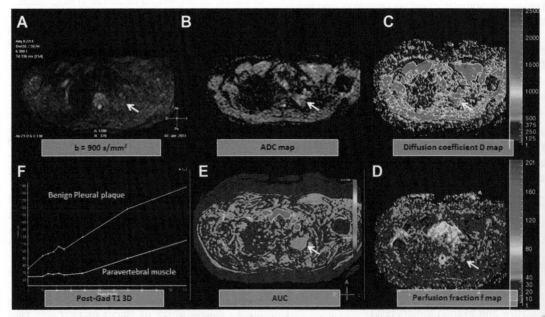

Fig. 11. Benign pleural plaque of tuberculous origin. The lesion (*white arrow*) does not show restriction on (*A*) DWI (b = 900 s/mm^2) and (*B*) ADC map (ADC = 2.03 × 10^{-3} mm^2/s), which is also confirmed in IVIM-derived (*C*) D map (D = 1.79 × 10^{-3} mm^2/s) (*D*) f map (f = 15%) (*white arrows*) shows low flow within the lesion. (*E*) Area under the curve (AUC) map shows a low-grade enhancement (*white arrow*). (*F*) TIC reveals a slow initial slope with progressive lineal enhancement over time.

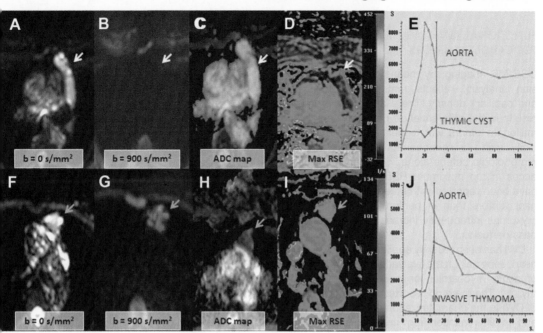

Fig. 12. Morphologic and functional MR imaging in a thymic cyst (*A–E; white arrow*) and an invasive thymoma (*F–I; gray arrow*). (*A–C*) and (*F–H*) DWI and corresponding ADC maps of both lesions demonstrate their different behavior, with absence of restriction of benign lesion (ADC = 4.11 × 10⁻³ mm²/s) and restriction of malignant one (ADC = 1.54 × 10⁻³ mm²/s). (*D, E*) and (*I, J*) RSE parametric map derived from DCE–MR imaging and corresponding TICs reveal the different vascular behavior of both nosologic entities.

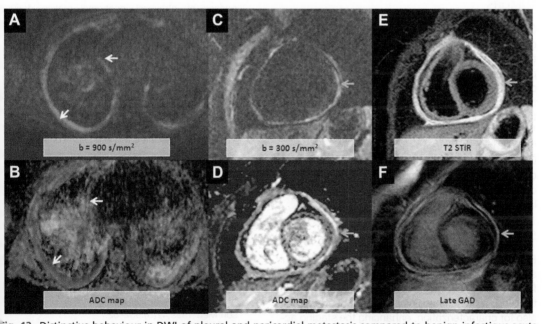

Fig. 13. Distinctive behaviour in DWI of pleural and pericardial metastasis compared to benign infectious acute pericarditis. (*A,B*) High b value chest DWI and ADC map of a 63 year-old patient with metastatic squamous cell carcinoma of the tongue showing hyperintensity of the pleura an pericardium at high b value and corresponding hypointensity on ADC map (*white arrows in A and B*) in keeping with pleural and pericardial metastasis. (*C-F*) Short axis oriented cardiac DWI (*C*) and corresponding ADC map (*D*), STIR (*E*) and late gadolinium enhacement (*F*) in a 28 year-old patient who presents with syncope and chest pain. Note the different behaviour of the pericardium at b=300 s/mm² gradient and ADC map (hyperintense in both; *gray arrows*), which correlates to hyperintensity of the pericardium in short axis STIR (*E; gray arrow*) and delayed uptake of contrast media in short axis late gadolinium enhancement sequence (*F; gray arrow*). This is compatible with acute infectious pericarditis.

FUNCTIONAL IMAGING OF CARDIAC AND PERICARDIAL TUMORS

DCE–MR imaging, by means of first-pass perfusion analysis, reflects tumor neoangiogenesis and capillary density. There are some promising results in the differentiation between benign and malignant tumors, with higher sensitivity and specificity using a semiquantitative approach than morphologic criteria alone.[85–87] Significant differences in the maximum RSE and slope of RSE have been reported with steeper slopes in malignant tumors than in benign ones.[86–88] Cardiac myxomas infrequently increase RSE during first-pass perfusion.[88]

DWI has been recently applied successfully in the heart, especially in the evaluation of edema in cases of acute myocarditis or ischemic cardiomyopathy.[89,90] There are no reported data about the role of DWI in the characterization of malignant lesions and its differentiation from nontumoral and benign ones. In the authors' experience, it is useful for distinguishing necrotic from solid areas inside tumors and for differentiating neoplastic lesions from cardiac thrombus and detection of recurrence (Fig. 13).

FUNCTIONAL IMAGING OF CHEST WALL TUMORS

Chest wall tumors include a heterogeneous group of entities originating from soft tissues of the thorax and bones. MR imaging is the preferred method for accurate delineation and delimitation of its boundaries. There is no literature regarding the use of functional MR imaging techniques in the evaluation of chest wall tumors; [18]FDG-PET/CT is the most widespread modality. "There is a promising potential role" because DWI has been described as providing better detection of soft tissue and bone lesions compared with morphologic sequences, particularly for bone metastasis.[91]

SUMMARY

Functional MR imaging of the chest provides useful and reproducible derived biomarkers not only for differentiation of benign versus malignant process in the lung, mediastinum, pleura, and chest wall but also for characterization, enhancing the staging accuracy, and displaying relevant information during treatment monitoring, with prognostic implications.

REFERENCES

1. Mittra E, Quon A. Positron emission tomography/computed tomography: the current technology and applications. Radiol Clin North Am 2009;47(1):147–60.

2. Padhani AR, Liu G, Koh DM, et al. Diffusion weighted magnetic resonance imaging as a cancer biomarker: consensus and recommendations. Neoplasia 2009;11(2):102–25.

3. García-Figueiras R, Padhani AR, Beer AJ, et al. Imaging of Tumor angiogenesis for radiologists part 1: biological and technical basis. Curr Probl Diagn Radiol 2015;44(5):407–24.

4. Le Bihan D, Breton E, Lallemand D, et al. Separation of diffusion and perfusion in intravoxel incoherent motion MR imaging. Radiology 1988;168(2):497–505.

5. Le Bihan D. Apparent diffusion coefficient and beyond: what diffusion MR imaging can tell us about tissue structure. Radiology 2013;268(2):318–22.

6. Raya JG, Dietrich O, Reiser MF, et al. Techniques for diffusion-weighted imaging of bone marrow. Eur J Radiol 2005;55(1):64–73.

7. Luna A, Sánchez-Gonzalez J, Caro P. Diffusion weighted imaging of the chest. Magn Reson Imaging Clin N Am 2011;19:69–94.

8. Rosenkrantz AB, Padhani AR, Chenevert TL, et al. Body diffusion kurtosis imaging: basic principles, applications, and considerations for clinical practice. J Magn Reson Imaging 2015. [Epub ahead of print].

9. Deng Y, Li X, Lei Y, et al. Use of diffusion-weighted magnetic resonance imaging to distinguish between lung cancer and focal inflammatory lesions: a comparison of intravoxel incoherent motion derived parameters and apparent diffusion coefficient. Acta Radiol 2015. [Epub ahead of print].

10. Heusch P, Köhler J, Wittsack H-J, et al. Hybrid [18F] FDG PET/MRI including non-Gaussian diffusion weighted imaging (DWI): preliminary results in non-small cell lung cancer (NSCLC). Eur J Radiol 2013;82(11):2055–60.

11. Wang L, Lin J, Liu K, et al. Intravoxel incoherent motion diffusion-weighted MR imaging in differentiation of lung cancer from obstructive lung consolidation: comparison and correlation with pharmacokinetic analysis from dynamic contrast-enhanced MR imaging. Eur Radiol 2014;24(8):1914–22.

12. Buonaccorsi GA, Roberts C, Cheung S, et al. Comparison of the performance of tracer kinetic model-driven registration for dynamic contrast enhanced MRI using different models of contrast enhancement. Acad Radiol 2006;13(9):1112–23.

13. Pruessmann KP, Weiger M, Scheidegger MB, et al. SENSE: sensitivity encoding for fast MRI. Magn Reson Med 1999;42(5):952–62.

14. Michoux N, Vallée J-P, Pechère-Bertschi A, et al. Analysis of contrast-enhanced MR images to assess renal function. MAGMA 2006;19(4):167–79.

15. Fujimoto K, Abe T, Müller NL, et al. Small peripheral pulmonary carcinomas evaluated with dynamic MR imaging: correlation with tumor vascularity and prognosis. Radiology 2003;227(3): 786–93.

16. Rijpkema M, Kaanders JH, Joosten FB, et al. Method for quantitative mapping of dynamic MRI contrast agent uptake in human tumors. J Magn Reson Imaging 2001;14(4):457–63.

17. Jemal A, Bray F, Center MM, et al. Global cancer statistics. CA Cancer J Clin 2011;61(2):69–90.

18. Regier M, Schwarz D, Henes FO, et al. Diffusion-weighted MR-imaging for the detection of pulmonary nodules at 1.5 Tesla: intraindividual comparison with multidetector computed tomography. J Med Imaging Radiat Oncol 2011;55(3):266–74.

19. Fricks BB, Meyer BC, Martus P, et al. MRI of the thorax during whole-body MRI: evaluation of different MR sequences and comparison to thoracic multidetector computed tomography (MDCT). J Magn Reson Imaging 2008;27(3):538–45.

20. Li B, Li Q, Chen C, et al. A systematic review and meta-analysis of the accuracy of diffusion-weighted MRI in the detection of malignant pulmonary nodules and masses. Acad Radiol 2014; 21(1):21–9.

21. Chen L, Zhang J, Bao J, et al. Meta-analysis of diffusion-weighted MRI in the differential diagnosis of lung lesions. J Magn Reson Imaging 2013;37(6): 1351–8.

22. Ohno Y, Koyama H, Onishi Y, et al. Non-small cell lung cancer: whole-body MR examination for M-stage assessment–utility for whole-body diffusion-weighted imaging compared with integrated FDG PET/CT. Radiology 2008;248(2):643–54.

23. Koyama H, Ohno Y, Nishio M, et al. Diffusion-weighted imaging vs STIR turbo SE imaging: capability for quantitative differentiation of small-cell lung cancer from non-small-cell lung cancer. Br J Radiol 2014;87(1038):20130307.

24. Usuda K, Zhao X-T, Sagawa M, et al. Diffusion-weighted imaging is superior to positron emission tomography in the detection and nodal assessment of lung cancers. Ann Thorac Surg 2011;91(6):1689–95.

25. Gümüştaş S, Inan N, Akansel G, et al. Differentiation of malignant and benign lung lesions with diffusion-weighted MR imaging. Radiol Oncol 2012;46(2):106–13.

26. Liu H, Liu Y, Yu T, et al. Usefulness of diffusion-weighted MR imaging in the evaluation of pulmonary lesions. Eur Radiol 2010;20(4):807–15.

27. Koyama H, Ohno Y, Seki S, et al. Value of diffusion-weighted MR imaging using various parameters for assessment and characterization of solitary pulmonary nodules. Eur J Radiol 2015;84(3):509–15.

28. Kono R, Fujimoto K, Terasaki H, et al. Dynamic MRI of solitary pulmonary nodules: comparison of enhancement patterns of malignant and benign small peripheral lung lesions. AJR Am J Roentgenol 2007;188(1):26–36.

29. Donmez FY, Yekeler E, Saeidi V, et al. Dynamic contrast enhancement patterns of solitary pulmonary nodules on 3D gradient-recalled echo MRI. AJR Am J Roentgenol 2007;189(6):1380–6.

30. Wu L-M, Xu J-R, Gu H-Y, et al. Preoperative mediastinal and hilar nodal staging with diffusion-weighted magnetic resonance imaging and fluorodeoxyglucose positron emission tomography/computed tomography in patients with non-small-cell lung cancer: which is better? J Surg Res 2012;178(1):304–14.

31. Kim YN, Yi CA, Lee KS, et al. A proposal for combined MRI and PET/CT interpretation criteria for preoperative nodal staging in non-small-cell lung cancer. Eur Radiol 2012;22(7):1537–46.

32. Schaefer JF, Vollmar J, Schick F, et al. Solitary pulmonary nodules: dynamic contrast-enhanced MR imaging–perfusion differences in malignant and benign lesions. Radiology 2004;232(2):544–53.

33. Coolen J, Vansteenkiste J, De Keyzer F, et al. Characterisation of solitary pulmonary lesions combining visual perfusion and quantitative diffusion MR imaging. Eur Radiol 2014;24(2):531–41.

34. Ohno Y, Koyama H, Takenaka D, et al. Dynamic MRI, dynamic multidetector-row computed tomography (MDCT), and coregistered 2-[fluorine-18]-fluoro-2-deoxy-D-glucose-positron emission tomography (FDG-PET)/CT: comparative study of capability for management of pulmonary nodules. J Magn Reson Imaging 2008;27(6):1284–95.

35. Sher T, Dy GK, Adjei AA. Small cell lung cancer. Mayo Clin Proc 2008;83(3):355–67.

36. Lee HY, Jeong JY, Lee KS, et al. Histopathology of lung adenocarcinoma based on new IASLC/ATS/ERS classification: prognostic stratification with functional and metabolic imaging biomarkers. J Magn Reson Imaging 2013;38(4):905–13.

37. Matoba M, Tonami H, Kondou T, et al. Lung carcinoma: diffusion-weighted mr imaging–preliminary evaluation with apparent diffusion coefficient. Radiology 2007;243(2):570–7.

38. Heusch P, Buchbender C, Köhler J, et al. Correlation of the apparent diffusion coefficient (ADC) with the standardized uptake value (SUV) in hybrid 18F-FDG PET/MRI in non-small cell lung cancer (NSCLC) lesions: initial results. Rofo 2013;185(11):1056–62.

39. Schaarschmidt BM, Buchbender C, Nensa F, et al. Correlation of the apparent diffusion coefficient (ADC) with the standardized uptake value (SUV) in lymph node metastases of non-small cell lung cancer (NSCLC) patients using hybrid 18F-FDG PET/MRI. PLoS One 2015;10(1):e0116277.

40. Tanaka R, Nakazato Y, Horikoshi H, et al. Diffusion-weighted imaging and positron emission tomography in various cytological subtypes of primary lung adenocarcinoma. Clin Imaging 2013;37(5):876–83.

41. Nomori H, Cong Y, Abe M, et al. Diffusion-weighted magnetic resonance imaging in preoperative assessment of non-small cell lung cancer. J Thorac Cardiovasc Surg 2015;149(4):991–6.

42. Usuda K, Sagawa M, Motono N, et al. Advantages of diffusion-weighted imaging over positron emission tomography-computed tomography in assessment of hilar and mediastinal lymph node in lung cancer. Ann Surg Oncol 2013;20(5):1676–83.

43. Baysal T, Mutlu DY, Yologlu S. Diffusion-weighted magnetic resonance imaging in differentiation of postobstructive consolidation from central lung carcinoma. Magn Reson Imaging 2009;27(10):1447–54.

44. Bourgouin PM, McLoud TC, Fitzgibbon JF, et al. Differentiation of bronchogenic carcinoma from postobstructive pneumonitis by magnetic resonance imaging: histopathologic correlation. J Thorac Imaging 1991;6(2):22–7.

45. Plathow C, Aschoff P, Lichy MP, et al. Positron emission tomography/computed tomography and whole-body magnetic resonance imaging in staging of advanced nonsmall cell lung cancer–initial results. Invest Radiol 2008;43(5):290–7.

46. Ohno Y, Koyama H, Yoshikawa T, et al. Lung cancer assessment using mr imaging: an update. Magn Reson Imaging Clin N Am 2015;23(2):231–44.

47. Nomori H, Mori T, Ikeda K, et al. Diffusion-weighted magnetic resonance imaging can be used in place of positron emission tomography for N staging of non-small cell lung cancer with fewer false-positive results. J Thorac Cardiovasc Surg 2008;135(4):816–22.

48. Chen W, Jian W, Li H, et al. Whole-body diffusion-weighted imaging vs. FDG-PET for the detection of non-small-cell lung cancer. How do they measure up? Magn Reson Imaging 2010;28(5):613–20.

49. Ohno Y, Koyama H, Nogami M, et al. STIR turbo SE MR imaging vs. coregistered FDG-PET/CT: quantitative and qualitative assessment of N-stage in non-small-cell lung cancer patients. J Magn Reson Imaging 2007;26(4):1071–80.

50. Sakurada A, Takahara T, Kwee TC, et al. Diagnostic performance of diffusion-weighted magnetic resonance imaging in esophageal cancer. Eur Radiol 2009;19(6):1461–9.

51. Takenaka D, Ohno Y, Matsumoto K, et al. Detection of bone metastases in non-small cell lung cancer patients: comparison of whole-body diffusion-weighted imaging (DWI), whole-body MR imaging without and with DWI, whole-body FDG-PET/CT, and bone scintigraphy. J Magn Reson Imaging 2009;30(2):298–308.

52. Yi CA, Shin KM, Lee KS, et al. Non-small cell lung cancer staging: efficacy comparison of integrated PET/CT versus 3.0-T whole-body MR imaging. Radiology 2008;248(2):632–42.

53. Ohno Y, Koyama H, Yoshikawa T, et al. Three-way Comparison of Whole-Body MR, Coregistered Whole-Body FDG PET/MR, and Integrated Whole-Body FDG PET/CT Imaging: TNM and Stage Assessment Capability for Non-Small Cell Lung Cancer Patients. Radiology 2015;275(3):849–61.

54. Schwenzer NF, Schraml C, Müller M, et al. Pulmonary lesion assessment: comparison of whole-body hybrid MR/PET and PET/CT imaging–pilot study. Radiology 2012;264(2):551–8.

55. Bains LJ, Zweifel M, Thoeny HC. Therapy response with diffusion MRI: an update. Cancer Imaging 2012;12:395–402.

56. Ohno Y, Koyama H, Yoshikawa T, et al. Diffusion-weighted MRI versus 18F-FDG PET/CT: performance as predictors of tumor treatment response and patient survival in patients with non-small cell lung cancer receiving chemoradiotherapy. AJR Am J Roentgenol 2012;198(1):75–82.

57. Yabuuchi H, Hatakenaka M, Takayama K, et al. Non-small cell lung cancer: detection of early response to chemotherapy by using contrast-enhanced dynamic and diffusion-weighted MR imaging. Radiology 2011;261:598–604.

58. Tsuchida T, Morikawa M, Demura Y, et al. Imaging the early response to chemotherapy in advanced lung cancer with diffusion-weighted magnetic resonance imaging compared to fluorine-18 fluorodeoxyglucose positron emission tomography and computed tomography. J Magn Reson Imaging 2013;38(1):80–8.

59. Okuma T, Matsuoka T, Yamamoto a, et al. Assessment of early treatment response after CT-guided radiofrequency ablation of unresectable lung tumours by diffusion-weighted MRI: a pilot study. Br J Radiol 2009;82(984):989–94.

60. Ohno Y, Nogami M, Higashino T, et al. Prognostic value of dynamic MR imaging for non-small-cell lung cancer patients after chemoradiotherapy. J Magn Reson Imaging 2005;21(6):775–83.

61. Figueiras RG, Padhani AR, Goh VJ, et al. Novel oncologic drugs: what they do and how they affect images. Radiographics 2011;31:2059–91.

62. Afaq A, Andreou A, Koh DM. Diffusion-weighted magnetic resonance imaging for tumour response assessment: why, when and how? Cancer Imaging 2010;10(Spec no A):S179–88.

63. Padhani AR, Koh D-M. Diffusion MR imaging for monitoring of treatment response. Magn Reson Imaging Clin N Am 2011;19(1):181–209.

64. Kelly RJ, Rajan A, Force J, et al. Evaluation of KRAS mutations, angiogenic biomarkers, and DCE-MRI in patients with advanced non-small-cell lung cancer receiving sorafenib. Clin Cancer Res 2011;17(5):1190–9.

65. Chang Y-C, Yu C-J, Chen C-M, et al. Dynamic contrast-enhanced MRI in advanced nonsmall-cell lung cancer patients treated with first-line bevacizumab, gemcitabine, and cisplatin. J Magn Reson Imaging 2012;36(2):387–96.

66. Padhani AR, Krohn KA, Lewis JS, et al. Imaging oxygenation of human tumours. Eur Radiol 2007;17(4):861–72.

7. Tatum JL, Kelloff GJ, Gillies RJ, et al. Hypoxia: importance in tumor biology, noninvasive measurement by imaging, and value of its measurement in the management of cancer therapy. Int J Radiat Biol 2006;82(10):699–757.

8. Robinson BW, Lake RA. Advances in malignant mesothelioma. N Engl J Med 2005;353(15):1591–603.

9. Gill RR, Gerbaudo VH, Jacobson FL, et al. MR imaging of benign and malignant pleural disease. Magn Reson Imaging Clin N Am 2008;16(2):319–39.

0. Bonomo L, Feragalli B, Sacco R, et al. Malignant pleural disease. Eur J Radiol 2000;34(2):98–118.

1. Coolen J, De Keyzer F, Nafteux P, et al. Malignant pleural disease: diagnosis by using diffusion-weighted and dynamic contrast-enhanced MR imaging–initial experience. Radiology 2012;263(3): 884–92.

2. Yildirim H, Metintas M, Entok E, et al. Clinical value of fluorodeoxyglucose-positron emission tomography/computed tomography in differentiation of malignant mesothelioma from asbestos-related benign pleural disease: an observational pilot study. J Thorac Oncol 2009;4(12):1480–4.

3. Coolen J, De Keyzer F, Nafteux P, et al. Malignant pleural mesothelioma: visual assessment by using pleural pointillism at diffusion-weighted MR imaging. Radiology 2015;274(2):576–84.

4. Sugarbaker DJ, Flores RM, Jaklitsch MT, et al. Resection margins, extrapleural nodal status, and cell type determine postoperative long-term survival in trimodality therapy of malignant pleural mesothelioma: results in 183 patients. J Thorac Cardiovasc Surg 1999;117(1):54–63 [discussion: 63–5].

5. Heelan RT, Rusch VW, Begg CB, et al. Staging of malignant pleural mesothelioma: comparison of CT and MR imaging. AJR Am J Roentgenol 1999; 172(4):1039–47.

6. Giesel FL, Bischoff H, von Tengg-Kobligk H, et al. Dynamic contrast-enhanced MRI of malignant pleural mesothelioma: a feasibility study of noninvasive assessment, therapeutic follow-up, and possible predictor of improved outcome. Chest 2006;129(6): 1570–6.

7. Ginat DT, Bokhari A, Bhatt S, et al. Imaging features of solitary fibrous tumors. AJR Am J Roentgenol 2011;196(3):487–95.

8. Inaoka T, Takahashi K, Miyokawa N, et al. Solitary fibrous tumor of the pleura: apparent diffusion coefficient (ADC) value and ADC map to predict malignant transformation. J Magn Reson Imaging 2007; 26(1):155–8.

9. Rosado-de-Christenson ML, Abbott GF, McAdams HP, et al. From the archives of the AFIP: localized fibrous tumor of the pleura. Radiographics 2003;23(3):759–83.

80. Weber MA, Bock M, Plathow C, et al. Asbestos-related pleural disease: value of dedicated magnetic resonance imaging techniques. Invest Radiol 2004;39(9):554–64.

81. Razek AA, Elmorsy A, Elshafey M, et al. Assessment of mediastinal tumors with diffusion-weighted single-shot echo-planar MRI. J Magn Reson Imaging 2009; 30(3):535–40.

82. Shin KE, Yi CA, Kim TS, et al. Diffusion-weighted MRI for distinguishing non-neoplastic cysts from solid masses in the mediastinum: problem-solving in mediastinal masses of indeterminate internal characteristics on CT. Eur Radiol 2014;24(3):677–84.

83. Lin C, Luciani A, Itti E, et al. Whole-body diffusion-weighted magnetic resonance imaging with apparent diffusion coefficient mapping for staging patients with diffuse large B-cell lymphoma. Eur Radiol 2010;20(8):2027–38.

84. Kwee TC, van Ufford HM, Beek FJ, et al. Whole-body MRI, including diffusion-weighted imaging, for the initial staging of malignant lymphoma: comparison to computed tomography. Invest Radiol 2009;44(10):683–90.

85. Bauner KU, Sourbron S, Picciolo M, et al. MR first pass perfusion of benign and malignant cardiac tumours-significant differences and diagnostic accuracy. Eur Radiol 2012;22(1):73–82.

86. Libicher M, Kauffmann GW, Hosch W. Dynamic contrast-enhanced MRI for evaluation of cardiac tumors. Eur Radiol 2006;16(8):1858–9.

87. Mohrs OK, Voigtlaender T, Petersen SE, et al. First experiences with contrast-enhanced first-pass MR perfusion imaging in patients with primary, benign cardiac masses and tumour-like lesions. Eur Radiol 2008;18(8):1617–24.

88. Fussen S, De Boeck BW, Zellweger MJ, et al. Cardiovascular magnetic resonance imaging for diagnosis and clinical management of suspected cardiac masses and tumours. Eur Heart J 2011; 32(12):1551–60.

89. Laissy JP, Gaxotte V, Ironde-Laissy E, et al. Cardiac diffusion-weighted MR imaging in recent, subacute, and chronic myocardial infarction: a pilot study. J Magn Reson Imaging 2013;38(6):1377–87.

90. Potet J, Rahmouni A, Mayer J, et al. Detection of myocardial edema with low-b-value diffusion-weighted echo-planar imaging sequence in patients with acute myocarditis. Radiology 2013;269(2):362–9.

91. Nagata S, Nishimura H, Uchida M, et al. Diffusion-weighted imaging of soft tissue tumors: usefulness of the apparent diffusion coefficient for differential diagnosis. Radiat Med 2008;26(5):287–95.

Multiparametric MR Imaging in Abdominal Malignancies

Antonio Luna, MD[a,b,*], Shivani Pahwa, MD[b], Claudio Bonini, MD[c],
Lidia Alcalá-Mata, MD[a], Katherine L. Wright, PhD[b], Vikas Gulani, MD, PhD[d,e,f]

KEYWORDS

- MR imaging • DWI • Perfusion MR imaging • MR elastography • [1]H-MR spectroscopy
- Hepatobiliary contrast agents • Multiparametric • Biomarker

KEY POINTS

- MR imaging provides different multiple imaging biomarkers for the assessment of hepatobiliary and pancreatic malignancies, which can be integrated in a comprehensive protocol using a multiparametric approach.
- Diffusion-weighted imaging is now fully embedded in clinical protocols in the evaluation of abdominal malignancies.
- Perfusion MR imaging is technically ready for the clinical arena, with a promising role in the assessment of response to targeted-therapies.
- Magnetic resonance (MR) elastography and [1]H-MR spectroscopy can be used to assess focal liver lesions, but are still limited to research centers.
- Hepatobiliary contrast agents are widely used in the detection of metastasis and in the assessment of hepatocellular carcinoma.

INTRODUCTION

Anatomic MR imaging is the most sensitive imaging tool in the detection of hepatobiliary and pancreatic (HBP) malignancies.[1] The combination of morphologic features and enhancement patterns provides an integral assessment of these tumors, including therapy monitoring using size criteria.[2] Recently, new MR imaging techniques are able to explore functional and molecular characteristics of abdominal cancers (Table 1). This functional information is very useful for overcoming limitations of morphologic MR imaging and has shown particular promise in the assessment of therapy response to novel targeted therapies.[3] These techniques are inherently quantitative and yield absolute or relative measurements of tissue properties, providing potential imaging biomarkers of disease severity.[4–7]

Dr V. Gulani has an NIH Grant: 1R01DK098503, and receives research support from Siemens Healthcare. Drs S. Pahwa and K.L. Wright receive research support from Siemens Healthcare. Dr A. Luna and Dr Bonini C has nothing to disclose.

[a] Department of Radiology, Health Time, Carmelo Torres 2, Jaén 23006, Spain; [b] Department of Radiology, University Hospitals of Cleveland, Case Western Reserve University, Cleveland, OH, USA; [c] Oroño Medical Diagnostic Center, Rosario, Argentina; [d] Department of Radiology, Case Comprehensive Cancer Center, University Hospitals of Cleveland, Case Western Reserve University, Cleveland, OH, USA; [e] Department of Urology, Case Comprehensive Cancer Center, University Hospitals of Cleveland, Case Western Reserve University, Cleveland, OH, USA; [f] Department of Biomedical Engineering, Case Comprehensive Cancer Center, University Hospitals of Cleveland, Case Western Reserve University, Cleveland, OH, USA
* Corresponding author.
E-mail address: aluna70@htime.org

Magn Reson Imaging Clin N Am 24 (2016) 157–186
http://dx.doi.org/10.1016/j.mric.2015.08.005
1064-9689/16/$ – see front matter © 2016 Elsevier Inc. All rights reserved.

Table 1
MR imaging functional techniques for abdominal tumor evaluation

Tumor Feature	MR Imaging Technique	Quantitative Parameters
Cellularity, necrosis, and apoptosis	DWI	ADC
Metabolism	^{1}H-MRS	Ratio of choline (ppm) to other metabolites
Angiogenesis	DCE-MR imaging	K^{trans}, v_e, K_{ep}, V_p AUC
Elasticity/stiffness	MRE	Young's modulus, shear modulus
Hepatic function	HB contrast agents	Lesion-to-liver enhancement ratio

Abbreviations: K_{ep}, rate constant; K^{trans}, efflux constant; v_e, volume of extravascular extracellular space; v_p, plasma volumen.

This review focuses on basic concepts behind these techniques, clinical applications, and levels of validation in the analysis of abdominal malignancies, and also the integration of these technologies into a multiparametric imaging (MPI) approach.

DIFFUSION-WEIGHTED MR IMAGING

Diffusion-weighted imaging (DWI) has gained ground in the upper abdomen, being included in state-of-the-art MR imaging protocols. This technique is easy to perform, relatively fast, and does not require administration of an extrinsic contrast agent. Its use facilitates lesion detection and characterization in the liver and pancreas. Furthermore, its role as a cancer biomarker of tissue cellularity and cell membrane integrity has been confirmed for HBP malignancies.[5]

DWI reflects the microscopic movement of water protons in different tissues. The net motion of water molecules is directly related to the movement of water in various tissue compartments. The presence of a dense cellular structure, many intact cell membranes, or viscous fluid with viscous content can reduce or restrict water mobility, which results in high signal on high b-value (heavily diffusion weighted) imaging and corresponds to low diffusivity on apparent diffusion coefficient (ADC) maps. Conversely, tissues with low cellularity show an increase in water diffusion, low signal intensity (SI) on high b-value images, and high diffusivity on ADC maps.

Technical Aspects of Diffusion-Weighted Imaging

Sequence design

An adequate sequence design of diffusion-weighted sequence in the upper abdomen is critical, because it has intrinsically limited spatial resolution. **Box 1** summarizes the list of scanning parameters to be optimized in a DWI sequence of the body. Most commonly, a single-shot spin-

echo echo-planar imaging sequence is performed, which has the advantage of a very fast readout, making it insensitive to macroscopic patient motion.[4] However, this family of sequences is prone to motion and magnetic susceptibility artifacts. The maintenance of echo time (TE) as short as possible, using parallel imaging, high bandwidth, and advanced suppression techniques, minimizes distortion artifacts, although diffusion requires intrinsically long TEs due to the time required to impart sufficient diffusion sensitivity. In order to reduce the effects of respiratory and cardiac motion, it is necessary to use gated acquisitions (**Fig. 1**). Most commonly, breath-hold or free-breathing sequences are used (**Box 2**). In addition, fat suppression must be used to avoid ghosting artifacts from the fat signal.

Modeling of diffusion signal

In order to use DWI as an oncological biomarker quantitative mapping is critical, especially in the

---

Box 1
Scanning parameters to optimize in diffusion-weighted imaging acquisitions

Increase SNR

Maintain TE as shortest as possible

Coarse matrix

Use parallel imaging

Simultaneous gradient application

Multiple signal averaging

Reduce artifacts

Optimize fat suppression

Increase bandwidth

Control eddy currents

Avoid areas with susceptibility artifacts

Use respiratory synchronism techniques

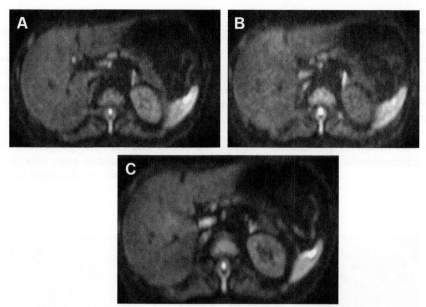

Fig. 1. Techniques of respiratory synchronization in DWI of the liver. Notice different SNR and acquisition time in (A) breath-hold (acquisition time: 120 seconds; 20 seconds per breath-hold), (B) free-breathing (acquisition time: 0 seconds), and (C) respiratory trigger (acquisition time: 220 seconds) acquisitions.

etting of therapy monitoring. The most widely used quantitative property is the ADC from a monocompartmental model of diffusion signal decay. ADC measurement minimizes the so-called T2 shine-through, referring to the high signal from long T2 species seen in DWI because of superimposed T2 weighting and permits evaluation of isolated diffusion effects.[4]

However, the ADC model does not distinguish between the different compartments where the water protons can move, such as intravascular, extravascular, extracellular, and intracellular spaces. If several b values are acquired less than and greater than 100 s/mm², it is possible to differentiate between the fast movement of intravascular water molecules with low b values (<100 s/mm²), and the slow signal decay of diffusion signal with b values greater than 100 s/mm², secondary to restricted water movement in the extracellular and intracellular compartments[8] (see Fig. 1 in the article by Broncano in this issue).[9] This model is known as Intra Voxel Incoherent Motion (IVIM) because it has been found useful in the characterization of focal liver and pancreatic lesions, with advantage over ADC measurements in some scenarios.[10,11] The contribution of true diffusion and perfusion toward signal loss is separated in this model and reflected in the following parameters: f (perfusion fraction) that represents the flowing water molecules within the capillaries; D (tissue diffusivity), a more reliable marker of tissue diffusion than ADC in organs with tissues with significant perfusion fraction; and finally, D* (pseudo-diffusion coefficient), related to the perfusion contribution to signal decay.

If ultrahigh b values greater than 1500 s/mm² are acquired, the remaining diffusion signal is related to a layer of polarized water molecules

---

Box 2
Main characteristics of breath-hold and free-breathing diffusion-weighted sequences

Breath-hold sequence

Limited SNR, spatial resolution, and slice thickness

Prone to distortion and ghosting artifacts

Limited number of b values (usually 2 or 3)

Limited quality of ADC map due to misregistration

Shorter acquisition time

Free breathing sequence

Increased SNR, spatial resolution, and slice thickness

Prone to respiratory artifacts, blurring, and volume averaging

Permit to acquire more b values

Better quality of ADC map

Usually longer acquisition time

near of the charges of the membranes. The measurement of this very slow diffusion pool requires the use of a non-Gaussian model, such as diffusional kurtosis imaging (DKI), which reflects the microstructural complexity of tissue (see Fig. 1 in the article by Broncano in this issue). Derived parameters from DKI can help in the characterization of focal liver lesions.[12] Compared with ADC, these models provide supplementary information of the diffusion signal from other compartments different to extracellular one (Fig. 2).

b-values selection

ADC calculation minimally requires the use of 2 b values, although the more b values obtained, the better the reliability of ADC maps. In the abdomen typically the ideal higher b value ranges between 600 and 1000 s/mm² in order to maintain a sufficient signal-to-noise ratio (SNR).[4] DKI requires a maximum b value in the range of 1500-2000 s/mm²,[12] and IVIM analysis requires several b values less than and greater than 100 s/mm² although it is feasible even with only 3 to 4 b values.[13] However, the optimum set of b values

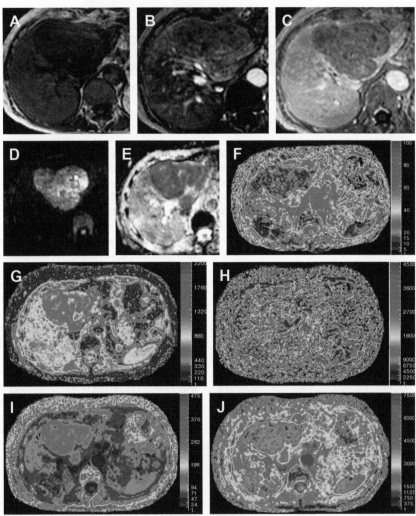

Fig. 2. DWI of HCC analyzed with different models of signal decay. (A–C) Precontrast, arterial, and venous phase of DCE-MR imaging show a large focal liver lesion with heterogeneous wash-in during arterial phase and posterior washout. (D) DWI with b value of 2000 s/mm² shows high SI of the lesion and (E) very low ADC value (0.65 × 10⁻³ mm²/s). IVIM model confirms the restriction of water diffusion of the lesion in the (F) D map with a value of 0.6 × 10⁻³ mm²/s. (G) Increased perfusion fraction (16%) and (H) pseudodiffusion value (D*: 28.8 × 10⁻³ mm²/s) demonstrate increased flow within the nodule. (I, J) Derived parameters from DKI show a kurtosis value of 1. and mean diffusion kurtosis of 1.4 × 10⁻³ mm²/s.

and diffusion model used for analysis for oncological applications in the body is still to be defined.

Clinical Applications of Diffusion-Weighted Imaging

Liver

Lesion detection DWI using a low b value around 50 s/mm^2, also known as black-blood diffusion, allows better detection of small focal liver lesions against a liver parenchyma without vessel signal[14] (**Fig. 3**). This type of approach has been shown to improve detection of metastases in comparison to fat-suppressed T2-weighted sequences and is of special interest for identifying metastases from colorectal cancer before surgery, with particular advantage in the detection of lesions smaller than 1 cm and those adjacent to vascular structures. Furthermore, in patients at risk for nephrogenic systemic fibrosis, DWI can be considered an alternative to contrast-enhanced imaging.[14] DWI in combination with gadoxetic acid (Gd-EOB-DTPA) improves detection of liver metastases compared with any individual technique alone, even after neoadjuvant chemotherapy.[15]

Lesion characterization The role of DWI in focal liver lesion characterization is controversial due to misregistration between images with different b values, caused by respiratory motion. Adequate reproducibility has been achieved for ADC, but lower for f and D*.[16] DWI has been shown to accurate differentiate between cystic and solid liver lesions. Benign lesions tend to show higher ADC values and lower SI with high b values than malignant ones (**Fig. 4**). However, there are no definitive data to support the use of ADC in the distinction between benign and malignant focal liver lesions, due to substantial overlap, particularly focal nodular hyperplasia (FNH) and adenomas with hepatocellular carcinoma (HCC) and metastasis. In addition, radiologists must be alert to potential pitfalls such as low ADC values seen in pyogenic abscess or high ADC values of necrotic or mucinous metastasis.[17]

IVIM-derived D and ADC show inconclusive results in the distinction of benign and malignant lesions, although with contradictory data about which of both parameters is more accurate.[10,13,18] D* and f are useful to differentiate hypervascular from hypovascular lesions.[10]

Hepatocellular nodules in cirrhosis DWI is of limited value in the evaluation of focal lesions in cirrhotic livers. DWI shows a lower sensitivity

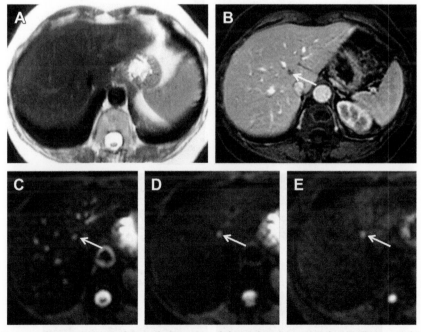

Fig. 3. Breast cancer liver metastasis (*arrows*) detection. (*A*) Axial turbo spin-echo (TSE) T2-weighted sequence does not depict a lesion in segment IVa, which was hardly visualized in (*B*) postcontrast portal phase of DCE-MR imaging sequence (*arrow*). (*C–E*) Axial DWI with b values of 0, 50 and 900 s/mm^2: notice how the lesion is better visualized (*arrows*) against a background liver parenchyma without vessel signal with b value of 50 s/mm^2. High SI on high b-value image suggests its malignant origin.

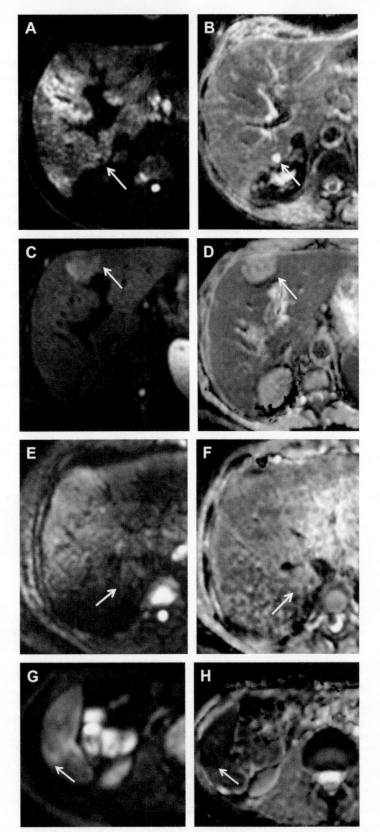

Fig. 4. Typical behavior on DWI of the most common focal liver lesions (*arrows*). Paired high b-value image and corresponding ADC map of (*A, B*) Simple cyst: ADC value: 2.1×10^{-3} mm^2/s. (*C, D*) Hemangioma: ADC value: 1.4×10^{-3} mm^2/s. (*E, F*) FNH ADC value: 1.5×10^{-3} mm^2/s. (*G, H*) Hepatocellular adenoma: ADC value: 0.9×10^{-3} mm^2/s. (*I, J*) HCC: ADC value: 0.65×10^{-3} mm^2/s. (*K, L*) Colorectal liver metastasis: ADC value: 0.8×10^{-3} mm^2/s. (*M, N*) CHC: ADC value: 0.9×10^{-3} mm^2/s. Notice the overlap in ADC values between benign and malignant solid lesions.

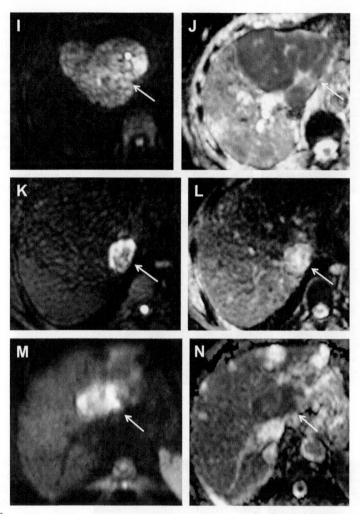

Fig. 4. (continued)

compared with dynamic contrast-enhanced MR imaging (DCE-MR imaging) and hepatobiliary (HB) phase in HCC detection.[19] It also does not allow differentiation between dysplastic nodules and early HCC.[20] However, DWI should be included in the protocol of detection of HCC, because it significantly improves sensitivity when used in combination with either technique.[20] Most commonly, HCC shows restriction of water diffusion, paralleling degree of cellularity and dedifferentiation. Furthermore, a recent meta-analysis concluded that DWI had excellent and moderately high diagnostic accuracy for the prediction of well-differentiated versus poorly differentiated HCC,[21] although overlap remains between different histologic grades.[22] Recently, IVIM-derived D values of HCC showed significantly better diagnostic performance than ADC values in differentiating high-grade from low-grade HCC. In addition, f demonstrated a

significant correlation with the percentage of arterial enhancement of HCC.[23] Interestingly, benign lesions associated with cirrhosis, such as confluent fibrosis or perfusion alterations, do not show increased signal with high b values.[24]

Therapy monitoring DWI has been used for early assessment of tumor response to treatment of both primary and secondary malignancies of the liver[4,5,25] (Figs. 5 and 6). The good reproducibility of ADC measurement means that any ADC changes after treatment can be related to treatment effects. In general, increases in ADC after 1 week of successful treatment can be detected in the liver.[5]

For example, DWI with ADC is useful in the early assessment of HCC response after transcatheter arterial chemoembolization (TACE), and differentiating between viable and necrotic portions of the treated HCCs.[26] Furthermore, DWI can detect

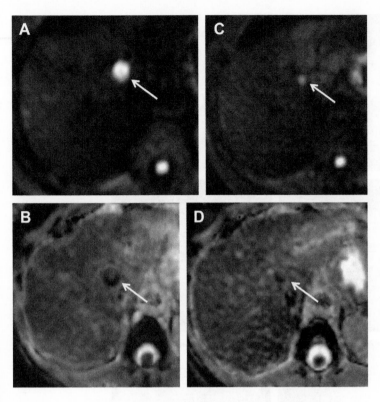

Fig. 5. Therapy monitoring of breast cancer liver metastasis (arrows) with DWI. (A, B) Pretreatment DWI with b value of 900 s/mm² and corresponding ADC map show lesions with true restriction of water motion in segment IVa. ADC value 0.48 × 10⁻³ mm²/s. (C, D) 4 months after chemotherapy DWI and ADC map demonstrate partial response with decrease in size and in SI in high b-value image, with increase in ADC value up to 1.1 × 10⁻³ mm²/s.

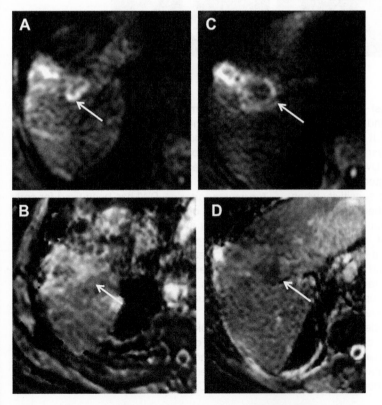

Fig. 6. Therapy monitoring of colorectal cancer liver metastasis (arrows) with DWI. (A, B) Pretreatment DWI with b value of 900 s/mm² and corresponding ADC map show a lesion with heterogeneous restriction of water motion in segment VIII. High pretreatment ADC value of 1.5 × 10⁻³ mm²/s suggests poor response to treatment. (C, D) 8 months after chemotherapy DWI and ADC map demonstrate progression with increase in size and in SI on high b-value image and decrease in ADC value: 0.73 × 10⁻³ mm²/s.

ecurrent tumor after treatment and predict HCC esponse to TACE using the monoexponential or biexponential models of analysis.[27,28]

DWI also can be used as a biomarker of treatment response of HCC to the antiangiogenic agent, sorafenib. First, ADC decreases probably related to hemorrhagic necrosis and, posteriorly, increases because of tumor necrosis. A delayed ADC decrease suggests tumor recurrence.[29] IVIM-related D and f have been shown also to be valuable markers of treatment response to sorafenib for HCC.[30]

For therapy monitoring of hepatic metastases, increases of ADC after the start of chemotherapy or radiotherapy have been related to responding metastases, although there is no defined threshold of increase in ADC to define response.[5,25] These changes can be detected during the first week after the start of treatment in colorectal and breast liver metastases and occur before changes in size.[31] In addition, DWI appears superior to positron emission tomography/computed tomography (PET/CT) for early response assessment of metastases of common solid tumors treated with Y90 radioembolization.[32] Lower pretreatment ADC value has been related to good response to chemotherapy in colorectal and gastric hepatic metastases, although these data were not confirmed in a prospective series including digestive tract and breast liver metastases.[31,33] Furthermore, low-pretreatment ADC value of colorectal

liver metastases has shown an association to shorter overall survival and progression-free survival.[34]

Biliary system and gallbladder malignancies
DWI detects intrahepatic and extrahepatic cholangiocarcinoma (CHC) with advantage over T2-weighted and in a similar manner to DCE-MR imaging. Because this lesion shows the lowest ADC of all hepatic malignancies, its differentiation from benign focal liver lesions using DWI is feasible. DWI also helps in the differentiation between mucus and viable intraductal CHC obstructing the bile duct. The lower the degree of tumor differentiation in CHC, the lower the ADC value is.[35] A target appearance on DWI, a hyperintense peripheral halo (viable tumor) with a hypointense central area (fibrosis), permits the accurate differentiation of small intrahepatic CHC from HCC, because this sign is superior to other morphologic, DCE-MR imaging, or HB phase features.[36]

As with other malignancies, gallbladder carcinoma typically demonstrates high signal on high b-value imaging, and low ADC values (**Fig. 7**). Acute cholecystitis may simulate a neoplastic process on DWI. For this reason, DWI must be evaluated along with the other morphologic images, increasing the accuracy in the differentiation of benign and malignant gallbladder lesions.[37]

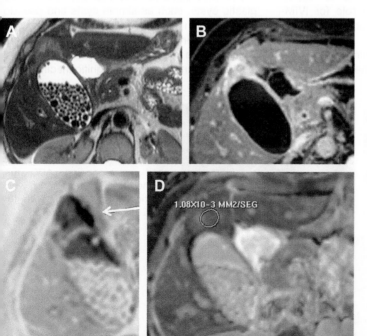

Fig. 7. Gallbladder carcinoma with DWI. (*A*) Axial TSE T2-weighted image and (*B*) delayed postcontrast T1 high resolution isotropic volume excitation (THRIVE) show a mural thickening of the fundus of the gallbladder invading the adjacent hepatic parenchyma. Notice the presence of multiple lithiasis. (*C, D*) High b-value DWI with inverted grayscale and corresponding ADC map demonstrates restriction of water motion of the mural lesion (*arrow*), with low ADC of 1.08×10^{-3} mm^2/s (ROI).

Pancreatic cancer and other pancreatic tumors
A recent meta-analysis demonstrates high performance of DWI in detection of pancreatic adenocarcinoma (PA), with similar sensitivity to fluorodeoxyglucose (18FDG) PET/CT, but better specificity.[38] Most commonly, PA shows high SI on high b-value imaging and lower ADC values than normal pancreas, related to dense fibrosis and increased cellular elements[39] (**Fig. 8**). However, PA can have different appearances on diffusion imaging depending on histologic characteristics. Edematous fibrosis and loose collagen fibers have been described in PA to yield higher ADC than normal parenchyma.[40] This heterogeneity in histologic content is probably the cause of contradictory data in the relationship between ADC values of PA and tumor grade.[41,42] Moreover, the association of acute pancreatitis and PA located in the pancreatic head has been reported. Both entities show a similar behavior in DWI, hampering cancer detection.[39] The use of IVIM-derived parameters, such as f, improves the differentiation between PA and normal pancreatic tissue.[43]

DWI is also helpful in the differentiation between PA and benign lesions, although with limitations in the distinction from mass-forming pancreatitis. There is an evident overlap in ADC values of both lesions, probably due to variable proportions of fibrosis and inflammation in mass-forming pancreatitis and different degrees of PA differentiation[39,41,42] (see **Fig. 8**; **Fig. 9**). However, initial data suggest a role for IVIM-derived perfusion parameters in this distinction.[11]

In the therapy monitoring setting, preliminary data suggest that lower pretreatment ADC values of advanced PA, treated with chemotherapy or chemoradiation, are related to poor response and early progression[44] (**Fig. 10**). DWI is also useful in the evaluation of autoimmune pancreatitis response to steroids. This entity shows high SI on high b value and lower ADC values than chronic pancreatitis and PA. However, with successful treatment, SI on high b value decreases, and ADC returns to normal values.[45]

Pancreatic neuroendocrine tumors (PNET) show a restrictive pattern in diffusion, in comparison with normal pancreatic parenchyma[46] (**Fig. 11**). However, the detection rate of PNETs with MR imaging including DWI was significantly lower than that of ^{68}Ga-DOTATATE PET/CT.[47] Most aggressive PNETs show lower ADC values than benign lesions. In addition, an inverse correlation between Ki-67 (cellular marker for proliferation) and ADC values has been established, which would allow for the evaluation of tumor aggressiveness.[46] Perfusion parameters from IVIM models are able to accurately differentiate PNET from PA.[11]

Pancreatic cystic lesions are a common incidental finding. It is important to differentiate cystic tumors from nonneoplastic lesions and identify malignant variants. Cystic tumors show different biological behavior and risk of malignancy[48] and can be classified as shown in **Box 3**. Cystic lesions greater than 2 cm in size are usually premalignant or malignant.[49]

DWI with high b value can differentiate nonneoplastic cysts, such as simple cysts and pseudocysts, which are usually isointense to the pancreas, from neoplastic cysts and abscesses, which remain hyperintense.[48] Boraschi and colleagues[50] found statistically significant differences

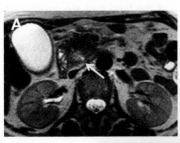
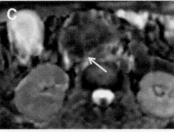
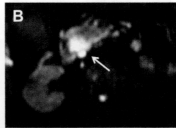

Fig. 8. Pancreatic carcinoma (*arrows*) with DWI. (*A*) Axial TSE T2-weighted image shows an ill-defined mass located in the pancreatic head. (*B, C*) High b-value DWI and corresponding ADC map demonstrate restriction of water motion of the lesion, with low ADC value: 0.9×10^{-3} mm^2/s.

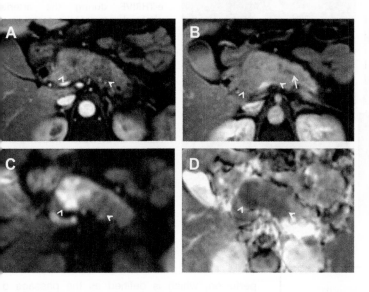

Fig. 9. Mass-forming chronic pancreatitis (*arrowheads*). (*A, B*) DCE-MR imaging during the portal and delayed phases show a large mass in the pancreatic head with peripheral enhancement during the portal phase and delayed heterogeneous wash-in. Notice the distal dilatation of main pancreatic duct due to obstruction (*arrow*). (*C, D*) High b-value DWI and corresponding ADC map demonstrate restriction of water motion of the lesion. Notice how the limits of the lesion are better depicted on DWI compared with DCE-MR imaging.

n ADC values of intraductal papillary mucinous neoplasms (IPMNs), mucinous cystic neoplasms (MCNs), serous cystadenomas, and pseudocysts, although other series have shown significant overlap in the ADC values of cystic pancreatic lesions.[48] More consistent data have shown significantly higher ADC values for IPMNs compared with MCNs.[51] Furthermore, ADC and D values of malignant IPMN are significantly lower than benign variants[11] (**Figs. 12 and 13**). Currently, the differentiation of cystic pancreatic lesions only based on

DWI remains limited, although integrated in a comprehensive MR protocol, diffusion is considered helpful.

PERFUSION MR IMAGING

A mainstay of tissue and lesion characterization in abdominal MR imaging is a DCE series, which assesses the enhancement of tissues at predetermined time points after contrast injection. The core physiology probed by this examination is

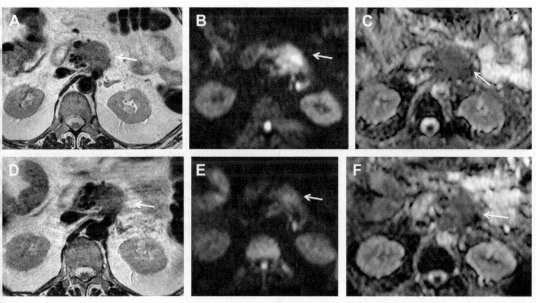

Fig. 10. Therapy monitoring of pancreatic carcinoma (*arrows*) with DWI. (*A*) Pretreatment axial TSE T2-weighted image depicts a large hyperintense lesion involving the distal aspect of the body and tail of the pancreas. (*B, C*) Pretreatment DWI with b value of 1000 s/mm^2 and corresponding ADC map show restriction of water motion of the pancreatic tumor with ADC value of 1.4 × 10^{-3} mm^2/s. (*D–F*) 5 months after chemotherapy TSE T2-weighted, DWI, and ADC map, respectively, demonstrate stable size of the mass, but with decrease in SI on high b-value image and increase in ADC value: 1.8 × 10^{-3} mm^2/s, indicating partial response.

168

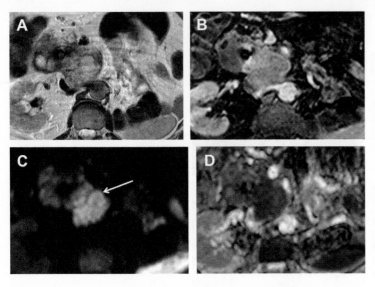

Fig. 11. PNET. (*A*) Axial TSE T2-weighted and (*B*) postcontrast e-THRIVE during the arterial phase demonstrate a large mass in pancreatic head with vessel involvement. The mass shows high SI on T2-weighted image and intense heterogeneous enhancement. (*C, D*) DWI with b value of 800 s/mm² (*arrow*) and corresponding ADC map confirm the aggressiveness of the lesion with intense restriction of water motion (ADC 1 × 10⁻³ mm²/s).

Box 3
Classification of pancreatic cystic lesions

Benign cystic tumors
Serous cystadenoma

Cystic tumors with malignant potential
Mucinous cystic neoplasms (MCN)
Intraductal papillary mucinous neoplasm (IPMN)

Frankly malignant cystic tumors
Cystadenocarcinoma
Intraductal papillary mucinous adenocarcinoma (Malignant IPMN)

Cystic-appearing pancreatic tumors
Solid pseudopapillary neoplasm
Acinar cell cystadenocarcinoma
Lymphangioma
Hemangioma
Paraganglioma

Solid pancreatic lesions with cystic degeneration
Pancreatic adenocarcinoma
Cystic pancreatic neuroendocrine neoplasm (PNET)
Metastasis
Cystic teratoma
Sarcoma

Nonneoplastic cystic lesions
True epithelial cyst
Mucinous nonneoplastic cyst
Pseudocyst
Abscess

---

perfusion, which is defined as the passage of blood through the capillary bed to deliver nutrients and oxygen to the tissue. The current clinical assessment uses 2 to 4 time points after contrast injection to visually assess enhancement patterns in organ parenchyma and lesions, which indirectly provide valuable information about tissue physiology and pathology. One limitation to this approach is that very few images are acquired to analyze a very complex enhancement curve. The arterial phase of enhancement, in particular, can be difficult to capture because of the transient and temporally variable nature of enhancement of lesions during this phase. Moreover, this assessment is qualitative, and factors, such as the radiologist's skill, accuracy of timing after injection, and the protocol used, can inordinately affect the clinical reading. A major frontier in abdominal MR imaging is the development of an accurate quantitative DCE-MR imaging examination that enables extraction of perfusion parameters, which reflect tissue properties. Recent literature suggests that this quantitative approach has potential applications in early diagnosis of liver cirrhosis,[52,53] noninvasive diagnosis of focal lesions,[54] assessment of response to novel antiangiogenic chemotherapeutic drugs,[55–57] and in predicting treatment response in tumors as HCC[56,58,59] and PA.[60]

Technical Design of Perfusion MR Imaging of Upper Abdomen

Image acquisition

The characteristics of an ideal DCE-MR imaging perfusion examination are listed in **Box 4.** Gadolinium-based contrast agents (GBCAs) are used as tracers and image acquisition aims to accurately capture changes in tissue SI, which is

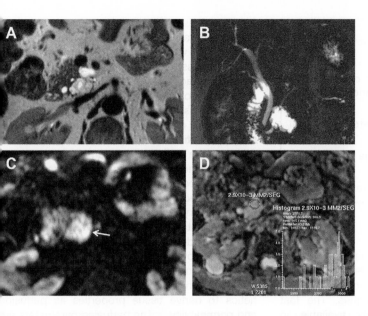

Fig. 12. Accessory-branch IPMN. (*A*, *B*) Axial TSE T2-weighted and coronal thick-slice 2-dimensional cholangiography demonstrate a cystic mass with small locules and septa in the pancreatic head. The mass is connected to a secondary branch of the pancreatic duct. (*C*, *D*) DWI with b value of 800 s/mm^2 and corresponding ADC map show high signal on high b-value image (*arrow*), but absence of true restriction of water motion of the pancreatic tumor with ADC value of 2.9×10^{-3} mm^2/s (ROI). This appearance is due to T2 shine-through effect.

elated to changes in concentration of the GBCA over time. Both extracellular and hepatobiliary contrast agents (HBCA; Gd-EOB-DTPA) have been used for perfusion MR imaging studies.[53,61–63] Before injecting the contrast agent, a T_1 quantification acquisition is performed to determine the baseline tissue signal. This T_1 quantification acquisition is done by using the variable flip angle technique[64]; flip angles in the range of 30° to 60° are recommended.[65,66] This T_1 quantification acquisition is followed by the actual DCE-MR imaging acquisition: a GBCA (0.1 mmol/kg body weight) is injected through a wide-bore

cannula (20 G or larger) placed in a large antecubital vein using a power injector at a flow rate of 2 to 4 mL/s, followed by a 20 to 30 mL saline flush. Repeated T_1-weighted gradient echo imaging of the tissue of interest is performed every few seconds. The capillary transit time in well-perfused organs such as the liver is on the order of 3 to 5 seconds; hence, a sampling interval of less than 2 seconds per volume is typically required.[64,67] Multiple volumes are acquired over a period of 3 to 5 minutes, starting 10 to 20 seconds before contrast injection, to capture the change in concentration of the GBCA with time.[52,53]

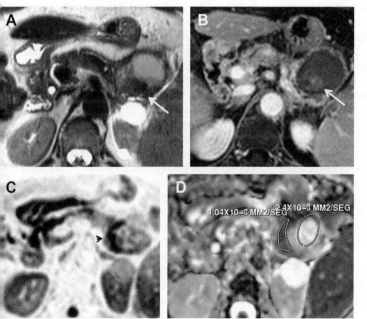

Fig. 13. Malignant MCN. (*A*, *B*) Axial TSE T2-weighted image and (*B*) axial postcontrast THRIVE during the venous phase show a complex cystic lesion with solid peripheral neoplastic component that shows enhancement and a mural nodule (*arrows*). (*C*, *D*) Diffusion-weighted image (*b*: 800 mm^2/s) with inverted grayscale and corresponding ADC map demonstrate restriction of water motion in the solid mural thickening (*arrowhead*), with ADC value of 1.04×10^{-3} mm^2/s. ADC of the cystic component is 2.4×10^{-3} mm^2/s (ROIs).

Meeting the high-spatial and temporal resolution and volumetric coverage goals in a perfusion DCE-MR imaging examination requires the use of ultrafast MR imaging techniques. The fast acquisition techniques currently available in clinical practice use combinations of acceleration technologies as partial Fourier acquisitions,[68] view sharing,[69,70] and parallel imaging.[71,72] Abdominal perfusion imaging based on these technologies has been applied to characterization of focal liver lesions[54,73,74] and in assessing response in liver tumors after antiangiogenic chemotherapy.[59,75] However, dynamic imaging performed with view-sharing techniques involves direct sharing of data across frames, and thus, each image has a broad temporal footprint. Motion can thus adversely affect the images, and at least theoretically, the accuracy of perfusion modeling can also be compromised. Thus, multiple acquisition strategies are under investigation in the research setting, using non-Cartesian acquisitions, non-Cartesian parallel imaging, and compressed sensing reconstructions.[76–83]

Images may be acquired during breath-hold or using respiratory triggering so that data are acquired at the same time in the respiratory cycle. A continuous breath-hold for 3 to 5 minutes of a perfusion scan is clearly impossible—and thus multiple breath-holds may be used.[79,80] However, this results in gaps in data acquisition, which affect perfusion calculations. Imaging using respiratory cycle triggering results in lower temporal resolution, which is inadequate for calculating perfusion parameters.[81] A more practical approach is acquiring data during quiet breathing, followed by use of postprocessing image registration techniques that align the images to the same level.[78,82–85] Thus, ultrafast 3-dimensional high-resolution techniques that enable free breathing perfusion examinations have become the subject of cutting-edge work in the field.[76,77,79–82,84–87]

Data analysis

The data obtained from a perfusion study can be analyzed in 3 ways: visual assessment, semiquantitative assessment, or a quantitative analysis.[68] These approaches are briefly described in **Table 2** along with pros and cons of each approach. Visual assessment is a qualitative evaluation of enhancement pattern of the lesion by the radiologist. The semiquantitative methods track change in tissue SI over time to provide parameters as time to peak enhancement, maximum enhancement, wash-in slope, washout slope, arterial perfusion index (defined as proportion of perfusion derived from an artery, for example, hepatic perfusion index for hepatic artery),[74] mean transit time (MTT), and area under the curve (AUC).[88,89] Quantitative methods allow conversion of SI-time curves to concentration-time curves, which are then modeled using knowledge of tracer pharmacokinetics to derive tissue properties as perfusion and permeability.[90] The perfusion parameters are finally calculated by voxel or region-of-interest (ROI) analysis.

Although multiple methods to model data have been described, most commonly used are compartment models,[65] which are discussed in this review. There is some variability in the literature regarding usage of the term compartment. Some authors consider vessels supplying the tissue as one compartment and the extravascular extracellular space (EES) in the tissue as a second compartment.[74,91] Others define vessels as an input and restrict the term compartment to the EES, where actual exchange of plasma occurs.[75,92] In this discussion, the latter convention is followed. The GBCAs diffuse freely across the blood vessel wall into the EES. The movement of GBCAs from circulation into the EES and then back into the venous system for clearance describes the physiologic properties of a tissue or vascular properties of a lesion. This movement is described in terms of compartment volumes and rate of transfer of GBCAs between the compartments. As most tracers are not taken up by cells, v_e represents volume of EES per unit volume of tissue. The transfer constant of GBCA from plasma into EES is called K^{trans} (forward volume transfer constant), and it depends on tissue permeability and flow. In high-permeability tissues such as liver, it measures the flow of contrast from the microvasculature into the EES; in high flow conditions, it represents the permeability.[93] Finally, the rate constant k_{ep} represents the return of contrast from the EES to the vessels and is obtained as a ratio of K^{trans} and v_e. In most tissues there is a single artery supplying the tissues—a single-input, single-compartment model is

Table 2
Methods of analyzing a perfusion MR imaging examination of the abdomen

Method	Description	Advantage	Disadvantage
Visual assessment	Images acquired in discrete breath-hold phases (early and/or late arterial, portal venous, and one or more delayed phases); enhancement patterns of the lesion and parenchyma analyzed by the radiologist	• No special technique required • Fairly accurate characterization of lesions	• Subjective • Intraobserver and interobserver variations • No quantitative parameters obtained, so difficult to follow-up lesions, assess treatment response after novel drug therapies
Semiquantitative assessment	Change in SI over time is tracked	• Easy to use • Provides semiquantitative metrics of perfusion	• Actual contrast concentration not calculated, hence affected by factors as rate of contrast injection • Not a true reflection of the tissue perfusion and permeability
Quantitative assessment	Change in concentration of GBCA with time is calculated; mathematical models used to derive tissue perfusion and permeability parameters	• Tissue properties as blood flow, interstitial volume, and permeability are derived • Potentially more objective	• Complex postprocessing required • Not available on standard clinical scanners • No universally agreed on mathematical models to calculate perfusion parameters

applied. The compartment model can be adapted according to variations in the arterial supply in organs and number of tissue compartments perfused: a dual-input, single-compartment model is often used in the liver where dual input is derived from hepatic artery and portal vein and the tissue perfused is liver parenchyma; a single-input, dual-compartment model is applied in the kidney where input is derived from renal artery, and glomeruli and tubules form the 2 tissue compartments. Based on the tissue evaluated and the model used, parameters such as arterial fraction, venous fraction, total blood flow, distribution volume (DV), MTT, and capillary permeability-surface area product (PS) can be derived (Fig. 14).

Although quantitative DCE-MR imaging methods have some advantages over visual assessment or semiquantitative methods, variations in physiologic assumptions made at the outset and the choice of mathematical models can influence the values of derived quantitative parameters. Another major limitation is that there are

no universally accepted acquisition methods, mathematical models, and software for calculation of perfusion parameters. Hence, these methods suffer from poor reproducibility, and it is difficult to compare results from different studies. Moreover, image acquisition, reconstruction, registration, and postprocessing techniques for most of the methods described thus far are complicated and time- and labor-intensive. Current efforts are geared toward development of standardized image acquisition and data analysis models so that these powerful techniques can gain wider acceptance in abdominal imaging.

Clinical Applications of Dynamic Contrast-Enhanced-MR Imaging

Liver

Both semiquantitative and quantitative methods have been applied for assessment of perfusion in liver in various disease states.[73] It has been shown that the hepatic perfusion index, that is, the fraction of perfusion derived from the hepatic artery,

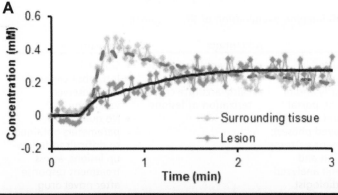

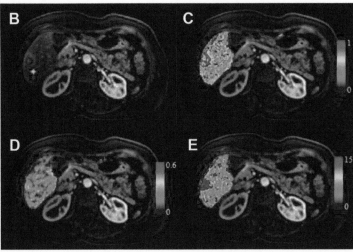

Fig. 14. Perfusion modeling in a patient with metastatic adenocarcinoma using 3-dimensional through-time spiral GRAPPA (generalized autocalibrating partially parallel acquisitions) acceleration technique with a temporal resolution of 2 seconds (A). Representative concentration time curves of both lesion and normal surrounding tissue as shown in the T_1-weighted image (B). Corresponding liver perfusion maps of (C) arterial fraction (AF should appear arterial fraction (AF), (D) DV, and (E) MTT. The AF, DV, and MTT for the lesion (76.3%, 29.7%, and 58.7 seconds respectively) were different from surrounding normal liver parenchyma (35%, 12.6%, and 5.6 seconds, respectively).

is different in patients with and without metastases[84,94] (see Fig. 14), even when the metastases are not macroscopically visible.[95] Also, metastases were found to have a finite PS and interstitial space volume, in contrast to normal liver, which has near zero PS and interstitial space volume.[63] Perfusion MR imaging in patients receiving bevacizumab-based chemotherapy for colorectal cancer metastases to liver revealed that a decrease in K^{trans} and k_{ep} ratios correlated with treatment response as early as 1 week after therapy.[96]

HCC is characterized by neoangiogenesis and derives most of its blood supply from the hepatic artery; this is reflected in the MR perfusion studies as increased hepatic arterial flow, total blood flow, and PS compared with metastases.[54,91] DCE-MR imaging has been used as an imaging biomarker to assess the effectiveness of various treatment modalities. These changes have been documented with standard cytotoxic therapies,[58,59] radiotherapy,[97] as well as with use of antiangiogenic drugs as bevacizumab[56] and antivascular endothelial growth factor tyrosine kinase inhibitor

sorafenib.[55,57] Various authors have reported significant changes in perfusion parameters that correlate with treatment response as well as disease outcome.[55–59,97] A decrease in K^{trans} was the most useful measure that predicted prolonged survival.[55,58] It has been suggested that a 40% decrease in K^{trans} correlates with significant drug effect.[98]

Pancreas

Perfusion MR imaging of the pancreas has been performed using radial k-space sampling gradient-echo sequence with k-space-weighted image contrast.[99,100] A significant difference ($P<.0001$) was found in K^{trans}, k_{ep}, and AUC values for pancreatic cancer, neuroendocrine tumors, chronic pancreatitis, and normal pancreas[100] (Fig. 15). In addition, it was found that K^{trans} values for pancreatic cancer, and for apparently normal pancreatic parenchyma adjacent to the tumor was significantly lower in patients who developed a recurrence than those who did not. This finding reflects the fact that pancreatic cancer is a hypovascular tumor and K^{trans} values reflect blood

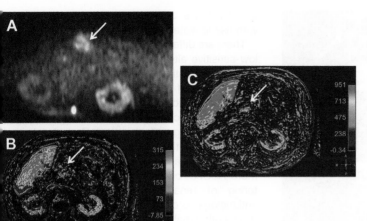

Fig. 15. DCE-MR imaging in 79 year-old man with pancreatic cancer (*arrows*). (*A*) DWI with b value of 800 s/mm2 shows a pancreatic mass with high signal intensity. (*B, C*) K^{trans} and k_{ep} parametric maps respectively, obtained using a bicompartmental model from DCE-MR imaging, show elevated values of both biomarkers, suggesting a potential good response of this tumor to antiangiogenic drugs.

low. Thus, perfusion MR imaging has a potential role in the characterization of solid pancreatic masses, which frequently have overlapping imaging features.

Perfusion MR imaging has also been studied in evaluating response after antiangiogenic chemotherapy in locally advanced pancreatic cancer; pretreatment K^{trans} and k_{ep} values were found to

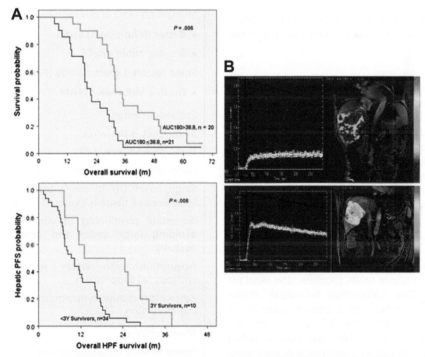

Fig. 16. Perfusion parameters predict survival in patients with unresectable intrahepatic CHC: (*A*) Survival curves. Overall survival in patients with AUC 180 above or below the median value and hepatic progression free survival (HPF) in 3-year versus less than 3-year survivors. (*B*) Prechemotherapy DCE-MR imaging with low AUC curve of gadolinium and corresponding MR imaging show poor contrast enhancement in a less than 3-year survivor, and high AUC curve of gadolinium and corresponding MR imaging showing greater contrast enhancement in a 3-year or greater survivor. PFS, progression-free survival. (*From* Konstantinidis IT, Do RKG, Gultekin DH, et al. Regional chemotherapy for unresectable intrahepatic cholangiocarcinoma: a potential role for dynamic magnetic resonance imaging as an imaging biomarker and a survival update from two prospective clinical trials. Ann Surg Oncol 2014;21(8):2675–83. with permission.)

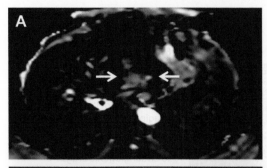

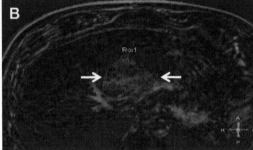

Fig. 17. HCC (*arrows*) shows flow in the subtraction image of FAIR-ASL sequence (*A*) in a similar manner to the enhancement showed during the arterial phase (subtraction image) of a DCE-MR imaging sequence (*B*).

be significantly higher in tumors that showed marked response compared with those that did not respond.[60]

Cholangiocarcinoma
The utility of perfusion MR imaging in assessing response to intra-arterial chemotherapy in patients with unresectable, intrahepatic CHC has been evaluated in a single clinical trial.[101] It was found that patients with a higher AUC at 90 and 180 seconds had a longer disease-free survival (**Fig. 16**). Hence, AUC can be an imaging biomarker that helps select patients who would benefit the most from intra-arterial chemotherapy.

ARTERIAL SPIN LABELING

Arterial spin labeling (ASL) has proven useful to quantify blood flow in brain, prostate, and renal tumors.[102,103] This noncontrast technique allows quantifying blood flow using arterial water as an endogenous contrast agent. A flow-sensitized image (labeled image) is subtracted from a control image in order to obtain a difference (subtraction) image, which reflects the tissue (and lesion) perfusion, as all the signal from the stationary tissue is the same in both images, and therefore, completely suppressed during the subtraction process. Water protons of the blood supplying the liver are saturated using a radiofrequency inversion pulse; when these labeled spins reach

the capillaries of the liver, they are exchanged with tissue water, originating the perfusion signal.

There are different technical approaches such as low-sensitive alternating inversion recovery (FAIR) and pseudocontinuous ASL acquisitions that permit the detection of flow and its quantification. Limited experience is accumulated in the upper abdomen because this technique is complex and very sensitive to breathing artifacts.[104–106] Recent data suggest a role for this technique in the differentiation between solid and cystic liver lesions.[107] Furthermore, ASL has been proven useful for therapy monitoring of renal cell carcinoma treated with antiangiogenic drugs, opening a window for their use for other malignancies of the upper abdomen[10] (**Fig. 17**).

¹H-MAGNETIC RESONANCE SPECTROSCOPY

MR spectroscopy (MRS) can explore in vivo the pathophysiology and metabolism of tumors.

Box 5
¹H-MR spectroscopy for liver tumor assessment

Techniques
Stimulated-echo acquisition mode (STEAM)
• Better definition of voxel
• Shorter minimum TE
Point-resolved spectroscopy (PRESS)
• Double SNR than STEAM

Sequence design
3T magnet is preferred
Torso phased-array coil
Automatic or manual shimming
Single-voxel (10–30 mm²) technique: Only a focal area of tissue is explored
Adequate positioning of voxel is critical to avoiding large vessel and areas of tumor necrosis
Acquisition with water suppression and without fat suppression
Respiratory motion synchronism or postprocessing correction

Shortcomings
Prone to field inhomogeneities
Prone to motion and other artifacts
Limited spectral resolution
Complex acquisition and postprocessing
Needs of T1 and T2 corrections
Limited clinical experience

This technique analyzes the tissue chemical composition of different molecules present in the voxel using nuclei such as phosphorus (^{31}P), carbon (^{13}C), and hydrogen (^{1}H). This last nucleus is the only nucleus that is readily analyzed in clinical practice, because it shows the highest sensitivity and SNR and does not require special hardware or equipment.[108] Box 5 summarizes the main technical characteristics of in vivo ^{1}H-MRS for liver tumor assessment, which is very challenging.

The detection of a choline peak at 3.2 ppm, a biomarker of tumor proliferation, is consistent with malignancy[109] (Fig. 18). In general, the greater the choline peak, the less differentiated the tumor. In vitro ^{1}H-MRS has shown excellent results in the differentiation of HCC from cirrhotic liver,[110] but these results have not been confirmed for in vivo ^{1}H-MRS of liver tumors. Increased choline resonances were found in malignant liver tumors compared with uninvolved liver or benign lesions, but without statistical difference in mean choline/lipid ratio.[109]

Conversely, the data from Fischbach and colleagues[111] showed reduced choline signal relative to that of water in metastatic lesions, without significant differences between malignant liver tumors and normal liver. These contradictory data can be due to multiple contributions to the total choline signal from choline, phosphocholine, glycerophosphocholine, and taurine, which are different in normal liver and malignant tumors, but not detectable with ^{1}H-MRS.[108] However, preliminary data suggest a possible role for ^{1}H-MRS in therapy monitoring of HCC, as an early drop in choline peak is identified in responding HCC to TACE.[109] The use of multivoxel acquisition, fat suppression, and 7-T magnets will probably improve these initial results.[112]

MAGNETIC RESONANCE ELASTOGRAPHY

MR elastography (MRE) has been applied mostly in the detection and grading of liver fibrosis because this technique allows the assessment of liver parenchyma stiffness. MRE requires

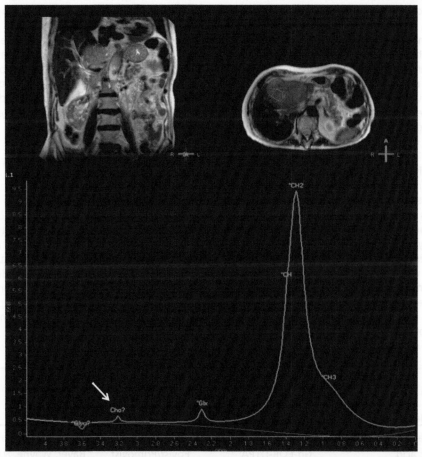

Fig. 18. Assessment of well-differentiated HCC with single-voxel PRESS ^{1}H-MRS, which shows a peak of choline (Cho) at 3.2 ppm (*arrow*) and an increase of lipids (peak at 1.3 ppm), consistent with a malignant lesion.

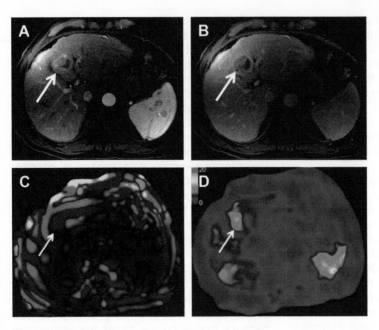

Fig. 19. MRE of HCC (*arrows*). (*A, B*) DCE-MR imaging during the arterial and venous phases shows a nodule with the typical pattern of wash-in/washout. (*C, D*) Wave and elastogram maps demonstrate increased stiffness of the lesion with a value of 8.33 kPa, consistent with a malignant origin. (*Courtesy of* Alvin C. Silva, MD, Mayo Clinic, Scottdale, AZ.)

specialized hardware and software, which has limited its clinical use. Low-frequency (50–60 Hz) mechanical shear waves are generated via an active audio driver outside the MR suite, which are transmitted to a passive driver placed over the liver. A modified phase-contrast sequence is used to image the propagating waves (wave image), which is then processed with an inversion algorithm to generate a quantitative image of shear stiffness (elastogram) measured in kilopascals. These shear waves propagate more rapidly in stiffer tissue and more slowly in softer tissue, and as they are applied continuously, the wavelength is longer in stiffer tissues.[6]

MRE has also been tested for characterization of liver tumors, because malignant tumors show significantly higher mean shear stiffness than benign ones (**Fig. 19**). Preliminary data suggest that cutoff values of 5 kPa accurately differentiated malignant tumors from benign tumors and normal liver parenchyma.[6] These results are similar to those obtained using acoustic radiation-forced imaging elastography. In addition, MRE can also differentiate the viscoelastic components of liver tumors by analyzing the complex-valued shear modules separately. Increased viscosity has been reported in malignant liver tumors. Moreover, a potential role for MRE in the early assessment of tumor response to vascular disrupting agents and chemotherapy in animal models has been proposed.[113] Larger studies are necessary to confirm these promising preliminary results.

HEPATOBILIARY CONTRAST AGENTS

HBCAs have both extracellular behavior and a hepatocyte-specific delayed phase, which improves detection and characterization of focal liver lesions.[25] There are 2 commercially available agents in the United States (**Table 3**). Gd-EOB-DTPA shows greater hepatocellular uptake and biliary excretion than gadobenate dimeglumine (Gd-BOPTA), which has resulted in more extended use and more reported clinical experience in recent years. **Table 4** summarizes some key characteristics of both contrast agents.

Table 3
Hepatobiliary contrast agents used for liver MR imaging

Generic Name	Abbreviated Name	Trade Name	Manufacturer
Gadobenate dimeglumine	Gd-BOPTA	Multihance	Bracco, Princeton, NJ, USA
Gadoxetic acid	Gd-EOB-DTPA	Eovist/Primovist	Bayer, Wayne, NJ, USA

Eovist is the trade name in the United States. Primovist is the trade name in the European Union, Australia, and Japan

Table 4
Main characteristics of hepatobiliary contrast agents used for liver MR imaging

	Dosage (mMol/kg)	Injection Rate (mL/s)	Elimination	Dynamic Phase	Hepatospecific Phase	Maximum Biliary Excretion (mn)	NSF Association*
Gd-BOPTA	0.05	2–3	1%–2% liver 98% kidney	Same as extracellular contrast agents	60–240 mn Patient should be scanned twice Delayed in cirrhotic livers	40	No
Gd-EOB-DTPA	0.025	1–2	50% liver 50% kidney	Less SI on arterial phase Overlap in venous and hepatospecific phase with limitations for hemangioma characterization	10–120 mn Delayed in cirrhotic livers	10–20	No

Abbreviation: NSF, nephrogenic systemic fibrosis.
* No unconfounded cases of NSF after single-agent injection have been reported in peer-reviewed literature for any of both HBCAs. Recent data support the safety of Gd-BOPTA in patients with impaired renal function.[119,120]

Boxes 6 and 7 summarize the normal appearance of common solid benign and malignant focal liver lesions (except hemangioma) and the current clinical applications in oncology of HBCA, respectively. Currently, HBCA have a defined role in the preoperative assessment of colorectal cancer liver metastasis, as they increase its detection compared with other imaging techniques, improving even more their results if they are used in combination with DWI[7,15,114] (Fig. 20). HB images do not rely on lesion vascularity, which is a significant advantage in the posttherapeutic setting, as after neoadjuvant chemotherapy the detection rates of metastases with MR imaging

are lowered, although they are still superior to other imaging methods.[15] Hence, the use of Gd-EOB-DTPA provides accurate preoperative staging and detection rates similar to pretreatment imaging.[15]

Both HBCA perform similarly in the detection of HCC,[115] with initial data supporting improvements compared with dynamic MR imaging with GBCAs for the detection of small HCC (<2 cm)[15,11] (Fig. 21). Furthermore, HBCAs help in the staging and histologic grading of this tumor, although there is still a need for larger multicenter trials to define their usefulness in this task.[7,15] Better defined is the role of these contrast agents in the

---

Box 6

Typical MR imaging characteristics of common solid benign and malignant focal liver lesions with hepatobiliary contrast agent

Focal nodular hyperplasia

Isointense to hypointense on T1-weighted images

Isointense to hyperintense on T2-weighted images

Intense arterial enhancement and isointense to hyperintense to liver in portal venous phase

Isointense to hyperintense to liver in HB phase

Central scar in 80%, which is hyperintense on T2-weighted sequence and shows delayed enhancement

Hepatocellular adenoma

Isointense to hyperintense with heterogeneous appearance on T1-weighted images

Variable signal intensity on T2-weighted images

Intense arterial enhancement

Absence of enhancement in HB phase, although in some cases can show variable enhancement with ga-doxetic acid

Fat and hemorrhage can be present

Hepatocellular carcinoma

Variable appearance on T1-weighted images

Isointense to hyperintense on T2-weighted images

Intense arterial enhancement and washout to liver in portal/delayed phases

Hypointense to liver in HB phase, although well-differentiated lesions can show enhancement

Hypovascular HCC cannot show intense arterial enhancement

Metastasis

Variable appearance on T1-weighted images

Isointense to hyperintense on T2-weighted images

Variable appearance on dynamic series, hypervascular to hypovascular on arterial phase, with washout in portal venous phase. Similar behavior to primary tumor on DCE-MR imaging

Absence of enhancement in HB phase

Modified from Lebedis C, Luna A, Soto JA. Use of magnetic resonance imaging contrast agents in the liver and biliary tract. Magn Reson Imaging Clin N Am 2012;20(4):715–37.

Box 7
Main clinical applications of hepatobiliary contrast agents in the assessment of focal liver lesions

Improved detection of colorectal cancer liver metastasis

- HBCAs have shown improved sensitivity and specificity than ultrasound, CT, and PET in the detection of liver metastasis
- These results are improved if they are used in combination with DWI
- In a recent meta-analysis including 1900 cases evaluating the detection of liver metastases, the sensitivity and specificity of gadoxetic acid were 93% and 95%, respectively[114]
- A recent consensus paper from a multidisciplinary expert panel stated that preoperative imaging with gadoxetic acid is of special interest in the assessment of patients with colorectal liver metastases who are going to be treated with chemotherapy[15]

Differentiation of FNH from adenoma

- Pooled sensitivities and specificities on this task are more than 83% and 95%, respectively, with both HBCAs[117,118]

Improved detection of HCC

- HBCAs improve diagnostic accuracy and sensitivity in the detection of HCC compared with multiphase CT
- HBCAs improves the detection of small HCC (<1 cm) compared with extracellular contrast agents according to preliminary results, although larger studies are needed to support these data
- According to initial data, the lesser the contrast enhancement during the HB phase, the higher the HCC aggressiveness
- Although dysplastic nodules mostly show enhancement on HB phase and not early HCC, there are not enough data to support the use of HBCAs for this task
- The role of HBCAs in the assessment of HCC and in its screening in cirrhotic livers has still to be defined and supported with cost-effectiveness studies or outcomes
- Hypointense nodules on HB phase, but with atypical enhancement pattern on DCE acquisition, should be considered suspicious for HCC and biopsy, or close surveillance is recommended

differentiation between adenoma and FNH, as their use improves the differentiation of these 2 entities compared with GBCAs[117,118] (**Figs. 22** and **23**). HBCAs are also of interest in the postoperative assessment of biliary or traumatic leaks.[7] More recently, decreased excretion of Gd-EOB-DTPA has been demonstrated in the setting of impaired HB function, which can be quantified. In this manner, this contrast agent has the potential

to assess the risk for liver failure after major liver resection.[113]

MULTIPARAMETRIC IMAGING

MR imaging explores different functional and molecular information of HBP malignancies in a single examination. Therefore, the combination of these different quantitative parameters can help gain

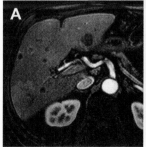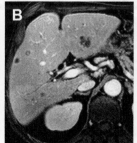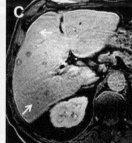

Fig. 20. Pancreatic cancer liver metastasis with Gd-BOPTA. (*A, B*) DCE-MR imaging during arterial and venous phases demonstrates multiple nodules with ring enhancement. (*C*) The HB phase permits the depiction of more millimetric metastases (*arrows*), which appear as hypointense nodules.

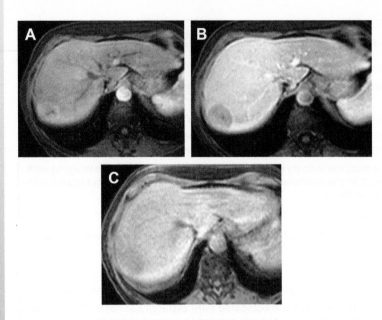

Fig. 21. Well-differentiated HCC with Gd-BOPTA. (*A*, *B*) DCE-MR imaging during arterial and venous phases demonstrates a nodule with homogeneous enhancement on arterial phase and delayed washout (*C*) The nodule is slightly hypointense to liver parenchyma during the HB phase.

insight into tumor biology. Measurement of changes in tumor characteristics with treatment can help in therapy monitoring, radiotherapy planning, and drug development. Furthermore, the combined use of MR imaging-derived parameters with other functional techniques such as CT perfusion or PET can improve results and will be enhanced with the use of new hybrid technology such as PET-MR imaging. MPI is in its infancy and further research is needed to enhance its role in the management of abdominal malignancies.

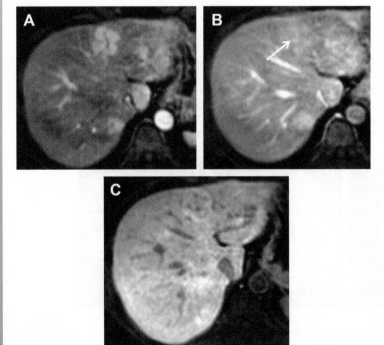

Fig. 22. FNH with Gd-EOB-DTPA (*A*, *B*) DCE-MR imaging during arterial and venous phases demonstrate a nodule with homogeneous enhancement on arterial phase, presenting a central hypovascular scar. The nodule becomes isointense to liver in the venous phase with enhancement of the scar (*arrow*). (*C*) Notice heterogeneous enhancement of the nodule during the HB phase.

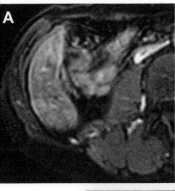
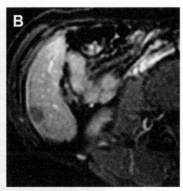
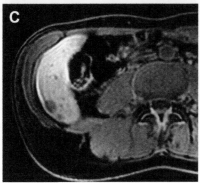

Fig. 23. Hepatocellular adenoma with Gd-BOPTA. (*A, B*) DCE-MR imaging during arterial and venous phases demonstrate a nodule with enhancement on arterial phase and delayed washout. (*C*) Notice the absence of enhancement during the HB phase.

SUMMARY

MR imaging provides multiple imaging biomarkers for the assessment of HBP malignancies, which can be integrated in a comprehensive protocol tailored to the clinical problem. These techniques are at various stages of clinical adoption, as many are technically demanding and lack sufficient standardization and still require further validation. The potential of all these techniques is enhanced if an MPI approach is used to assess tumor behavior.

REFERENCES

1. Bartolozzi C, Lencioni R, Donati F, et al. liver and pancreas. Eur Radiol 1999;9(8):1496–551.
2. Eisenhauer EA, Therasse P, Bogaerts J, et al. New response evaluation criteria in solid tumours: revised RECIST guideline (version 1.1). Eur J Cancer 2009;45(2):228–47.
3. Wahl RL, Jacene H, Kasamon Y, et al. From RECIST to PERCIST: evolving considerations for PET response criteria in solid tumors. J Nucl Med 2009;50(Suppl 1):122–50.
4. Padhani AR, Liu G, Koh DM, et al. Diffusion-weighted magnetic resonance imaging as a cancer biomarker: consensus and recommendations. Neoplasia 2009;11(2):102–25.
5. Goh V, Gourtsoyianni S, Koh DM. Functional imaging of the liver. Semin Ultrasound CT MR 2013; 34(1):54–65.
6. Venkatesh SK, Yin M, Glockner JF, et al. MR elastography of liver tumors: preliminary results. AJR Am J Roentgenol 2008;190(6):1534–40.
7. Lebedis C, Luna A, Soto JA. Use of magnetic resonance imaging contrast agents in the liver and biliary tract. Magn Reson Imaging Clin N Am 2012;20(4):715–37.
8. Luciani A, Vignaud A, Cavet M, et al. Liver cirrhosis: intravoxel incoherent motion MR imaging—pilot study. Radiology 2008;249(3):891–9.
9. Broncano J, Alcalá AL, González J, et al. Functional MR Imaging in Chest Malignancies. Magn Reson Imaging Clin N Am 2016, in press.
10. Yoon JH, Lee JM, Yu MH, et al. Evaluation of hepatic focal lesions using diffusion-weighted MR imaging: comparison of apparent diffusion coefficient and intravoxel incoherent motion-derived parameters. J Magn Reson Imaging 2014;39(2):276–85.
11. Kang KM, Lee JM, Yoon JH, et al. Intravoxel incoherent motion diffusion-weighted MR imaging for characterization of focal pancreatic lesions. Radiology 2014;270(2):444–53.
12. Rosenkzrantz AB, Padhani AR, Chevenert TL, et al. Body diffusion kurtosis imaging: Basic principles, applications, and considerations for clinical practice. J Magn Reson Imaging 2015.

13. Penner AH, Sprinkart AM, Kukuk GM, et al. Intra-voxel incoherent motion model-based liver lesion characterisation from three b-value diffusion-weighted MRI. Eur Radiol 2013;23(10):2773–83.

14. Hardie AD, Naik M, Hecht EM, et al. Diagnosis of liver metastases: value of diffusion-weighted MRI compared with gadolinium-enhanced MRI. Eur Radiol 2010;20(6):1431–41.

15. Jhaveri K, Cleary S, Audet P, et al. Consensus statements from a multidisciplinary expert panel on the utilization and application of a liver-specific MRI contrast agent (gadoxetic acid). AJR Am J Roentgenol 2015;204(3):498–509.

16. Kakite S, Dyvorne H, Besa C, et al. Hepatocellular carcinoma: short-term reproducibility of apparent diffusion coefficient and intravoxel incoherent motion parameters at 3.0T. J Magn Reson Imaging 2015;41(1):149–56.

17. Bittencourt LK, Matos C, Coutinho AC Jr. Diffusion-weighted magnetic resonance imaging in the upper abdomen: technical issues and clinical applications. Magn Reson Imaging Clin N Am 2011;19(1):111–31.

18. Doblas S, Wagner M, Leitao HS, et al. Characterizing focal hepatic lesions by free-breathing intravoxel incoherent motion MRI at 3.0 T. Invest Radiol 2013;48(10):722–8.

19. Faletti R, Cassinis MC, Fonio P, et al. Multiparametric Gd-EOB-DTPA magnetic resonance in diagnosis of HCC: dynamic study, hepatobiliary phase, and diffusion-weighted imaging compared to histology after orthotopic liver transplantation. Abdom Imaging 2015;40(1):46–55.

20. Hwang J, Kim YK, Kim JM, et al. Pretransplant diagnosis of hepatocellular carcinoma by gadoxetic acid-enhanced and diffusion-weighted magnetic resonance imaging. Liver Transpl 2014;20(12):1436–46.

21. Chen J, Wu M, Liu R, et al. Preoperative evaluation of the histological grade of hepatocellular carcinoma with diffusion-weighted imaging: a meta-analysis. PLoS One 2015;10(2):e0117661.

22. Nishie A, Tajima T, Asayama Y, et al. Diagnostic performance of apparent diffusion coefficient for predicting histological grade of hepatocellular carcinoma. Eur J Radiol 2011;80(2):29–33.

23. Woo S, Lee JM, Yoon JH, et al. Intravoxel incoherent motion diffusion-weighted MR imaging of hepatocellular carcinoma: correlation with enhancement degree and histologic grade. Radiology 2014;270(3):758–67.

24. Motosugi U, Ichikawa T, Sou H, et al. Distinguishing hypervascular pseudolesions of the liver from hypervascular hepatocellular carcinomas with gadoxetic acid-enhanced MR imaging. Radiology 2010;256(1):151–8.

25. deSouza DA, Parente DB, de Araújo AL, et al. Modern imaging evaluation of the liver: emerging MR imaging techniques and indications. Magn Reson Imaging Clin N Am 2013;21(2):337–63.

26. Chung JC, Naik NK, Lewandowski RJ, et al. Diffusion-weighted magnetic resonance imaging to predict response of hepatocellular carcinoma to chemoembolization. World J Gastroenterol 2010 16(25):3161–7.

27. Mannelli L, Kim S, Hadju CH, et al. Serial diffusion weighted MRI in patients with hepatocellular carcinoma: prediction and assessment of response to transarterial chemoembolization. Preliminary experience. Eur J Radiol 2013;82(4):577–82.

28. Park YS, Lee CH, Kim JH, et al. Using intravoxel incoherent motion (IVIM) MR imaging to predict lipiodol uptake in patients with hepatocellular carcinoma following transcatheter arterial chemoembolization: a preliminary result. Magn Reson Imaging 2014;32(6):638–46.

29. Schraml C, Schwenzer NF, Martirosian P, et al. Diffusion-weighted MRI of advanced hepatocellular carcinoma during sorafenib treatment: initial results. AJR Am J Roentgenol 2009;193(4):W301–7

30. Lewin M, Fartoux L, Vignaud A, et al. The diffusion weighted imaging perfusion fraction f is a potential marker of sorafenib treatment in advanced hepatocellular carcinoma: a pilot study. Eur Radiol 2011 21(2):281–90.

31. Koh DM, Scurr E, Collins D, et al. Predicting response of colorectal hepatic metastasis: value of pretreatment apparent diffusion coefficients. AJR Am J Roentgenol 2007;188(4):1001–8.

32. Barabasch A, Kraemer NA, Ciritsis A, et al. Diagnostic accuracy of diffusion-weighted magnetic resonance imaging versus positron emission tomography/computed tomography for early response assessment of liver metastases to y90-radioembolization. Invest Radiol 2015;50(6) 409–15.

33. Mungai F, Pasquinelli F, Mazzoni LN, et al. Diffusion-weighted magnetic resonance imaging in the prediction and assessment of chemotherapy outcome in liver metastases. Radiol Med 2014 119(8):625–33.

34. Heijmen L, ter Voert EE, Oyen WJ, et al. Multimodality imaging to predict response to systemic treatment in patients with advanced colorectal cancer. PLoS One 2015;10(4):e0120823.

35. Cui XY, Chen HW, Cai S, et al. Diffusion-weighted MR imaging for detection of extrahepatic cholangiocarcinoma. Eur J Radiol 2012;81(11):2961–5.

36. Park HJ, Kim YK, Park MJ, et al. Small intrahepatic mass-forming cholangiocarcinoma: target sign on diffusion weighted imaging for differentiation from hepatocellular carcinoma. Abdom Imaging 2013 38(4):793–801.

37. Kim SJ, Lee JM, Kim H, et al. Role of diffusion weighted magnetic resonance imaging in the

diagnosis of gallbladder cancer. J Magn Reson Imaging 2013;38(1):127–37.

38. Wu LM, Hu JN, Hua J, et al. Diagnostic value of diffusion-weighted magnetic resonance imaging compared with fluorodeoxyglucose positron emission tomography/computed tomography for pancreatic malignancy: a meta-analysis using a hierarchical regression model. J Gastroenterol Hepatol 2012;27(6):1027–35.

39. Muraoka N, Uematsu H, Kimura H, et al. Apparent diffusion coefficient in pancreatic cancer: characterization and histopathological correlations. J Magn Reson Imaging 2008;27(6):1302–8.

40. Fukukura Y, Takumi K, Kamimura K, et al. Pancreatic adenocarcinoma: variability of diffusion-weighted MR imaging findings. Radiology 2012; 263(3):732–40.

41. Rosenkrantz AB, Matza BW, Sabach A, et al. Pancreatic cancer: lack of association between apparent diffusion coefficient values and adverse pathological features. Clin Radiol 2013;68(4):e191–7.

42. Wang Y, Chen ZE, Nikolaidis P, et al. Diffusion-weighted magnetic resonance imaging of pancreatic adenocarcinomas: association with histopathology and tumor grade. J Magn Reson Imaging 2011; 33(1):136–42.

43. Lemke A, Laun FB, Klauss M, et al. Differentiation of pancreas carcinoma from healthy pancreatic tissue using multiple b-values: comparison of apparent diffusion coefficient and intravoxel incoherent motion derived parameters. Invest Radiol 2009;44(12):769–77.

44. Cuneo KC, Chenevert TL, Ben-Josef E, et al. A pilot study of diffusion-weighted MRI in patients undergoing neoadjuvant chemoradiation for pancreatic cancer. Transl Oncol 2014;7(5):644–9.

45. Muhi A, Ichikawa T, Motosugi U, et al. Mass-forming autoimmune pancreatitis and pancreatic carcinoma: differential diagnosis on the basis of computed tomography and magnetic resonance cholangiopancreatography, and diffusion-weighted imaging findings. J Magn Reson Imaging 2012;35(4):827–36.

46. Wang Y, Chen ZE, Yaghmai V, et al. Diffusion-weighted MR imaging in pancreatic endocrine tumors correlated with histopathologic characteristics. J Magn Reson Imaging 2011;33(5):1071–9.

47. Schmid-Tannwald C, Schmid-Tannwald CM, Morelli JN, et al. Comparison of abdominal MRI with diffusion-weighted imaging to ^{68}Ga-DOTATATE PET/CT in detection of neuroendocrine tumors of the pancreas. Eur J Nucl Med Mol Imaging 2013; 40(6):897–907.

48. Wang Y, Miller FH, Chen ZE, et al. Diffusion-weighted MR imaging of solid and cystic lesions of the pancreas. Radiographics 2011; 31(3):47–64.

49. Karatzas T, Dimitroulis D, Charalampoudos P, et al. Management of cystic and solid pancreatic incidentalomas: a review analysis. J BUON 2013; 18(1):17–24.

50. Boraschi P, Donati F, Gigoni R, et al. Diffusion-weighted MRI in the characterization of cystic pancreatic lesions: usefulness of ADC values. Magn Reson Imaging 2010;28(10):1447–55.

51. Fatima Z, Ichikawa T, Motosugi U, et al. Magnetic resonance diffusion-weighted imaging in the characterization of pancreatic mucinous cystic lesions. Clin Radiol 2011;66(2):108–11.

52. Chen B-B, Hsu C-Y, Yu C-W, et al. Dynamic contrast-enhanced magnetic resonance imaging with Gd-EOB-DTPA for the evaluation of liver fibrosis in chronic hepatitis patients. Eur Radiol 2012;22(1):171–80.

53. Annet L, Materne R, Danse E, et al. Hepatic flow parameters measured with MR imaging and Doppler US: correlations with degree of cirrhosis and portal hypertension. Radiology 2003;229(2):409–14.

54. Abdullah SS, Pialat JB, Wiart M, et al. Characterization of hepatocellular carcinoma and colorectal liver metastasis by means of perfusion MRI. J Magn Reson Imaging 2008;28(2):390–5.

55. Hsu C-Y, Shen Y-C, Yu C-W, et al. Dynamic contrast-enhanced magnetic resonance imaging biomarkers predict survival and response in hepatocellular carcinoma patients treated with sorafenib and metronomic tegafur/uracil. J Hepatol 2011; 55(4):858–65.

56. Yopp AC, Schwartz LH, Kemeny N, et al. Antiangiogenic therapy for primary liver cancer: correlation of changes in dynamic contrast-enhanced magnetic resonance imaging with tissue hypoxia markers and clinical response. Ann Surg Oncol 2011;18(8):2192–9.

57. Zhu AX, Sahani DV, Duda DG, et al. Efficacy, safety, and potential biomarkers of sunitinib monotherapy in advanced hepatocellular carcinoma: a phase II study. J Clin Oncol 2009;27:3027–35.

58. Jarnagin WR, Schwartz LH, Gultekin DH, et al. Regional chemotherapy for unresectable primary liver cancer: results of a phase II clinical trial and assessment of DCE-MRI as a biomarker of survival. Ann Oncol 2009;20(9):1589–95.

59. Wang J, Chen LT, Tsang YM, et al. Dynamic contrast-enhanced MRI analysis of perfusion changes in advanced hepatocellular carcinoma treated with an antiangiogenic agent: a preliminary study. AJR Am J Roentgenol 2004;183:713–9.

60. Akisik MF, Sandrasegaran K, Bu G, et al. Pancreatic cancer: utility of dynamic contrast-enhanced MR imaging in assessment of antiangiogenic therapy. Radiology 2010;256(2):441–9.

61. Scharf J, Zapletal C, Hess T, et al. Assessment of hepatic perfusion in pigs by pharmacokinetic

analysis of dynamic MR images. J Magn Reson Imaging 1999;9:568–72.

62. Sourbron S, Sommer WH, Reiser MF, et al. Combined quantification of liver perfusion and function with dynamic gadoxetic acid-enhanced MR imaging. Radiology 2012;263: 874–83.

63. Koh TS, Thng CH, Lee PS, et al. Hepatic metastases: in vivo assessment of perfusion parameters at dynamic contrast-enhanced MR imaging with dual-input two-compartment tracer kinetics model. Radiology 2008;249:307–20.

64. Wang HZ, Riederer SJ, Lee JN. Optimizing the precision in T1 relaxation estimation using limited flip angles. Magn Reson Med 1987;5:399–416.

65. Sourbron S. Technical aspects of MR perfusion. Eur J Radiol 2010;76:304–13.

66. Judd RM, Reeder SB, Atalar E, et al. A magnetization-driven gradient echo pulse sequence for the study of myocardial perfusion. Magn Reson Med 1995;34: 276–82.

67. Goh V, Liaw J, Bartram CI, et al. Effect of temporal interval between scan acquisitions on quantitative vascular parameters in colorectal cancer: implications for helical volumetric perfusion CT techniques. AJR Am J Roentgenol 2008;191(6):W288–92.

68. Margosian P, Schmitt F. Faster MR imaging: imaging with half the data. Heal Care Instrum 1986;1: 195–7.

69. Jones RA, Haraldseth O, Müller TB, et al. K-space substitution: a novel dynamic imaging technique. Magn Reson Med 1993;29:830–4.

70. Song T, Laine AF, Chen Q, et al. Optimal k-space sampling for dynamic contrast-enhanced MRI with an application to MR renography. Magn Reson Med 2009;61:1242–8.

71. Griswold MA, Jakob PM, Heidemann RM, et al. Generalized autocalibrating partially parallel acquisitions (GRAPPA). Magn Reson Med 2002;47: 1202–10.

72. Pruessmann KP, Weiger M, Scheidegger MB, et al. SENSE: sensitivity encoding for fast MRI. Magn Reson Med 1999;42:952–62.

73. Rao S-X, Chen C-Z, Liu H, et al. Three-dimensional whole-liver perfusion magnetic resonance imaging in patients with hepatocellular carcinomas and colorectal hepatic metastases. BMC Gastroenterol 2013;13:53.

74. Thng CH, Koh TS, Collins DJ, et al. Perfusion magnetic resonance imaging of the liver. World J Gastroenterol 2010;16:1598–609.

75. Chandarana H, Taouli B. Diffusion and perfusion imaging of the liver. Eur J Radiol 2010;76:348–58.

76. Bultman EM, Brodsky EK, Horng DE, et al. Quantitative hepatic perfusion modeling using DCE-MRI with sequential breatholds. J Magn Reson Imaging 2014;39:853–65.

77. Salmani Rahimi M, Korosec FR, Wang K, et al. Combined dynamic contrast-enhanced liver MR and MRA using interleaved variable density sampling. Magn Reson Med 2015;73(3):973–83.

78. Feng L, Grimm R, Block KT, et al. Golden-angle radial sparse parallel MRI: combination of compressed sensing, parallel imaging, and golden-angle radial sampling for fast and flexible dynamic volumetric MRI. Magn Reson Med 2014; 72(3):707–17.

79. Hagiwara M, Rusinek H, Lee VS, et al. Advanced liver fibrosis: diagnosis with 3D whole-liver perfusion MR imaging–initial experience. Radiology 2008;246:926–34.

80. Miyazaki K, Orton MR, Davidson RL, et al. Neuroendocrine tumor liver metastases: use of dynamic contrast-enhanced MR imaging to monitor and predict radiolabeled octreotide therapy response. Radiology 2012;263:139–48.

81. Michaely HJ, Sourbron SP, Buettner C, et al. Temporal constraints in renal perfusion imaging with a 2-compartment model. Invest Radiol 2008;43: 120–8.

82. Materne R, Smith AM, Peeters F, et al. Assessment of hepatic perfusion parameters with dynamic MRI. Magn Reson Med 2002;47:135–42.

83. Chandarana H, Feng L, Block TK, et al. Free-breathing contrast-enhanced multiphase MRI of the liver using a combination of compressed sensing, parallel imaging, and golden-angle radial sampling. Invest Radiol 2013;48(1):10–6.

84. Mendichovszky IA, Cutajar M, Gordon I. Reproducibility of the aortic input function (AIF) derived from dynamic contrast-enhanced magnetic resonance imaging (DCE-MRI) of the kidneys in a volunteer study. Eur J Radiol 2009;71(3):576–81.

85. Chen Y, Lee GR, Wright KL, et al. Free-breathing liver perfusion imaging using 3-dimensional through-time spiral generalized autocalibrating partially parallel acquisition acceleration. Invest Radiol 2015;50(6):367–75.

86. Michoux N, Montet X, Pechère A, et al. Parametric and quantitative analysis of MR renographic curves for assessing the functional behaviour of the kidney. Eur J Radiol 2005;54(1):124–35.

87. Brodsky EK, Bultman EM, Johnson KM, et al. High spatial and high-temporal resolution dynamic contrast-enhanced perfusion imaging of the liver with time-resolved three-dimensional radial MRI. Magn Reson Med 2014;71(3):934–41.

88. Ho VB, Allen SF, Hood MN, et al. Renal masses: quantitative assessment of enhancement with dynamic MR imaging. Radiology 2002;224(3): 695–700.

89. Scharf J, Kemmling A, Hess T, et al. Assessment of hepatic perfusion in transplanted livers by pharmacokinetic analysis of dynamic magnetic

resonance measurements. Invest Radiol 2007; 42(4):224–9.

90. Brix G, Lucht R, Griebel J. Tracer kinetic analysis of signal time series from dynamic contrast-enhanced MR imaging. Biomed Tech (Berl) 2006;51(5-6): 325–30.

91. Chen B-B, Shih TT-F. DCE-MRI in hepatocellular carcinoma-clinical and therapeutic image biomarker. World J Gastroenterol 2014;20(12):3125–34.

92. Sourbron SP, Buckley DL. Tracer kinetic modelling in MRI: estimating perfusion and capillary permeability. Phys Med Biol 2011;57(2):R1–33.

93. Tofts PS, Brix G, Buckley DL, et al. Estimating kinetic parameters from dynamic contrast-enhanced T1-weighted MRI of a diffusable tracer: standardized quantities and symbols. J Magn Reson Imaging 1999;10(3):223–32.

94. Totman JJ, O'Gorman RL, Kane PA, et al. Comparison of the hepatic perfusion index measured with gadolinium-enhanced volumetric MRI in controls and in patients with colorectal cancer. Br J Radiol 2005;78(926):105–9.

95. Tsushima Y, Blomley MJK, Yokoyama H, et al. Does the presence of distant and local malignancy alter parenchymal perfusion in apparently disease-free areas of the liver? Dig Dis Sci 2001;46(10):2113–9.

96. Hirashima Y, Yamada Y, Tateishi U, et al. Pharmacokinetic parameters from 3-Tesla DCE-MRI as surrogate biomarkers of antitumor effects of bevacizumab plus FOLFIRI in colorectal cancer with liver metastasis. Int J Cancer 2012;130(10): 2359–65.

97. Liang P-C, Ch'ang H-J, Hsu C, et al. Dynamic MRI signals in the second week of radiotherapy relate to treatment outcomes of hepatocellular carcinoma: a preliminary result. Liver Int 2007;27(4):516–28.

98. Murphy P, Koh D-M. Imaging in clinical trials. Cancer Imaging 2010;10 Spec no:S74–82.

99. Song HK, Dougherty L. Dynamic MRI with projection reconstruction and KWIC processing for simultaneous high spatial and temporal resolution. Magn Reson Med 2004;52(4):815–24.

100. Kim JH, Lee JM, Park JH, et al. Solid pancreatic lesions: characterization by using timing bolus dynamic contrast-enhanced MR imaging assessment–a preliminary study. Radiology 2013;266(1): 185–96.

101. Konstantinidis IT, Do RKG, Gultekin DH, et al. Regional chemotherapy for unresectable intrahepatic cholangiocarcinoma: a potential role for dynamic magnetic resonance imaging as an imaging biomarker and a survival update from two prospective clinical trials. Ann Surg Oncol 2014;21(8):2675–83.

102. Sánchez-González J, Luna A, da Cruz LC. Perfusion imaging by magnetic resonance. In: Luna A, Vilanova JC, da Cruz LC, et al, editors. Functional imaging in oncology: biophysical basis and technical approaches, vol. 1. Berlin: Springer; 2014. p. 341–76.

103. Cai W, Li F, Wang J, et al. A comparison of arterial spin labeling perfusion MRI and DCE-MRI in human prostate cancer. NMR Biomed 2014;27(7): 817–25.

104. Bazelaire C De, Rofsky NM, Duhamel G, et al. Arterial spin labeling blood flow magnetic resonance imaging for the characterization of metastatic renal cell carcinoma(1). Acad Radiol 2005;12(3):347–57.

105. Aguirre-Reyes DF, Sotelo JA, Arab JP, et al. Intrahepatic portal vein blood volume estimated by non-contrast magnetic resonance imaging for the assessment of portal hypertension. Magn Reson Imaging 2015;33(8):970–7.

106. Schraml C, Schwenzer NF, Martirosian P, et al. Perfusion imaging of the pancreas using an arterial spin labeling technique. J Magn Reson Imaging 2008;28(6):1459–65.

107. Luna A, Martin T, Alcala-Mata L, et al. Feasibility of arterial spin label to differentiate solid and cystic focal liver lesions. Scientific poster gastrointestinal (MR technique). RSNA; 2014. SSQ08–2.

108. ter Voert EG, Heijmen L, van Laarhoven HW, et al. In vivo magnetic resonance spectroscopy of liver tumors and metastases. World J Gastroenterol 2011;17(47):5133–49.

109. Kuo YT, Li CW, Chen CY, et al. In vivo proton magnetic resonance spectroscopy of large focal hepatic lesions and metabolite change of hepatocellular carcinoma before and after transcatheter arterial chemoembolization using 3.0-T MR scanner. J Magn Reson Imaging 2004;19(5):598–604.

110. Soper R, Himmelreich U, Painter D, et al. Pathology of hepatocellular carcinoma and its precursors using proton magnetic resonance spectroscopy and a statistical classification strategy. Pathology 2002;34(5):417–22.

111. Fischbach F, Schirmer T, Thormann M, et al. Quantitative proton magnetic resonance spectroscopy of the normal liver and malignant hepatic lesions at 3.0 Tesla. Eur Radiol 2008; 18(11):2549–58.

112. Xu L, Liu B, Huang Y, et al. 3.0 T proton magnetic resonance spectroscopy of the liver: quantification of choline. World J Gastroenterol 2013;19(9):1472–7.

113. Van Beers BE, Daire JL, Garteiser P. New imaging techniques for liver diseases. J Hepatol 2015; 62(3):690–700.

114. Chen L, Zhang J, Zhang L, et al. Meta-analysis of gadoxetic acid disodium (Gd-EOB-DTPA)-enhanced magnetic resonance imaging for the detection of liver metastases. PLoS One 2012; 7(11):e48681.

115. Park Y, Kim SH, Kim SH, et al. Gadoxetic acid (Gd-EOB-DTPA)-enhanced MRI versus gadobenate dimeglumine (Gd-BOPTA)-enhanced MRI for pre-operatively detecting hepatocellular carcinoma: an initial experience. Korean J Radiol 2010;11(4): 433–40.

116. Marin D, Di Martino M, Guerrisi A, et al. Hepatocellular carcinoma in patients with cirrhosis: qualitative comparison of gadobenate dimeglumine-enhanced MR imaging and multiphasic 64-section CT. Radiology 2009;251(1):85–95.

117. Grazioli L, Morana G, Kirchin MA, et al. Accurate differentiation of focal nodular hyperplasia from hepatic adenoma at gadobenate dimeglumine-enhanced MR imaging: prospective study. Radiology 2005;236(1):166–77.

118. Grazioli L, Bondioni MP, Haradome H, et al. Hepatocellular adenoma and focal nodular hyperplasia: value of gadoxetic acid-enhanced MR imaging in differential diagnosis. Radiology 2012;262(2): 520–9.

119. Soulez G, Bloomgarden DC, Rofsky NM, et al. Prospective cohort study of nephrogenic systemic fibrosis in patients with stage 3-5 chronic kidney disease undergoing MRI with injected gadobenate dimeglumine or gadoteridol. AJR Am J Roentgenol 2015;205(3):469–78.

120. Nandwana SB, Moreno CC, Osipow MT, et al. Gadobenate dimeglumine administration and nephrogenic systemic fibrosis: Is there a real risk in patients with impaired renal function? Radiology 2015;276(3):741–7.

Role of Multiparametric MR Imaging in Malignancies of the Urogenital Tract

Alberto Diaz de Leon, MD, Daniel Costa, MD,
Ivan Pedrosa, MD*

KEYWORDS

- MR imaging • Diffusion-weighted imaging • Dynamic contrast-enhanced MR imaging
- Arterial spin labeling • Kidney cancer • Prostate cancer • Urothelial carcinoma

KEY POINTS

- Multiparametric MR imaging (mpMRI) protocols include standard sequences tailored for the morphologic evaluation of urogenital tract malignancies that take into account specific needs, such as spatial resolution, respiratory compensation strategies versus breath-hold imaging, and anatomic coverage.
- mpMRI also includes acquisitions that provide information about the tumor microenvironment and that extend beyond their morphologic assessment, such as diffusion-weighted imaging (DWI), dynamic contrast-enhanced (DCE) MR imaging, and arterial spin-labeled (ASL) strategies.
- mpMRI may offer detailed preoperative insight into renal cell carcinoma (RCC) histologic subtype and grade and provide an opportunity to quantitatively assess tumor response to targeted therapies in patients with metastatic disease.
- DWI and apparent diffusion coefficient (ADC) values may play a role in predicting histologic grade and potential treatment response of urothelial carcinoma.
- The role of mpMRI in the evaluation of prostate cancer extends beyond tumor staging and now includes disease identification/localization prior to targeted biopsy as well as follow-up of patients on active surveillance.

INTRODUCTION

The term, *mpMRI*, is increasingly used in reference to an approach that takes advantage of the added value of different MR imaging acquisitions to evaluate patients with different tumors, including genitourinary (GU) malignancies. These approaches often include anatomic T1-weighted and T2-weighted images of the region of interest combined with other acquisitions, such as DWI and/or DCE imaging, to provide information about the tumor microenvironment beyond what can be achieved with any single sequence alone. Appropriately performed, these mpMRI protocols offer anatomic insight and possibly qualitative, semi-quantitative, and fully quantitative imaging biomarkers, which attempt to reflect the underlying tumor histopathology and biological behavior. This is best illustrated in the characterization and risk stratification of renal and prostate masses, grading of ureteral malignancies, and staging of bladder cancer, settings where the radiologist

The authors have nothing to disclose.
Department of Radiology, University of Texas Southwestern Medical Center, 2201 Inwood Road, 2nd Floor, Suite 202, Dallas, TX, USA
* Corresponding author.
E-mail address: ivan.pedrosa@UTSouthwestern.edu

has the opportunity to influence clinical management. Moreover, these methods can be applied to quantitatively monitoring tumor response to therapy.

This review discusses technical aspects and the clinical role of mpMRI protocols in the evaluation of malignancies of the urogenital tract, including the kidney, ureter, bladder, and prostate.

MULTIPARAMETRIC MR IMAGING— TECHNIQUES

Most mpMRI protocols share similar imaging strategies, although different sequences may be applied depending on the body part imaged due to anatomic and practical considerations. Imaging the kidneys has inherent challenges resulting from large degree of motion associated with respiration compared with imaging the prostate, for example, which does not move as much. The size of these organs also influences the spatial resolution of the mpMRI acquisitions. Thus, fast, motion-insensitive sequences or motion-compensated strategies with modest spatial resolution are preferred in the abdomen compared with longer, high-resolution scans in the pelvis.

The MR imaging protocols used for the evaluation of renal masses have been discussed elsewhere.[1–5] Examinations can be performed at either 1.5T or 3T, although use of a phased-array body coil is mandatory for an optimal examination. Both 2-D and 3-D acquisitions are used in most renal mass protocols.

Although standard MR imaging protocols for abdominal imaging allow for evaluation of the ureters, a dedicated magnetic resonance (MR) urography (MRU) protocol[4,6–8] offers advantages in the assessment of primary and secondary malignancies involving the ureters. The MRU protocol at the authors' institution is similar to the mpMRI protocol for evaluation of renal masses with the addition of several sequences to optimize visualization of the collecting systems, ureter, and bladder (discussed later).

Dedicated mpMRI protocols for assessment of bladder tumors are less broadly adopted in clinical practice, although they are described elsewhere.[9–12] Optimal evaluation requires high spatial resolution images with a phased-array surface coil. Dedicated pelvic coils or those with larger number of coil elements over a small anatomic area, such as a cardiac coil, tend to provide better image quality for targeted imaging of the pelvis. The use of an endorectal coil (ERC) for evaluation of bladder base and posterior bladder tumors has also been described elsewhere, although it is not routinely used at the authors' institution.[13]

There are a few unique issues that must be considered when imaging the bladder. Small tumors may be obscured in an underdistended bladder. Bladder overdistention may lead to discomfort, which might result in increased voluntary motion and decreased sensitivity to flat and small tumors. Optimal bladder distention can be achieved by asking the patient to void 2 hours prior to imaging.[9] Assessment of small lesions before and after contrast can be further challenged by progressive filling of the bladder during the MR imaging examination, making the image coregistration difficult. Motion artifacts as a result of bowel peristalsis can degrade images, although administering hyoscyamine (oral or sublingual) or glucagon (intramuscular or intravenous) prior to imaging can be helpful.[14] Finally, chemical shift artifacts at the fat-water interface are commonly encountered when imaging the bladder and can limit evaluation of the bladder wall. Increasing the receiving bandwidth and changing the direction of the frequency-encoding gradient are ways to reduce or displace this artifact, respectively.[15]

The standard sequences in the mpMRI protocol for the evaluation of the prostate have been described elsewhere[16] and are now widely accepted.[17] Currently, there is, however, no consensus regarding the appropriate choice of hardware when imaging the prostate, specifically regarding whether an ERC should be used.[17] At 1.5T, the use of an ERC is generally supported and is superior to an external coil alone for evaluation of prostate cancer.[18–21] 3T imaging without an ERC is supported by the superior signal-to-noise ratio (SNR) compared with 1.5T scanners as well as lower costs, improved patient work flow, and presumed patient acceptance due to discomfort associated with the ERC.[22,23] The reported image quality of 3T MR imaging without ERC is similar that of 1.5T MR imaging using an ERC[24]; however, comparisons of diagnostic performance with both 1.5T and 3T strategies with and without the ERC are lacking.[25]

Prostate imaging is optimized by adequate patient preparation. Patients are asked to avoid ejaculation at least 3 days prior to imaging to increase seminal vesicle distention. In postbiopsy patients, imaging should be avoided, if possible, for at least 6 weeks after the procedure because hemorrhage and architectural distortion may mimic or obscure tumors as well as capsular disruption.[17]

T2-Weighted Sequences

Depending on the organ of interest, T2-weighted spin-echo acquisitions can be obtained using either multishot or single-shot techniques, with or without at suppression. The authors prefer half-Fourier single-shot turbo spin-echo (HASTE)/single-shot fast spin-echo (SSFSE)/single-shot turbo spin-echo (SSTSE) sequences for T2-weighted imaging of the kidneys and upper GU tract. The fast, sequential acquisitions enabled by these sequences are particularly useful in the upper abdomen where diaphragmatic motion can result in significant image degradation. The addition of fat-suppression strategies helps improve image contrast.

T2-weighted multishot sequences provide the additional benefits of greater image contrast, SNR, and spatial resolution compared with single-shot techniques, although they are more vulnerable to motion artifacts. Multishot techniques can be combined with a variety of respiratory compensation strategies to eliminate or improve motion artifacts, although imaging times are further increased. Novel acquisition strategies, such as those using rotating blades during k-space acquisition (eg, Propeller [GE Healthcare, Waukesha, WI], Blade [Siemens Healthcare, Erlangen, Germany], MultiVane [Philips Healthcare, Best, The Netherlands]), are particularly effective in eliminating respiratory-associated artifacts.

Heavily T2-weighted images using long echo times and thick-slice profile acquired in the coronal plane are useful in the evaluation of the collecting system and ureters. These rely on the intrinsic long T2 relaxation time of urine to display hyperintense signal in the GU track against the dark, suppressed background on a single 2-D image. Evaluation of the GU tract is feasible using a variety of 2-D breath-held, thick-slab acquisitions, such as HASTE/SSFSE/SSTSE or rapid acquisition with relaxation enhancement, as well as respiratory-triggered 3-D fast spin-echo (FSE)/turbo spin-echo sequences. Fat saturation techniques can provide additional optimization in the background suppression. Volumetric acquisitions help evaluate complex anatomy and pathology using multiplanar reconstructions and 3-D reformations, such as maximum intensity projection and volume rendering. In contrast, the short acquisition time (ie, approximately 2 seconds per image) of 2-D acquisitions offer the opportunity to create cinelike acquisitions, which can be helpful in distinguish areas of ureteral peristalsis from true pathology (ie, stenosis).

Multiplanar high-resolution, free-breathing, T2-weighted multishot FSE images are preferred for evaluation of malignancies in the bladder. A saturation band placed over the subcutaneous fat in the anterior abdominal wall can help mitigate respiratory ghosting artifacts, although caution must be taken to avoid obscuring the anterior bladder. Other respiratory compensation strategies and alternative k-space acquisitions, such as rotating blades in k-space, may be useful although usually require longer acquisition times. Patient motion artifacts can still be problematic in some cases and may necessitate use of motion-insensitive SSFSE techniques. Steady-state free-precession sequences provide images with very high SNR where fluid and blood vessels are hyperintense, although limited by off-resonance artifacts when applied to a large field of view. The addition of fluid-attenuated inversion recovery strategies has been advocated to achieve T2-weighted evaluation of tumors while suppressing hyperintense urine signal.[26]

Assessment of patients with known or suspected prostatic cancer requires high-resolution, small field of view (eg, 180–220 mm) multiplanar T2-weighted FSE images, with axial images considered the workhorse for depiction of anatomy with optimal distinction between the intermediate-to-high signal intensity of the peripheral zone and the heterogeneous, high and low signal intensity of the central gland in most patients. These images are also the most important to assess extraprostatic extension in most patients. Coronal and sagittal images can be included to help distinguish nodular features of benign prostatic hypertrophy (BPH) from ill-defined tumors as well as wedge-shaped abnormalities in prostatitis. These can also help in the assessment of areas suspicious for extraprostatic or seminal vesicle invasion. An FSE acquisition with an echo time between 90 to 120 ms provides optimal soft-tissue contrast for delineation of prostatic cancers against the hyperintense peripheral zone.[27,28] Detection of extraprostatic extension may be improved with the utilization of a 3-D FSE acquisition with isotropic voxel resolution.[29] A quantitative approach has been recently proposed with a whole-gland T2 mapping using a multiecho T2-weighted FSE sequence in approximately 6 minutes.[30] Although the role of this type of acquisition has not been yet established, it provides an opportunity to explore additional quantitative measures of tumor characteristics in the context of mpMRI of the prostate.

T1-Weighted Sequences

When imaging the abdomen, the use of gradient-recalled echo (GRE) techniques for the acquisition of T1-weighted images provides rapid imaging (ie, full renal coverage in 15–20 seconds) with an adequate SNR. Depending on the selection of imaging parameters, these images can serve a variety of roles, including, but not limited to, the detection of lipids and noncontrast assessment for vessel patency.

2-D GRE T1-weighted in-phase (IP) and opposed-phase (OP) images, or chemical shift imaging, of the abdomen are used in the renal mass and MRU protocols for the detection of intravoxel lipids. Recently developed 3-D dual-echo Dixon-based acquisitions allow for acquisition of thinner, contiguous slices in a single breath-hold that can then be reconstructed into water, fat, IP, and OP imaging data sets. The thinner slices allow for detection of smaller amounts of intratumoral lipids. Alternatively, Dixon-based sequences with multiple echoes (eg, 6 echoes) offer a way to not only detect but also quantify intralesional lipids, which may provide additional information about tumor biology (**Fig. 1**).

Determination of the tissue T1-relaxation time (T1-mapping) may be necessary when performing quantitative analysis of DCE data sets. There are different strategies to accomplish this, such as separate T1 acquisitions obtained with the same parameters as those for the DCE protocol but with variable flip angles (eg, 2°, 5°, and 10°), Look-Locker acquisitions, and modified Look-Locker acquisitions.[31]

Contrast-Enhanced Imaging

Although the terms, *DCE MR imaging* and *multiphasic contrast-enhanced (MCE) MR imaging*, are often used interchangeably, these refer to different imaging acquisition strategies. MCE MR imaging and CT are analogous in that images are acquired during specific phases, usually at 2 to 4 specific times after the contrast administration. MCE MR imaging protocols are based on lower temporal, higher spatial-resolution acquisitions, which provide some level of temporal information while maintaining the high spatial resolution needed for characterization of disease and treatment planning in clinical practice. This method is best typified by renal imaging (ie, corticomedullary, nephrographic, and excretory phases) and is used to provide a qualitative assessment of enhancement characteristics of a specific organ and/or pathophysiologic condition.

DCE MR imaging involves a lower spatial, higher temporal resolution strategy during the acquisition of multiple serial images before, during, and after intravenous injection of gadolinium to provide a more detailed, quantitative, and/or semiquantitative pharmacokinetic assessment of enhancement. This technique is most often used in the evaluation of prostate masses and, to a lesser extent, renal masses and bladder tumors. Accurate quantitative assessment of enhancement characteristics in a tumor usually requires high temporal resolution imaging, because it allows for the acquisition of a greater number of images. This may be dependent, however, on the intrinsic pathophysiologic characteristics of the tumor.

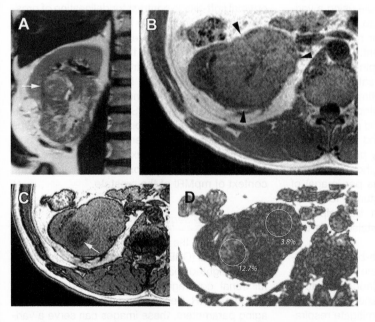

Fig. 1. Heterogeneous lipid accumulation in high-grade clear cell renal cell carcinoma (Fuhrman grade 3). (*A*) Coronal T2-weighted SSTSE image shows a large heterogeneous right renal mass with a more focal nodule in the superolateral aspect of the mass (*arrow*). (*B*) Axial T1-weighted in-phase gradient-echo image through the level of the nodule (*A*) shows near uniform moderately hyperintense signal intensity relative to renal cortex in the mass (*arrowheads*). (*C*) Axial T1-weighted gradient-echo opposed-phase image, at the same anatomic level as in (*B*), shows marked diffuse drop in signal intensity in the region well defined nodule (*arrow*), indicating the presence of intravoxel fat. (*D*) Fat fraction map calculated from a 3-D T1-weighted, multiecho, multipoint Dixon technique confirms and quantifies the presence of intravoxel fat within the mass. Note the high fat fraction (12.7%) in the nodule compared with the lower fat level in rest of the mass (3.8%). The tumor showed histopathologic features consistent with the presence of greater fat content within the nodule.

For example, the vascularity in the prostate and in prostate cancer is low compared with that of the kidneys and renal cancer, respectively. Thus, a higher temporal resolution may be necessary for assessment of renal masses than that of prostate cancer. MCE MR imaging with high spatial resolution offers a semiquantitative, although potentially less accurate, description of enhancement characteristics.[32]

Kidney

At the authors' institution, 3-D fat-suppressed spoiled gradient echo (SPGR) T1-weighted sequences are acquired in the coronal plane. The water reconstruction of Dixon-based acquisitions is preferred because of the more robust, homogeneous fat suppression compared with frequency-selective fat saturation strategies, particularly at high field strength (ie, 3T). A semiquantitative assessment of renal mass enhancement is accomplished by an acquisition during the corticomedullary phase (timed to the arrival of contrast to the kidneys with an MR imaging fluoroscopic technique) followed by images obtained during the early (ie, 40 s) and late (ie, 90 s) nephrographic phase. Sagittal oblique images of each kidney and axial images are obtained during the excretory phase.

A more quantitative assessment of vascularity in renal masses is feasible using a DCE MR imaging protocol, although respiratory motion and the needs for anatomic coverage may dictate the acquisition strategy. An acquisition of a single slice through the renal mass with a saturation prepared 2-D T1-weighted acquisition provides a motion-insensitive (ie, free breathing) and a very fast (<2 s) temporal resolution[33]; however, this approach provides limited tumor coverage. Alternatively, a 3-D acquisition with a SPGR sequence provides an assessment of the entire tumor although with lower temporal resolution and, thus, generally incompatible with free-breathing acquisitions. The authors prefer the whole-tumor assessment using a 3-D SPGR acquisition with a 5-second temporal resolution acquired in groups of 3 sets of images within a 15-second breath-hold. These are alternated with 15-second periods for breathing over a 6-minute total acquisition time. Newer acquisitions using alternative k-space filling approaches, such as different versions of k-hole, radial, spiral, and view-sharing strategies, may provide the opportunity to obtain high-quality, free-breathing, whole-tumor DCE data sets.

Ureter

Neoplasms arising from or involving the ureters are usually evaluated with an MCE MR imaging protocol and qualitative assessment of enhancement

characteristics. The authors use an magnetic resonance urography (MRU) protocol, which comprises the same MCE acquisitions as that of the renal mass protocol, with the addition of an excretory phase acquisition, which is typically obtained 5 minutes after intravenous contrast administration. When using a standard dose of contrast, concentrated gadolinium in urine results in dark signal intensity due to T2* effects. The intravenous administration of 5 to 10 mg of furosemide prior to injection of gadolinium facilitates the evaluation of the collecting system by increasing water excretion and distention of the collecting system as well as dilution of the concentrated gadolinium, which becomes hyperintense.[34,35] Although administration of a low-dose of gadolinium has also been suggested, MRU in the absence of a pharmacologic diuresis is limited by lack of distention of the collecting system.[36]

Bladder

The use of DCE MR imaging or MCE MR imaging approaches for assessment of bladder tumors varies among institutions, because the utility remains controversial.[37] MCE MR imaging acquisitions may provide a better delineation of the tumor extension in some patients, although local staging is usually based on high-resolution T2-weighted images. A single-slice, high-temporal resolution DCE protocol has been proposed for the characterization and staging of bladder cancer.[38] This approach is not widely used, however, in clinical practice, mainly due to limited anatomic coverage to assess the entire tumor. Again, the newly developed 3-D T1-weighted acquisitions may offer an opportunity to assess the whole-tumor with quantitative DCE MR imaging, although the experience with these techniques is still limited.

Prostate

A detailed discussion of DCE imaging of the prostate and the various means of analysis (ie, kinetic compartmental modeling) is beyond the scope of this review. DCE MR imaging of the prostate is accomplished with a 3-D T1-weighted SPGR sequence covering the entire prostate and acquired before, during, and after the administration of a single dose of a gadolinium-based contrast agent administered at 2 to 4 mL/s followed by a 20-mL saline flush.[39] Images are acquired repeatedly for at least 5 minutes. There is debate about the optimal temporal resolution of DCE MR imaging acquisitions. A temporal resolution of 5 to 10 seconds (no more than 15 seconds) has been proposed for quantitative assessment of DCE data sets.[39] Faster 3-D acquisitions are possible and may provide an improved delineation of prostate tumors.[40]

Several models have been proposed to analyze DCE image data sets, with the 2-compartment Tofts model representing the most commonly applied.[41] There is no consensus, however, regarding the best approach to analyze DCE MR imaging results.[17] The authors use a commercially available postprocessing software for qualitative, quantitative, and semiquantitative analysis, for expedited review and increased consistency.[16] Optimal results have been reported using a 3-D acquisition with higher spatial resolution but much slower temporal resolution using a semiquantitative 3 time-point approach for data analysis.[42]

Diffusion-Weighted Imaging

The technical parameters for DWI, including method of acquisition (FSE, gradient-echo, line scan, echo-planar imaging [EPI], and so forth), breath-hold versus respiratory compensated versus free-breathing imaging, and optimal number of b-values, vary depending on the anatomic region of interest. In general, fat suppression is considered essential to avoid chemical shift artifacts for all body applications. Additionally, parallel imaging is often used to achieve a shorter echo time, thereby increasing SNR and decreasing the echo train, thus reducing geometric distortion related to susceptibility artifacts.[43]

Breath-hold DWI with a single-shot EPI technique allows for rapid image acquisition and reduction in motion artifact. Only a few b-values and/or number of signal averages can be obtained within the duration of a breath-hold; thus, these acquisitions suffer from poor SNR, which only worsens with higher b-values. Limited SNR frequently results in poor fitting of the data when calculating ADC maps.

Free-breathing techniques with multiple signal averages are associated with longer acquisition times, although there are benefits from greater SNR, contrast-to-noise ratio, and the ability to acquire a greater number of b-values. Alternatively, images can be acquired with respiratory compensation strategies, such as respiratory triggering with abdominal bellows or pencil-beam navigators. For clinical MR imaging examinations, the authors rely on abdominal bellows for respiratory compensation because of the time efficiency of this approach compared with navigator-triggered acquisitions. Although navigator-triggered acquisitions tend to offer more robust slice registration, the inherent long acquisition times prohibit their broad implementation in clinical practice.

As is true for many other applications, there are no standardized protocols for DWI of the urinary tract. Free-breathing, breath-hold, and respiratory triggered sequences have been proposed and a wide range of number and levels of b-values reported. The number of b-values acquired is based on a balance between the total acquisition time and the need for reliable fitting of the data for generating ADC maps. In general, a larger number of b-values may improve the quality of the fitting for the ADC calculation, although other factors such as respiratory motion and SNR (ie, at higher b-values), must be taken into consideration. The selection of b-values is also influenced by the type of acquisition and body part. As the b-value increases, signal from water molecules decreases as does the SNR. Most manufacturers allow for a different number of signal averages(NSA)/excitations (NEX) for each b-value permitting them to increase the SNR for the higher b-values by adding more averages while obtaining less averages for lower b-values, thus maintaining the total acquisition time as short as possible. The authors use the following strategy to select the number of signal averages for each b-value: 1 acquisition for b-values between 0 and 499; 2 acquisitions for b-values between 500 and 999; 3 acquisitions for b-values between 1000 and 1499; and 4 acquisitions for b-values between 1500 and 2000. In some cases the number of averages may need to be modified depending on the clinical indication, magnet field strength (ie, 1.5T vs 3T), and coil characteristics (ie, endorectal plus phased array coil vs phased-array alone).

Regarding the selection of b-values, the authors use a respiratory-triggered DWI acquisition with 4 b-values when imaging the upper abdomen 0 s/mm^2, 50 s/mm^2, 400 s/mm^2, and 800 s/mm^2. Many variations of this protocol have been reported and may be considered in specific applications. Similarly, for evaluation of the prostate, an optimal b-value has not been established. The European Society of Urogenital Radiology suggests the use of 3 b-values: 0 s/mm^2, 100 s/mm^2, and 800 to 1000 s/mm^2.[44] It has recently been suggested that higher b-values (1000–2000 s/mm^2) allow for improved cancer detection, particularly in the transitional zone.[45–47] Parallel imaging and a higher bandwidth are recommended when using a single-shot EPI DWI technique to help overcome spatial distortion related to magnetic field inhomogeneities caused by air in the rectum or in the ERC.[48–50]

Arterial Spin-Labeled MR imaging

ASL is a method for quantitatively assessing blood flow to a region of interest by using arterial water

is an endogenous contrast agent.[15] Arterial hydrogen protons are labeled using a radiofrequency inversion pulse and allowed to enter the imaging plane. Quantitative ASL perfusion maps can be created after subtraction of images acquired without and with labeling and provide a measurement of tissue perfusion in milliliters per 100 g of tissue per minute.[51–54] Because the signal difference between label and control images is usually small (ie, approximately 2% for brain studies), ASL acquisitions are relatively SNR poor and relay on multiple signal averages. ASL has been extensively studied in brain applications, although its use in GU pathology is increasing and discussed in detail later. Different versions of ASL imaging have been implemented and applied in the kidneys with different labeling strategies. Among these are pulsed ASL acquisitions, such as flow-sensitive alternating inversion recovery and pseudocontinuous ASL acquisitions, the latter offering a more efficient labeling strategy and therefore superior SNR compared with pulsed ASL approaches. Similarly, different ASL readout strategies are available for assessment of renal perfusion and diseases, such as single-slice, multislice, and 3-D acquisitions.

Blood Oxygen Level–Dependent MR Imaging

Blood oxygen level–dependent (BOLD) MR imaging is a type of acquisition used to assess tissue oxygenation by using the paramagnetic properties of deoxyhemoglobin.[55,56] Changes in deoxyhemoglobin concentration result in generation of phase incoherence of magnetic spins and signal attenuation, and this difference in signal is reflected on T2*-weighted gradient-echo sequences. The utility of BOLD MR imaging has recently been reported for the characterization of renal masses and subtyping of RCC,[57,58] although differences among various histopathologic subtypes may be related to T2* effects associated, for example, with iron (ie, hemosiderin) deposition in the tumor instead of differences in oxygenation levels. Data regarding the use of BOLD to evaluate urinary tract malignancies before and after chemotherapeutic interventions are still lacking.

Magnetic Resonance Spectroscopy

In MR spectroscopy (MRS), resonant frequencies unique for protons in different metabolites are reflected by its respective position on an output graph. The strength of the MR signal is proportional to the number of protons at that frequency. Its role in the evaluation of the urinary tract remains largely investigational. In the kidney, studies have shown that MRS in metastatic RCC (mRCC)

demonstrate a significantly lower ratio of signal at a 5.4-ppm frequency shift to that at 1.3 ppm (the latter may be correlated with the lipid content in the voxel) compared with that in healthy tissue.[59,60] In the prostate, the primary metabolites of interest are choline and citrate. Normal prostatic epithelial cells synthesize and secrete citrate.[61] Accordingly, citrate is decreased in the setting of prostate cancer, which is thought to be due to both loss of normal cellular function and luminal morphology/organization.[62,63] Choline, a marker of cell turnover, is elevated in prostate cancer.[64] Despite its potential as a metabolic biomarker in GU cancer, MRS is rarely used in clinical practice due to difficult implementation (eg, common technical failures) with the exception of a few centers with specific expertise in this technique.

CLINICAL APPLICATIONS
Kidney

MR imaging can play an important role in the evaluation of renal masses by providing an opportunity to reliably diagnose benign tumors, such as classic angiomyolipomas, containing bulk adipose tissue. MR imaging can also narrow the differential diagnosis in patients with suspected angiomyolipomas without visible fat, facilitating the recommendation to proceed with a diagnostic percutaneous biopsy and thereby avoid an unnecessary surgery. In some instances, MR imaging allows for a specific histopathologic diagnosis and even tumor grading in patients with RCC. Because of the lack of ionizing radiation, MR imaging may play an important role also in patients on active surveillance and those followed with serial imaging after treatment.

Mass characterization and subtyping of renal cell carcinoma
The noninvasive determination of a tumor subtype can have considerable therapeutic implications. Chemotherapeutic options can be appropriately tailored in those who are poor surgical candidates or have metastatic disease.[65,66] Alternatively, subtyping may be helpful to the urologist for operative planning in surgical candidates.

The 3 most common subtypes of RCC include clear cell RCC (ccRCC, 65%–80%), papillary RCC (pRCC, 10%–15%), and chromophone RCC (chrRCC, 4%–11%).[67,68] These subtypes can be differentiated based on certain imaging characteristics using an mpMRI protocol.[7,69]

ccRCC is a heterogeneous tumor with variable signal intensity on T1-weighted and T2-weighted images, although it frequently displays hyperintense signal on T2-weighted images. ccRCC is a hypervascular tumor and can be differentiated from other histopathologic forms of RCC based on the enhancement characteristics.[70] The average enhancement of ccRCC during the corticomedullary phase is approximately 200% compared with 30% for pRCC and 110% of chrRCC.[70] ccRCC tends to exhibit enhancement similar to or higher than that of the renal cortex (ie, tumor-to-cortex ratio 1.4).[70] On ASL, ccRCC demonstrates high blood flow levels (171.6 mL/min/100 g ± 61.2) (Fig. 2).[71] The presence of a central area of no enhancement, retroperitoneal collateral vessels, and venous invasion is associated with high-grade tumor.[69] Intracytoplasmic deposition of lipids is distinctive of ccRCC and results in a characteristic appearance on IP/OP imaging with moderately high signal intensity on T1-weighted images relative to the renal cortex demonstrating a decrease in signal intensity on OP imaging.[4,7,69] The combination of intravoxel lipids on OP imaging, a central area of no enhancement, and avid corticomedullary enhancement is highly specific of ccRCC. Cystic

variants of ccRCC do occur and manifest as a complex, predominantly cystic mass with irregular, nodular and septal avid enhancement, a presentation shown to be highly specific (94%) for low-grade ccRCC.[69] Interruption of the tumor pseudocapsule suggests locally advanced disease and a high nuclear grade.[72]

pRCC shows a lower signal intensity relative to the renal cortex on T2-weighted in the viable (ie, vascularized) portions of the tumor and favors a peripheral location in the kidney.[7,69,73,74] This subtype of RCC enhances to a lesser degree and progressively after contrast administration compared to ccRCC and chrRCC.[70] Tumor hemorrhage is common and illustrated by hyperintense signal on T1-weighted images. Like ccRCC, pRCC can manifest as a complex cystic mass, though the presence of hemorrhagic contents and peripheral hypoenhancing nodules favor the papillary subtype.

pRCC is classified histopathologically into type 1 (basophilic) and type 2 (eosinophilic), with the latter demonstrating worse prognosis.[74] Two

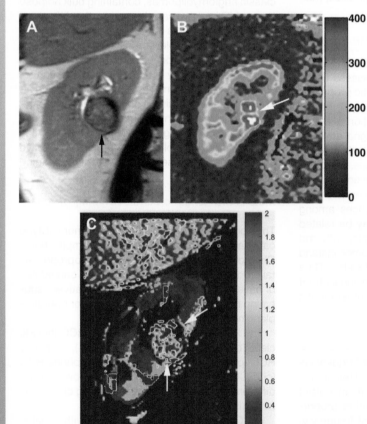

Fig. 2. Low-grade (Fuhrman grade 2). (A) Coronal T2-weighted SSTSE image shows a central, partially exophytic mass (arrow), heterogeneously isointense to hypointense to renal cortex, arising from the mid–right kidney. (B) ASL perfusion map shows high levels of perfusion (ie, >300 mL/100 g/min) within the mass (arrow). (C) K^{trans} map generated from a DCE acquisition confirms high vascularity in the mass (arrows).

distinct imaging subtypes of pRCC have also been described, focal and infiltrating.[75] Infiltrating pRCC is a subtype of type 2 pRCC that carries a much worse prognosis than that of focal pRCC tumors (i.e. both pathologic type 1 or 2), and the association of an infiltrative phenotype with worse prognosis is independent of tumor size and stage.[75] Infiltrating type 2 pRCC is frequently associated with venous invasion. Regardless of its presentation, viable portions of the tumor in pRCC are almost always hypoenhancing during the corticomedullary phase (ie, approximately 20% of that of the renal cortex),[70] with rare exceptions showing enhancement approaching 50% or higher. Similarly, the blood flow levels of pRCC on ASL are lower (27.0 mL/min/100 g $\pm$ 15.1) than that of other RCC subtypes (**Fig. 3**).

The variable, nonspecific imaging characteristics of chrRCC complicates accurate presurgical diagnosis. chrRCC may be hypointense to hyperintense to renal cortex on T2-weighted images and should be suspected in the setting of a large (>4 cm) renal mass, which shows moderate corticomedullary (ie, approximately 50–60% of that of the renal cortex) homogeneous enhancement

during the corticomedullary phase[70] without a central area of no enhancement.

Evaluation for therapeutic response in metastatic renal cell carcinoma

Traditional means for evaluating treatment response are based on size criteria (for example, response evaluation criteria in solid tumors (RECIST), version 1.1]).[76] Optimal response to newer systemic, antiangiogenic agents can manifest, however, as changes in tumor vascularity with or without obvious size change.[77,78] This is further complicated by the occurrence of pseudo-progression, the phenomenon of transient, subacute imaging changes in a tumor mimicking progression. MCE MR imaging is well suited for the evaluation of these unusual patterns of treatment response and provides an opportunity for qualitative assessment of the degree of enhancement.

Quantitative measurements of tumor perfusion in DCE MR imaging are also possible, including intratumoral vascular fraction, tumor blood flow, vascular permeability-surface area product and accessible extravascular-extracellular space.

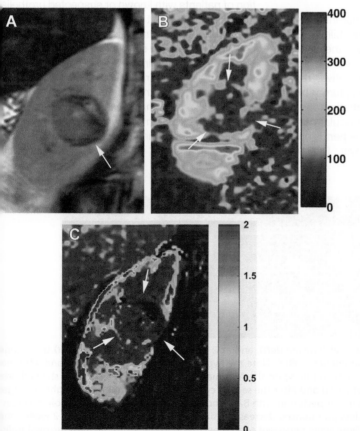

Fig. 3. Papillary renal cell carcinoma (Fuhrman grade 3). (*A*) Coronal T2-weighted SSTSE image shows a hypointense renal mass (*arrow*) in the central, mid–right kidney. (*B*) ASL perfusion map shows low levels of perfusion in the mass (*arrows*). (*C*) K^{trans} map generated from DCE acquisition demonstrate expected hypovascularity within the mass (*arrows*).

K^{trans} is a commonly cited measure of interest, a parameter describing the transfer constant between the intravascular and extravascular space. A change greater than 40% in K^{trans} from baseline to follow-up has been proposed as consistent with a drug effect in pharmacodynamic studies.[79] Two reports evaluating K^{trans} in sorafenib-treated mRCC patients have offered somewhat divergent conclusions. In 15 patients treated with sorafenib in a phase II study, K^{trans} decreased significantly during treatment (60.3%) and both K^{trans} at baseline and the decrease in K^{trans} after therapy were significantly associated with progression-free survival.[80] These patients had higher response rates and time to progression, however, than the overall rates in phase II studies. In another report, changes in K^{trans} and the area under the contrast concentration versus time curve 90 seconds after contrast injection in mRCC patients correlated with the administered dose of sorafenib, indicating its usefulness as a pharmacodynamic biomarker, although these 2 variables did not correlate with progression-free survival and, therefore, were not considered predictive biomarkers.[81] The investigators indicated, however, a potential association between high baseline K^{trans} and a prolonged time to progression or death.[81]

The relative contribution to signal intensity of both blood flow and vascular permeability in DCE MR imaging, however, complicates the assessment of tumor response to targeted therapies. ASL provides an alternative quantitative, reproducible means for directly assessing tumor blood flow. The lack of contrast administration and the virtually negligible contribution of vascular permeability to the measurements of tissue perfusion are potential advantages of ASL over DCE MR

imaging.[82] In a trial of patients with mRCC receiving an antiangiogenic drug (Vatalanib, Novartis Pharmaceuticals, East Hanover, New Jersey, and Schering AG, Berlin, Germany), early changes at 1 month in blood flow on ASL and tumor size were compared with tumor size changes at 4 months. ASL blood flow changes at 1 month were correlated significantly with time to progression, whereas tumor size changes were not.[83] No correlation was observed between blood flow changes and tumor size changes at 1 month. Similar changes in tumor vascularity can be seen with other antiangiogenic drugs (**Fig. 4**).

Ureter and Collecting System

The role of MR imaging in screening patients at risk for urothelial neoplasms has not yet been systematically studied. MR imaging remains infrequently used as the primary diagnostic test for hematuria and assessment for upper tract urothelial carcinoma due to its insensitivity to reliably detect and distinguish urinary tract calculi and air.

Nevertheless, MRU continues to evolve and remains a viable option due to its excellent contrast resolution and lack of ionizing radiation for evaluation of patients with known or suspected urothelial carcinoma, the most common primary malignant ureteral neoplasm. In patients unable to receive contrast, it has been suggested that the combination of T2-weighted images and DWI alone are as sensitive as a contrast-enhanced MRU for the detection of undiagnosed upper tract urothelial carcinoma.[84] MRU has been shown more sensitive and specific than noncontrast CT for the diagnosis of causes of urinary tract obstruction other than urolithiasis.[85,86] In a single report of patients

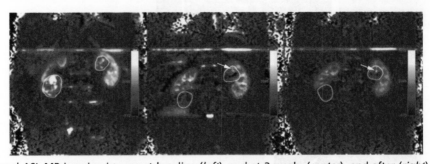

Fig. 4. Coronal ASL MR imaging images at baseline (*left*), and at 2 weeks (*center*), and after (*right*) the second cycle of therapy with sunitinib in a patient with mRCC. Note the hypervascular nature of the right and left renal masses (*circles*) showing high signal (ie, blood flow) on the ASL image at baseline. The right mass showed progressive decrease in size at 2 weeks of (28%) and after the second cycle (40%) on anatomic T2-weighted image (not shown) and marked decrease in tumor perfusion with 82% and 93% decrease at these time points, respectively. The left renal mass showed a less pronounced decrease in size (6.5% and 20% decrease at 2 weeks and after the second cycle, respectively). Note some persistent central perfusion in the left renal mass (*arrows*) indicative of lack of response in that portion of the tumor.

with known urothelial carcinoma, MR imaging was found superior to CT for staging these tumors.[87]

Urothelial carcinoma can be multifocal and can present as a sessile intraluminal filling defect or a focus of irregular wall thickening and enhancement.[88,89] Compared with skeletal muscle, urothelial carcinoma is isointense on T1-weighted images and hyperintense on T2-weighted images and is lower in signal intensity relative to urine on T2-weighted images, allowing for its identification in a dilated collecting system/ureter.

In the setting of urothelial carcinoma, proliferation of benign fibrous tissue in the wall of the ureter results in ureteral wall thickening. MR imaging is able to distinguish this reactive, benign wall thickening from malignant invasion, because the latter is relatively hypoenhancing compared with avidly enhancing fibrous tissue.[87,89] Disruption, or fragmentation, of this rim of avid enhancement is helpful in tumor staging because it suggests invasion beyond the muscularis layer (ie, at least T3).[90]

The ADC value of urothelial carcinoma may serve as a potential predictor of its histopathologic grade (Fig. 5). Prior studies have shown an inverse relationship between ADC values and histologic grade and likelihood of metastatic potential.[91,92] ADC values of upper urinary tract urothelial carcinoma have also been shown to be inversely correlated with Ki-67, a marker of cell proliferation and prognostic biomarker for bladder cancer described in detail later.[92]

Bladder

The role of MR imaging in the evaluation of bladder cancer is primarily in local staging. MR imaging has been shown more accurate than CT in demonstrating intramural invasion and extravesicular extension.[12] Bladder carcinoma is staged using the TNM staging system, and T staging is based on the degree of bladder wall invasion. Preoperative distinction between T1 and T2, or greater, stages of disease is vital in guiding management. For T1 disease, a transurethral resection is performed; for stages T2 and above, a partial or total cystectomy and adjuvant therapies are provided.

Bladder carcinoma can present as a sessile or pedunculated endoluminal soft tissue mass of variable signal intensity, although typically hyperintense to detrusor muscle on T2-weighted images. On early postcontrast images, tumor, mucosa, and submucosa enhance to a similar degree; tumor can be distinguished from the surrounding hypointense urine and relatively hypoenhancing detrusor during this phase.[12,37]

Tumor staging is primarily based on high-resolution T2-weighted images although both DCE and DWI may be helpful. Alone, T2-weighted images and DCE images have limited sensitivity of 40% to 67% and 52% to 85%, respectively.[12,37,93–95] In patients with T1 disease, tumor presents as a superficial sessile or papillary mass. On T2-weighted images, the hypointense muscular layer remains uninterrupted, smooth, and hypointense. Tenting of the surrounding bladder wall may or may not be present. Submucosal thickening often accompanies these findings, although it confounds accurate staging, because this finding may be reactive (ie, inflammatory change and/or fibrosis) or represent muscle invasion.

On postcontrast images, however, inflammatory tissue and fibrosis enhance similarly to detrusor muscle, after peak tumor enhancement. In patients who have undergone a bladder biopsy, high temporal resolution DCE imaging may assist in differentiating bladder cancer from postbiopsy inflammatory/granulation tissue because tumors enhanced faster than the latter.[38] Additionally, DWI has been shown to accurately delineate tumor from normal detrusor muscle and distinguish benign submucosal thickening from tumor; cancer is hyperintense compared with muscle and benign inflammatory change or fibrosis.[93,94,96,97] Hyperintense detrusor muscle signal underlying tumor on T2-weighted and/or DWIs suggests muscle invasion.[98] Muscle invasion can also be inferred when there is ureteral dilatation to the level of an ureteropelvic junction bladder tumor.

Similar to urothelial carcinoma of the ureter, DWI and ADC values may play a role in predicting histologic grade and potential treatment response. ADC values correlate inversely with tumor size,

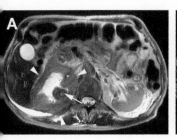
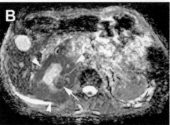

Fig. 5. Upper tract urothelial carcinoma. (A) Axial T2-weighted SSTSE image of the upper abdomen shows a large, infiltrative mass encompassing the right renal collecting system (arrowheads) with a more focal, peripheral nodular component (arrow). (B) Axial ADC image shows restricted diffusion in the mass (arrowheads) and nodule (arrow). Biopsy confirmed high-grade urothelial carcinoma.

histologic grade, and T stage in bladder cancer, in addition to Ki-67, a marker of cell proliferation and prognostic biomarker for bladder cancer.[99] The latter may be a more significant prognostic indicator than histologic grade and pathologic nodal status.[100,101] Prior studies have also shown an association between a higher Ki-67 level and favorable chemoradiosensitivity in bladder cancer, suggesting that lower ADC values may indicate a greater likelihood for treatment response.[102] Similarly, primary bladder tumors with earlier and more avid enhancement on DCE MR imaging are associated with a greater risk of local recurrence after resection.[103]

Prostate

The role of mpMRI in the evaluation of prostate cancer has rapidly evolved since its original inception. Initially limited to disease staging in patients with a known diagnosis of prostate cancer, MR imaging is now accepted as the most accurate imaging technique for detection and localization of cancer in the prostate.[104,105] Preoperative imaging for disease localization may help determine whether nerve-sparing surgery or focal therapies can be pursued.[106–108] The development of MR imaging–transrectal ultrasound (TRUS) image fusion software has further expanded the utility of MR imaging in evaluating patients with rising prostate-specific antigen (PSA) levels and prior negative systematic TRUS biopsies.[109,110] MR imaging–TRUS fusion biopsy of the prostate increases detection of clinically significant prostate cancer while reducing detection of insignificant disease, allowing for a more reliable risk stratification of biopsy-naïve patients and those with known cancer (eg, active surveillance patients).[111]

Prostate carcinoma occurs more commonly in the peripheral zone (70%) than the transitional

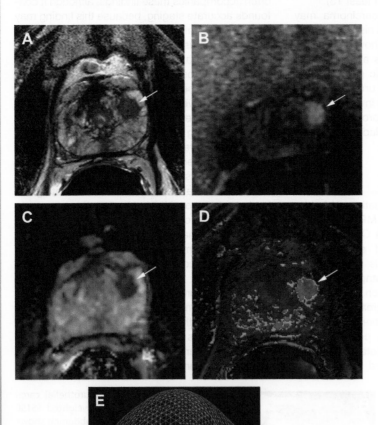

Fig. 6. Prostate cancer diagnosed with mpMRI and targeted MR imaging–TRUS fusion biopsy. A 57-year old man with elevated PSA (11 ng/mL) and 2 previous negative biopsies underwent MR imaging for biopsy planning. (A) Axial T2 weighted image shows a focal area of low signal intensity in the anterior left midgland (arrow). (B) The lesion shows restricted diffusion manifested by high signal intensity (arrow) on the DWI (b-value = 2000) and (C) low signal intensity (arrow) on the ADC map as well as rapid enhancement and washout on DCE, (D) illustrated by red color (arrow) on the kinetic map. (E) Targeted MR imaging–TRUS fusion biopsy revealed Gleason score 3 + 4 prostate cancer in 5 of 5 cores with up to 55% of core length involved by tumor.

20%) and central zones (10%). On T2-weighted images prostate cancer is visualized as an apparent focus of hypointensity relative to the background high signal intensity peripheral zone.[112] On T1-weighted images, prostate cancer is isointense to surrounding prostatic tissue. T1-weighted images are also helpful in distinguishing hyperintense postbiopsy hematoma (commonly hypointense on T2-weighted images) from tumor. On DCE images, rapid enhancement and washout are characteristic of prostate carcinoma.

On DWI, tumors show restricted diffusion with ADC values lower than benign or normal prostatic tissue (Fig. 6).[113] A few studies have shown an inverse relationship between ADC values and tumor aggressiveness. ADC values less than 0.6 10^{-3} mm²/s increase the likelihood of aggressive disease (Gleason 4) (Fig. 7), although substantial overlap in ADC values exists among tumors with different Gleason scores.[114,115] Additionally, in patients undergoing active surveillance, ADC values may serve as a biomarker of tumor progression and likelihood of the need for treatment intervention.[116,117]

When staging prostate cancer, the primary question to answer is whether the tumor is organ confined (stage T1 or T2) or has extended beyond the prostate pseudocapsule (stage T3 and above).

Findings characterizing organ-confined and extracapsular disease have been discussed extensively.[16]

Standardization

The general framework for radiology reporting is said to consist of structured format, consistent content, and standard language.[118] This framework is best typified in breast imaging, where report vocabulary and organization are strongly influenced by the Breast Imaging Reporting and Data System (BI-RADS) lexicon. Lack of guidelines and significant variability in interpretation, however, continue to represent challenges for prostate MR imaging.[119] Efforts to improve consistency of interpretation include the development of Prostate Imaging Reporting and Data System (PI-RADS),[17] endorsed by the European Society of Urogenital Radiology and the American College of Radiology, and implementation of Likert scales.[119,120] In short, PI-RADS version 2 is a scoring scheme that assigns a value, between 1 and 5, to a focal prostate lesion based on strict criteria about the appearance of the lesion on T2-weighted imaging, DWI, and DCE to convey the likelihood of malignancy.[17] The larger the score, the greater the likelihood of malignancy. The authors use a Likert scale scoring system and report templates dividing the

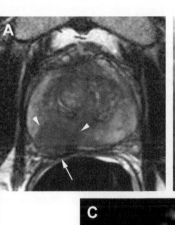
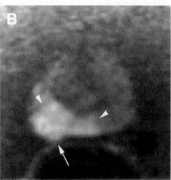
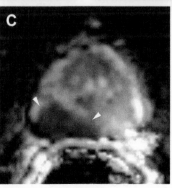

Fig. 7. Inverse relationship between ADC values and Gleason score. A 64-year-old man with elevated PSA (36 ng/mL) and recently diagnosed prostate cancer underwent MR imaging for local staging. (A) Axial T2-weighted image shows a large, ill-defined mass predominantly involving the right midgland peripheral zone (arrowheads). (B) The mass exhibits marked increased signal intensity (arrowheads) on the diffusion image (b-value = 2000). Note the larger tumor extension demonstrated by DWI compared with the T2-weighted image. Posterior bulging of the prostate contour on both T2- and diffusion-weighted images (arrows in [A] and [B]) is consistent with extraprostatic extension. (C) The ADC map confirms marked restriction in the mass (arrowheads) with low ADC values (0.5 10^{-3} mm²/s), which increases the risk of high Gleason score (ie, aggressive tumor) in this patient. Biopsy confirmed the presence of clinically significant cancer with Gleason score 4 + 3 prostate cancer in 4 cores of the right midgland with up to 95% of core length involved by tumor.

peripheral zone in 12 sectors (base, midgland, or apex—medial or lateral and right or left) and the anterior gland in 6 sectors (base, midgland, or apex—right or left).[121]

SUMMARY

mpMRI is a useful tool to depict and accentuate biophysical contrasts to yield anatomic and pathophysiologic information about GU malignancies. The role of mpMRI continues to grow due to its ability to detect and characterize GU tumors as well as assess response to treatment. Familiarity with the various imaging techniques and findings allows radiologists to have a significant impact on clinical management of patients with GU malignancies.

REFERENCES

1. Allen BC, Tirman P, Jennings Clingan M, et al. Characterizing solid renal neoplasms with MRI in adults. Abdom Imaging 2014;39(2):358–87.
2. Nikken JJ, Krestin GP. MRI of the kidney-state of the art. Eur Radiol 2007;17(11):2780–93.
3. Ramamurthy NK, Moosavi B, McInnes MD, et al. Multiparametric MRI of solid renal masses: pearls and pitfalls. Clin Radiol 2015;70(3):304–16.
4. Sun MR, Pedrosa I. Magnetic resonance imaging of renal masses. Semin Ultrasound CT MR 2009; 30(4):326–51.
5. Zhang J, Pedrosa I, Rofsky NM. MR techniques for renal imaging. Radiol Clin North Am 2003;41(5): 877–907.
6. Lee KS, Zeikus E, DeWolf WC, et al. MR urography versus retrograde pyelography/ureteroscopy for the exclusion of upper urinary tract malignancy. Clin Radiol 2010;65(3):185–92.
7. Pedrosa I, Sun MR, Spencer M, et al. MR imaging of renal masses: correlation with findings at surgery and pathologic analysis. Radiographics 2008; 28(4):985–1003.
8. Rothpearl A, Frager D, Subramanian A, et al. MR urography: technique and application. Radiology 1995;194(1):125–30.
9. Barentsz JO, Ruijs SH, Strijk SP. The role of MR imaging in carcinoma of the urinary bladder. AJR Am J Roentgenol 1993;160(5):937–47.
10. Mallampati GK, Siegelman ES. MR imaging of the bladder. Magn Reson Imaging Clin N Am 2004; 12(3):545–55, vii.
11. Teeger S, Sica GT. MR imaging of bladder diseases. Magn Reson Imaging Clin N Am 1996; 4(3):565–81.
12. Tekes A, Kamel I, Imam K, et al. Dynamic MRI of bladder cancer: evaluation of staging accuracy. AJR Am J Roentgenol 2005;184(1):121–7.
13. Sugimura Y, Hayashi N, Yamashita A, et al. Endorectal magnetic resonance imaging of the prostate and bladder. Hinyokika Kiyo 1994;40(1):31–6.
14. Winkler ML, Hricak H. Pelvis imaging with MR technique for improvement. Radiology 1986; 158(3):848–9.
15. Lawler LP. MR imaging of the bladder. Radiol Clin North Am 2003;41(1):161–77 (0033-8389 (Print)).
16. Costa DN, Pedrosa I, Roehrborn C, et al. Multiparametric magnetic resonance imaging of the prostate: technical aspects and role in clinical management. Top Magn Reson Imaging 2014; 23(4):243–57.
17. ACR. MR Prostate Imaging Reporting and Data System version 2.0. Available at: http://www.acr.org/Quality-Safety/Resources/PIRADS/. Accessed June 12, 2015.
18. Amis ES Jr, Bigongiari LR, Bluth EI, et al. Pretreatment staging of clinically localized prostate cancer. American College of Radiology. ACR Appropriateness Criteria. Radiology 2000; 215(Suppl):703–8.
19. Engelbrecht MR, Jager GJ, Laheij RJ, et al. Local staging of prostate cancer using magnetic resonance imaging: a meta-analysis. Eur Radiol 2002; 12(9):2294–302.
20. Hricak H, Jager GJ, Laheij RJ, et al. Carcinoma of the prostate gland: MR imaging with pelvic phased-array coils versus integrated endorectal-pelvic phased-array coils. Radiology 1994;193(3): 703–9.
21. Schnall MD, Imai Y, Tomaszewski J, et al. Prostate cancer: local staging with endorectal surface coil MR imaging. Radiology 1991;178(3):797–802.
22. Heijmink SW, Fütterer JJ, Hambrock T, et al. Prostate cancer: body-array versus endorectal coil MR imaging at 3 T–comparison of image quality, localization, and staging performance. Radiology 2007;244(1):184–95.
23. Lee SH, Park KK, Choi KH, et al. Is endorectal coil necessary for the staging of clinically localized prostate cancer? Comparison of non-endorectal versus endorectal MR imaging. World J Urol 2010;28(6):667–72.
24. Sosna J, Pedrosa I, Dewolf WC, et al. MR imaging of the prostate at 3 Tesla: comparison of an external phased-array coil to imaging with an endorectal coil at 1.5 Tesla. Acad Radiol 2004;11(8): 857–62.
25. Turkbey B, Merino MJ, Gallardo EC, et al. Comparison of endorectal coil and nonendorectal coil T2W and diffusion-weighted MRI at 3 Tesla for localizing prostate cancer: correlation with whole-mount histopathology. J Magn Reson Imaging 2014;39(6): 1443–8.
26. Daniel BL, Shimakawa A, Blum MR, et al. Single shot fluid attenuated inversion recovery (FLAIR)

magnetic resonance imaging of the bladder. J Magn Reson Imaging 2000;11(6):673–7.

27. Kier R, Wain S, Troiano R. Fast spin-echo MR images of the pelvis obtained with a phased-array coil: value in localizing and staging prostatic carcinoma. AJR Am J Roentgenol 1993;161(3):601–6.

28. Liney GP, Knowles AJ, Manton DJ, et al. Comparison of conventional single echo and multi-echo sequences with a fast spin-echo sequence for quantitative T2 mapping: application to the prostate. J Magn Reson Imaging 1996;6(4):603–7.

29. Itatani R, Namimoto T, Takaoka H, et al. Extracapsular extension of prostate cancer: diagnostic value of combined multiparametric magnetic resonance imaging and isovoxel 3-dimensional T2-weighted imaging at 1.5 T. J Comput Assist Tomogr 2015;39(1):37–43.

30. Yamauchi FI, Penzkofer T, Fedorov A, et al. Prostate cancer discrimination in the peripheral zone with a reduced field-of-view T2-mapping MRI sequence. Magn Reson Imaging 2015;33(5):525–30.

31. Treier R, Steingoetter A, Fried M, et al. Optimized and combined T1 and B1 mapping technique for fast and accurate T1 quantification in contrast-enhanced abdominal MRI. Magn Reson Med 2007;57(3):568–76.

32. McMahon CJ, Bloch BN, Lenkinski RE, et al. Dynamic contrast-enhanced MR imaging in the evaluation of patients with prostate cancer. Magn Reson Imaging Clin N Am 2009;17(2):363–83.

33. de Bazelaire C, Rofsky NM, Duhamel G, et al. Combined T2* and T1 measurements for improved perfusion and permeability studies in high field using dynamic contrast enhancement. Eur Radiol 2006;16(9):2083–91.

34. El-Diasty T, Mansour O, Farouk A. Diuretic contrast-enhanced magnetic resonance urography versus intravenous urography for depiction of nondilated urinary tracts. Abdom Imaging 2003;28(1):135–45.

35. Ergen FB, Hussain HK, Carlos RC, et al. 3D excretory MR urography: improved image quality with intravenous saline and diuretic administration. J Magn Reson Imaging 2007;25(4):783–9.

36. Hagspiel KD, Butty S, Nandalur KR, et al. Magnetic resonance urography for the assessment of potential renal donors: comparison of the RARE technique with a low-dose gadolinium-enhanced magnetic resonance urography technique in the absence of pharmacological and mechanical intervention. Eur Radiol 2005;15(11):2230–7.

37. Kim B, Semelka RC, Ascher SM, et al. Bladder tumor staging: comparison of contrast-enhanced CT, T1- and T2-weighted MR imaging, dynamic gadolinium-enhanced imaging, and late gadolinium-enhanced imaging. Radiology 1994; 193(1):239–45.

38. Barentsz JO, Jager GJ, van Vierzen PB, et al. Staging urinary bladder cancer after transurethral biopsy: value of fast dynamic contrast-enhanced MR imaging. Radiology 1996;201(1):185–93.

39. Verma S, Turkbey B, Muradyan N, et al. Overview of dynamic contrast-enhanced MRI in prostate cancer diagnosis and management. AJR Am J Roentgenol 2012;198(6):1277–88.

40. Rosenkrantz AB, Geppert C, Grimm R, et al. Dynamic contrast-enhanced MRI of the prostate with high spatiotemporal resolution using compressed sensing, parallel imaging, and continuous golden-angle radial sampling: preliminary experience. J Magn Reson Imaging 2015;41(5):1365–73.

41. Tofts PS, Brix G, Buckley DL, et al. Estimating kinetic parameters from dynamic contrast-enhanced T(1)-weighted MRI of a diffusable tracer: standardized quantities and symbols. J Magn Reson Imaging 1999;10(3):223–32.

42. Bloch BN, Genega EM, Costa DN, et al. Prediction of prostate cancer extracapsular extension with high spatial resolution dynamic contrast-enhanced 3-T MRI. Eur Radiol 2012;22(10): 2201–10.

43. Skare S, Newbould RD, Clayton DB, et al. Clinical multishot DW-EPI through parallel imaging with considerations of susceptibility, motion, and noise. Magn Reson Med 2007;57(5):881–90.

44. Barentsz JO, Richenberg J, Clements R, et al. ESUR prostate MR guidelines 2012. Eur Radiol 2012;22(4):746–57.

45. Kim CK, Park BK, Kim B. High-b-value diffusion-weighted imaging at 3 T to detect prostate cancer: comparisons between b values of 1,000 and 2,000 s/mm2. AJR Am J Roentgenol 2010; 194(1):W33–7.

46. Katahira K, Takahara T, Kwee TC, et al. Ultra-high-b-value diffusion-weighted MR imaging for the detection of prostate cancer: evaluation in 201 cases with histopathological correlation. Eur Radiol 2011;21(1):188–96.

47. Ohgiya Y, Suyama J, Seino N, et al. Diagnostic accuracy of ultra-high-b-value 3.0-T diffusion-weighted MR imaging for detection of prostate cancer. Clin Imaging 2012;36(5):526–31.

48. Rosen Y, Bloch BN, Lenkinski RE, et al. 3T MR of the prostate: reducing susceptibility gradients by inflating the endorectal coil with a barium sulfate suspension. Magn Reson Med 2007;57(5): 898–904.

49. Scherrer B, Gholipour A, Warfield SK. Super-resolution reconstruction to increase the spatial resolution of diffusion weighted images from orthogonal anisotropic acquisitions. Med Image Anal 2012; 16(7):1465–76.

50. Donato F Jr, Costa DN, Yuan Q, et al. Geometric distortion in diffusion-weighted MR imaging

of the prostate-contributing factors and strategies for improvement. Acad Radiol 2014;21(6):817–23.

51. Alsop DC, Detre JA. Multisection cerebral blood flow MR imaging with continuous arterial spin labeling. Radiology 1998;208(2):410–6.

52. Fenchel M, Martirosian P, Langanke J, et al. Perfusion MR imaging with FAIR true FISP spin labeling in patients with and without renal artery stenosis: initial experience. Radiology 2006;238(3):1013–21.

53. Lanzman RS, Wittsack HJ, Martirosian P, et al. Quantification of renal allograft perfusion using arterial spin labeling MRI: initial results. Eur Radiol 2010;20(6):1485–91.

54. Martirosian P, Klose U, Mader I, et al. FAIR true-FISP perfusion imaging of the kidneys. Magn Reson Med 2004;51(2):353–61.

55. Ogawa S, Lee TM, Nayak AS, et al. Oxygenation-sensitive contrast in magnetic resonance image of rodent brain at high magnetic fields. Magn Reson Med 1990;14(1):68–78.

56. Prasad PV, Edelman RR, Epstein FH. Noninvasive evaluation of intrarenal oxygenation with BOLD MRI. Circulation 1996;94(12):3271–5.

57. Choi YA, Kim CK, Park SY, et al. Subtype differentiation of renal cell carcinoma using diffusion-weighted and blood oxygenation level-dependent MRI. AJR Am J Roentgenol 2014;203(1):W78–84.

58. Min JH, Kim CK, Park BK, et al. Assessment of renal lesions with blood oxygenation level-dependent MRI at 3 T: preliminary experience. AJR Am J Roentgenol 2011;197(3):W489–94.

59. Katz-Brull R, Rofsky NM, Morrin MM, et al. Decreases in free cholesterol and fatty acid unsaturation in renal cell carcinoma demonstrated by breath-hold magnetic resonance spectroscopy. Am J Physiol Renal Physiol 2005;288(4):F637–41.

60. Tugnoli V, Bottura G, Fini G, et al. 1H-NMR and 13C-NMR lipid profiles of human renal tissues. Biopolymers 2003;72(2):86–95.

61. Costello LC, Franklin RB. Concepts of citrate production and secretion by prostate. 1. Metabolic relationships. Prostate 1991;18(1):25–46.

62. Costello LC, Franklin RB. Concepts of citrate production and secretion by prostate: 2. Hormonal relationships in normal and neoplastic prostate. Prostate 1991;19(3):181–205.

63. Kahn T, Bürrig K, Schmitz-Dräger B, et al. Prostatic carcinoma and benign prostatic hyperplasia: MR imaging with histopathologic correlation. Radiology 1989;173(3):847–51.

64. Kurhanewicz J, Swanson MG, Nelson SJ, et al. Combined magnetic resonance imaging and spectroscopic imaging approach to molecular imaging of prostate cancer. J Magn Reson Imaging 2002;16(4):451–63.

65. Motzer RJ, Hutson TE, Tomczak P, et al. Sunitinib versus interferon alfa in metastatic renal-cell carcinoma. N Engl J Med 2007;356(2):115–24.

66. Schrader AJ, Olbert PJ, Hegele A, et al. Metastatic non-clear cell renal cell carcinoma: current therapeutic options. BJU Int 2008;101(11):1343–5.

67. Bostwick DG, Murphy GP. Diagnosis and prognosis of renal cell carcinoma: highlights from an international consensus workshop. Semin Urol Oncol 1998;16(1):46–52.

68. Leroy X, Zini L, Leteurtre E, et al. Morphologic subtyping of papillary renal cell carcinoma: correlation with prognosis and differential expression of MUC1 between the two subtypes. Mod Pathol 2002;15(11):1126–30.

69. Pedrosa I, Chou MT, Ngo L, et al. MR classification of renal masses with pathologic correlation. Eur Radiol 2008;18(2):365–75.

70. Sun MR, Ngo L, Genega EM, et al. Renal cell carcinoma: dynamic contrast-enhanced MR imaging for differentiation of tumor subtypes–correlation with pathologic findings. Radiology 2009;250(3):793–802.

71. Lanzman RS, Robson PM, Sun MR, et al. Arterial spin-labeling MR imaging of renal masses: correlation with histopathologic findings. Radiology 2012;265(3):799–808.

72. Roy C Sr, El Ghali S, Buy X, et al. Significance of the pseudocapsule on MRI of renal neoplasms and its potential application for local staging: a retrospective study. AJR Am J Roentgenol 2005;184(1):113–20.

73. Mejean A, Hopirtean V, Bazin JP, et al. Prognostic factors for the survival of patients with papillary renal cell carcinoma: meaning of histological typing and multifocality. J Urol 2003;170(3):764–7.

74. Sasiwimonphan K, Takahashi N, Leibovich BC, et al. Small (<4 cm) renal mass: differentiation of angiomyolipoma without visible fat from renal cell carcinoma utilizing MR imaging. Radiology 2012;263(1):160–8.

75. Rosenkrantz AB, Sekhar A, Genega EM, et al. Prognostic implications of the magnetic resonance imaging appearance in papillary renal cell carcinoma. Eur Radiol 2013;23(2):579–87.

76. Eisenhauer EA, Therasse P, Bogaerts J, et al. New response evaluation criteria in solid tumours: revised RECIST guideline (version 1.1). Eur J Cancer 2009;45(2):228–47.

77. Baccala A Jr, Hedgepeth R, Kaouk J, et al. Pathological evidence of necrosis in recurrent renal mass following treatment with sunitinib. Int J Urol 2007;14(12):1095–7 [discussion: 1097].

78. Ratain MJ, Eckhardt SG. Phase II studies of modern drugs directed against new targets: if you are not fazed, too, then resist RECIST. J Clin Oncol 2004;22(22):4442–5.

79. Rosen MA, Schnall MD. Dynamic contrast-enhanced magnetic resonance imaging for assessing tumor vascularity and vascular effects of targeted therapies in renal cell carcinoma. Clin Cancer Res 2007;13(2 Pt 2):770s–6s.

80. van der Veldt AA, Meijerink MR, van den Eertwegh AJ, et al. Targeted therapies in renal cell cancer: recent developments in imaging. Target Oncol 2010;5(2):95–112.

81. Hahn OM, Yang C, Medved M, et al. Dynamic contrast-enhanced magnetic resonance imaging pharmacodynamic biomarker study of sorafenib in metastatic renal carcinoma. J Clin Oncol 2008; 26(28):4572–8.

82. Wolf RL, Wang J, Wang S, et al. Grading of CNS neoplasms using continuous arterial spin labeled perfusion MR imaging at 3 Tesla. J Magn Reson Imaging 2005;22(4):475–82.

83. de Bazelaire C, Alsop DC, George D, et al. Magnetic resonance imaging-measured blood flow change after antiangiogenic therapy with PTK787/ ZK 222584 correlates with clinical outcome in metastatic renal cell carcinoma. Clin Cancer Res 2008; 14(17):5548–54.

84. Akita H, Jinzaki M, Kikuchi E, et al. Preoperative T categorization and prediction of histopathologic grading of urothelial carcinoma in renal pelvis using diffusion-weighted MRI. AJR Am J Roentgenol 2011;197(5):1130–6.

85. Shokeir AA, El-Diasty T, Eassa W, et al. Diagnosis of ureteral obstruction in patients with compromised renal function: the role of noninvasive imaging modalities. J Urol 2004;171(6 Pt 1):2303–6.

86. Shokeir AA, El-Diasty T, Eassa W, et al. Diagnosis of noncalcareous hydronephrosis: role of magnetic resonance urography and noncontrast computed tomography. Urology 2004;63(2):225–9.

87. Weeks SM, Brown ED, Brown JJ, et al. Transitional cell carcinoma of the upper urinary tract: staging by MRI. Abdom Imaging 1995;20(4):365–7.

88. O'Connor OJ, McLaughlin P, Maher MM. MR urography. AJR Am J Roentgenol 2010;195(3):W201–6.

89. Browne RF, Meehan CP, Colville J, et al. Transitional cell carcinoma of the upper urinary tract: spectrum of imaging findings. Radiographics 2005;25(6): 1609–27.

90. Obuchi M, Ishigami K, Takahashi K, et al. Gadolinium-enhanced fat-suppressed T1-weighted imaging for staging ureteral carcinoma: correlation with histopathology. AJR Am J Roentgenol 2007; 188(3):W256–61.

91. Uchida Y, Yoshida S, Kobayashi S, et al. Diffusion-weighted MRI as a potential imaging biomarker reflecting the metastatic potential of upper urinary tract cancer. Br J Radiol 2014;87(1042):20130791.

92. Yoshida S, Kobayashi S, Koga F, et al. Apparent diffusion coefficient as a prognostic biomarker of upper urinary tract cancer: a preliminary report. Eur Radiol 2013;23(8):2206–14.

93. Takeuchi M, Sasaki S, Ito M, et al. Urinary bladder cancer: diffusion-weighted MR imaging–accuracy for diagnosing T stage and estimating histologic grade. Radiology 2009;251(1):112–21.

94. Watanabe H, Kanematsu M, Kondo H, et al. Preoperative T staging of urinary bladder cancer: does diffusion-weighted MRI have supplementary value? AJR Am J Roentgenol 2009;192(5):1361–6.

95. Tanimoto A, Yuasa Y, Imai Y, et al. Bladder tumor staging: comparison of conventional and gadolinium-enhanced dynamic MR imaging and CT. Radiology 1992;185(3):741–7.

96. Matsuki M, Inada Y, Tatsugami F, et al. Diffusion-weighted MR imaging for urinary bladder carcinoma: initial results. Eur Radiol 2007;17(1):201–4.

97. El-Assmy A, Abou-El-Ghar ME, Mosbah A, et al. Bladder tumour staging: comparison of diffusion- and T2-weighted MR imaging. Eur Radiol 2009; 19(7):1575–81.

98. Takeuchi M, Sasaki S, Naiki T, et al. MR imaging of urinary bladder cancer for T-staging: a review and a pictorial essay of diffusion-weighted imaging. J Magn Reson Imaging 2013;38(6):1299–309.

99. Kobayashi S, Koga F, Kajino K, et al. Apparent diffusion coefficient value reflects invasive and proliferative potential of bladder cancer. J Magn Reson Imaging 2014;39(1):172–8.

100. Margulis V, Lotan Y, Karakiewicz PI, et al. Multi-institutional validation of the predictive value of Ki-67 labeling index in patients with urinary bladder cancer. J Natl Cancer Inst 2009;101(2):114–9.

101. Margulis V, Shariat SF, Ashfaq R, et al. Ki-67 is an independent predictor of bladder cancer outcome in patients treated with radical cystectomy for organ-confined disease. Clin Cancer Res 2006; 12(24):7369–73.

102. Yoshida S, Koga F, Kobayashi S, et al. Role of diffusion-weighted magnetic resonance imaging in predicting sensitivity to chemoradiotherapy in muscle-invasive bladder cancer. Int J Radiat Oncol Biol Phys 2012;83(1):e21–7.

103. Tuncbilek N, Kaplan M, Altaner S, et al. Value of dynamic contrast-enhanced MRI and correlation with tumor angiogenesis in bladder cancer. AJR Am J Roentgenol 2009;192(4):949–55.

104. Cornud F, Delongchamps NB, Mozer P, et al. Value of multiparametric MRI in the work-up of prostate cancer. Curr Urol Rep 2012;13(1):82–92.

105. Kurhanewicz J, Vigneron D, Carroll P, et al. Multiparametric magnetic resonance imaging in prostate cancer: present and future. Curr Opin Urol 2008;18(1):71–7.

106. Labanaris AP, Zugor V, Takriti S, et al. The role of conventional and functional endorectal magnetic resonance imaging in the decision of whether to

preserve or resect the neurovascular bundles during radical retropubic prostatectomy. Scand J Urol Nephrol 2009;43(1):25–31.

107. Sciarra A, Barentsz J, Bjartell A, et al. Advances in magnetic resonance imaging: how they are changing the management of prostate cancer. Eur Urol 2011;59(6):962–77.

108. Muller BG, van den Bos W, Pinto PA, et al. Imaging modalities in focal therapy: patient selection, treatment guidance, and follow-up. Curr Opin Urol 2014;24(3):218–24.

109. Sonn GA, Chang E, Natarajan S, et al. Value of targeted prostate biopsy using magnetic resonance-ultrasound fusion in men with prior negative biopsy and elevated prostate-specific antigen. Eur Urol 2014;65(4):809–15.

110. Zhang ZX, Yang J, Zhang CZ, et al. The value of magnetic resonance imaging in the detection of prostate cancer in patients with previous negative biopsies and elevated prostate-specific antigen levels: a meta-analysis. Acad Radiol 2014;21(5): 578–89.

111. Mendhiratta N, Rosenkrantz AB, Meng X, et al. MRI-ultrasound fusion-targeted prostate biopsy in a consecutive cohort of men with no previous biopsy: reduction of over-detection through improved risk stratification. J Urol 2015. [Epub ahead of print].

112. Hoeks CM, Barentsz JO, Hambrock T, et al. Prostate cancer: multiparametric MR imaging for detection, localization, and staging. Radiology 2011; 261(1):46–66.

113. Hricak H, Choyke PL, Eberhardt SC, et al. Imaging prostate cancer: a multidisciplinary perspective. Radiology 2007;243(1):28–53.

114. Hambrock T, Somford DM, Huisman HJ, et al. Relationship between apparent diffusion coefficients at 3.0-T MR imaging and Gleason grade in peripheral zone prostate cancer. Radiology 2011;259(2):453–61.

115. Vargas HA, Akin O, Franiel T, et al. Diffusion-weighted endorectal MR imaging at 3 T for prostate cancer: tumor detection and assessment of aggressiveness. Radiology 2011;259(3):775–84.

116. van As NJ, de Souza NM, Riches SF, et al. A study of diffusion-weighted magnetic resonance imaging in men with untreated localised prostate cancer on active surveillance. Eur Urol 2009;56(6):981–7.

117. Giles SL, Morgan VA, Riches SF, et al. Apparent diffusion coefficient as a predictive biomarker of prostate cancer progression: value of fast and slow diffusion components. AJR Am J Roentgenol 2011;196(3):586–91.

118. Sistrom CL, Langlotz CP. A framework for improving radiology reporting. J Am Coll Radiol 2005;2(2):159–67.

119. Dickinson L, Ahmed HU, Allen C, et al. Scoring systems used for the interpretation and reporting of multiparametric MRI for prostate cancer detection, localization, and characterization: could standardization lead to improved utilization of imaging within the diagnostic pathway? J Magn Reson Imaging 2013;37(1):48–58.

120. Rosenkrantz AB, Haghighi M, Horn J, et al. Utility of quantitative MRI metrics for assessment of stage and grade of urothelial carcinoma of the bladder: preliminary results. AJR Am J Roentgenol 2013; 201(6):1254–9.

121. Muller BG, Shih JH, Sankineni S, et al. Prostate cancer: interobserver agreement and accuracy with the revised prostate imaging reporting and data system at multiparametric MR imaging. Radiology 2015;142818.

Functional MR Imaging in Gynecologic Cancer

Nandita M. deSouza, MD, FRCR, FRCP[a],*, Andrea Rockall, MRCP, FRCR[b,c],
Susan Freeman, FRCR[d]

KEYWORDS

- Gynecologic cancer • Dynamic contrast-enhanced • Diffusion-weighted • Detection • Staging
- Characterization • Response • Recurrence

KEY POINTS

- Diffusion-weighted MR imaging improves detection, staging, characterization, and response monitoring in gynecologic malignancy.
- Dynamic contrast-enhanced MR imaging is equivalent to diffusion-weighted MR imaging for detecting and staging gynecologic malignancy, but adds complexity and cost.
- Where implemented, functional MR imaging techniques should always be used as an adjunct to morphologic T2-weighted MR imaging for assessing gynecologic tumors.
- Quantitative assessments derived from functional MR imaging have largely been trialed in single-center studies; multicenter use in clinical trials requires their standardization.

INTRODUCTION

Imaging has a major role to play in all phases of assessment of gynecological cancer, including disease detection, characterization, prognostication, staging, response assessment, and monitoring, and in the assessment of recurrent disease. Because of its superior soft tissue contrast, MR imaging is the modality of choice. Recently, a number of functional MR imaging techniques using diffusion-weighted (DW-) MR imaging, dynamic contrast enhanced (DCE-) MR imaging and MR spectroscopy (MRS) have been exploited to further improve the imaging information provided (**Box 1**). More information on each of these topics can be found in Body diffusion-weighted MR imaging in Oncology: Imaging at 3T by Dr Koh et al, Assessment of angiogenesis with MR imaging: DCE-MR imaging and beyond by Drs Salem and O'Connor, and Imaging of tumor metabolism: MR spectroscopy by Drs Noguerol, et al. The current article details the use of each technique for gynecological cancer at each stage of the clinical pathway.

ENDOMETRIAL CANCER
Detection

Endometrial cancer, the commonest gynecologic malignancy in the developed world, occurs predominantly after menopause with more than 90% of patients presenting over the age of 50 years.[1] Transvaginal ultrasonography accurately evaluates the endometrial thickness and guides the requirement for endometrial biopsy, if the endometrial thickness is greater than 4 mm.[2] Where available, the excellent soft tissue contrast of T2-

The authors have nothing to disclose.
[a] Division of Radiotherapy & Imaging, The Institute of Cancer Research, The Royal Marsden Hospital, Fulham Road, London SW3 6JJ, UK; [b] Department of Radiology, Hammersmith Hospital, Imperial College Healthcare NHS Trust, DuCane Road, London W12 0HS, UK; [c] Department of Radiology, Imperial College, South Kensington, London SW7 2AZ, UK; [d] Department of Radiology, Cambridge University Hospitals NHS Foundation Trust, Hills Road, Cambridge CB2 0QQ, UK
* Corresponding author. MRI Unit, The Royal Marsden Hospital, Downs Road, Sutton, Surrey SM2 5PT, UK.
E-mail address: Nandita.Desouza@icr.ac.uk

Magn Reson Imaging Clin N Am 24 (2016) 205–222
http://dx.doi.org/10.1016/j.mric.2015.08.008
1064-9689/16/$ – see front matter © 2016 Elsevier Inc. All rights reserved.

mri.theclinics.com

Box 1
Pearls and pitfalls

- Functional techniques such as dynamic contrast-enhanced MR imaging and diffusion-weighted MR imaging must always be used in conjunction with conventional morphologic MR imaging.
- Diffusion-weighted MR imaging is easy to implement but suffers from low signal-to-noise ratio, and thus may be noncontributory for detecting small lesions unless methods to increase signal-to-noise ratio are addressed.
- Air in the bowel and hemorrhage cause B1 field in homogeneities and result in significant geometric distortion on diffusion-weighted images, particularly at high b-values.
- Detection and staging of small cervical tumors is enhanced using endovaginal MR imaging.
- Detection of metastatic lymph nodes even with functional techniques is related to size, and 18-fluorodeoxyglucose ([18]FDG) PET-CT currently remains the imaging modality of choice for their identification.
- Visualization of peritoneal metastases may be improved on high b-value diffusion-weighted images

---

weighted (T2-W) MR imaging provides the most accurate method of visualizing endometrial tumors. In some circumstances, the endometrium can be difficult to assess by T2-W MR imaging alone, particularly in cases where the endometrium is distorted by the presence of leiomyomas or adenomyosis. This visualization can be improved by the addition of DW-MR imaging (83% of tumors successfully identified compared with T2-W imaging alone, compared with 96% on fused DW-MR imaging and T2-W images).[3]

Apparent diffusion coefficient (ADC) values derived from DW-MR imaging can be used to differentiate benign from malignant endometrial lesions.[4] In 2 separate studies, the use of a cutoff ADC value proved useful in distinguishing benign from malignant lesions with an 85% to 87% sensitivity and 100% specificity.[4,5] This is valuable in patients when preoperative endometrial sampling is not possible or when the endometrial pipelle does not adequately sample a tumor.[6] Additionally, the detection of peritoneal dissemination improved with the combination of DW-MR imaging and conventional imaging (sensitivity, 84%; specificity, 91%), which enables preoperative treatment planning. MRS also has been explored in differentiating benign and malignant endometrial lesions largely through the assessment or quantification of the choline resonance.[7] Lipid peaks may also be present in endometrial carcinomas, which are absent in benign endometrial lesions[8] likely owing to cytosolic lipid droplets.

Staging

Federation Internationale Gynecologie Obstetrique (FIGO) staging remains surgically based after total abdominal hysterectomy, bilateral salpingooophorectomy, peritoneal washings, and retroperitoneal lymph node dissection. MR imaging is not currently included within the FIGO staging system. Both the National Cancer Institute in France and the European Society of Urogenital Radiology recommend preoperative MR imaging in the management of endometrial carcinoma particularly those of high-risk histologic subtypes,[9,10] because the information provided guides management and surgical planning.

Multiple studies have investigated the additional role of DCE-MR imaging for evaluating the depth of myometrial invasion in patients with endometrial carcinoma. Many found that the overall staging accuracy of T2-W imaging improved with the use of DCE-MR imaging,[11–16] although this is improvement has not been seen in other series[17,18] and is particularly important where fibroids and adenomyosis are present. A recent metaanalysis confirmed that DCE-MR imaging MR imaging is superior to T2-W imaging for both deep and superficial myometrial invasion, with a pooled specificity of DCE-MR imaging of 72% compared with 58% for T2-W imaging, but without a difference in sensitivity.[19] Moreover, DCE-MR imaging improves confidence in staging accuracy in the presence of fibroids, adenomyosis,[20,21] and in detecting cervical involvement thus distinguishing stage I and II disease.[18,22] However, even with DCE-MR imaging, tumor extension into the cornua limits assessment of myometrial invasion[18] and peritumoral inflammation may further overestimate it.

The accuracy of DW-MR imaging in assessing the depth of myometrial invasion ranges from 62% to 90%[23] and so may be used where intravenous contrast medium is contraindicated (Fig. 1).[21,2] DW-MR imaging may also improve detection of drop metastases in the cervix or metastatic spread outside the uterus, such as in the adnexa or peritoneum (Fig. 2).[21,23,24] The conspicuity of lymph node

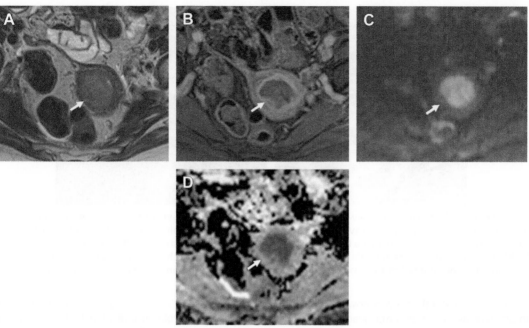

Fig. 1. Local staging of endometrial cancer. Transverse T2-weighted image (A) shows a tumor within the endometrial cavity that has ill-defined margins with likely extension into the outer half of the myometrium (arrow). After intravenous gadolinium (B), there is marked peritumoral enhancement (arrow). The depth of myometrial invasion is clearly delineated on diffusion-weighted imaging (b = 1000 s/mm^2; C, arrow) and the corresponding ADC map (D, arrow) as less than 50% of the myometrial thickness, thus confirming a FIGO stage IA.

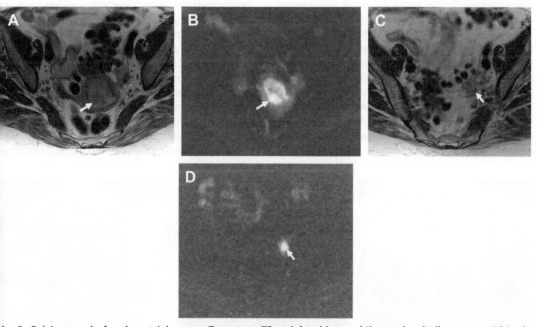

Fig. 2. Pelvic spread of endometrial cancer. Transverse T2-weighted image (A) reveals a bulky tumor within the endometrial cavity (arrow) with corresponding restricted diffusion on diffusion-weighted imaging (DWI; b = 1000 s/mm^2; B, arrow). However, the left ovary also seems to be prominent on the T2-weighted image (C, arrow), and its marked restricted diffusion on DWI (b = 1000 s/mm^2; D, arrow) confirms the presence of an adnexal metastasis, upstaging the disease to FIGO stage IIIA.

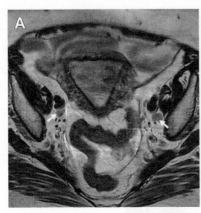
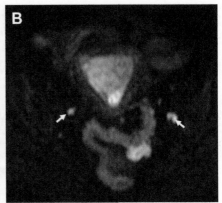

Fig. 3. Endometrial carcinosarcoma with metastatic spread. Transverse T2-weighted image (A) demonstrates an intermediate signal intensity tumor within the endometrial cavity and small bilateral obturator lymph nodes (arrows). The diffusion-weighted image (B; b = 1000 s/mm²) demonstrates restricted diffusion within the tumor and highlights a peritoneal metastasis abutting the sigmoid colon (arrow). Both lymph nodes seems to be restricted although this does not definitively indicate metastatic involvement; the one on the left retains a fatty hilum.

improves with DW-MR imaging; however, the ability to differentiate benign and malignant lymph nodes remains controversial (Fig. 3).[25,26]

An increase in the choline/water ratio on MRS with tumor stage has been reported[7] with differentiation of FIGO stage I tumors from stage II and III tumors (P = .029), but this is less accurate than MR imaging.

Characterization and Prognostication

The histologic grade and subtype of endometrial carcinoma on histology from biopsy is subject to sampling error. The ADC value has been interrogated to assess the aggressiveness of endometrial carcinoma. Rechichi and colleagues[27] reported no correlation with tumor grade, depth of myometrial invasion, or the presence of lymph node involvement. The interquartile range of ADC indicative of tumor heterogeneity has also been shown to increase in deep myometrial invasion, lymphovascular space invasion, and lymph node

metastases.[28] ADC histogram analysis from the entire tumor volume indicated that the standard deviation, quartile, 75th, 90th, and 95th percentiles of ADC showed significant differences between all grades (P≤.03) and between high and low grades.[29] The mean choline/water ratios do not differ between tumor grades.[7]

Sarcomas do not seem to be different from carcinomas on conventional T2-W MR imaging. The vast majority of leiomyosarcomas arise de novo within the myometrium. Compared with their benign counterparts, leiomyosarcomas have an ill-defined and irregular margin, internal hemorrhage and necrosis and demonstrate rapid growth. In addition, they often present with local and distant spread including extrauterine tumor nodules, lymph node metastases, and liver, lung, and bone metastases.[30] Both densely cellular leiomyomas and uterine sarcomas demonstrate restricted diffusion on DW-MR imaging, although the majority of benign leiomyomas do not demonstrate this marked restricted

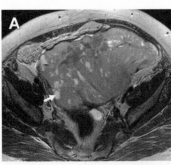
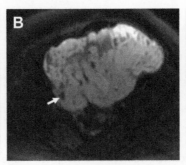
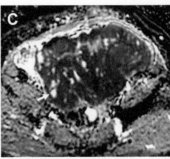

Fig. 4. Leiomyosarcoma. Transverse T2-weighted image (A), diffusion-weighted imaging, (B) and apparent diffusion coefficient map (C) images through the mid pelvis showing a large, heterogeneous mass arising from the uterine body with lobulated margins (arrow). The irregular appearance and marked restricted diffusion in B and C with focal necrosis (arrows) is highly suggestive of leiomyosarcoma.

diffusion[31] so that the mean ADC value of sarcomas is significantly lower (Fig. 4). Endometrial stromal sarcomas are a rare entity and also show diffusion restriction, although also the evidence base is limited to case reports.[32]

On MRS, uterine tumors characteristically show increased lipids[33]; lipid peaks were identified in 100% of uterine sarcomas, but not in the majority of benign leiomyomas. The choline peak is less reliable; it was demonstrated in all leiomyomas and 10 out of 12 sarcomas (the other 2 being markedly necrotic).[34] The identification of lipids merits further investigation as a biomarker for differentiating benign leiomyomas from uterine sarcomas, particularly where management with hysterectomy versus uterine artery embolization or myomectomy is considered.

Monitoring Treatment Response

Because the majority of patients with endometrial carcinoma are treated and cured with surgery, there is a limited role for DCE- and DW-MR imaging in treatment response.

Follow-up and Detection of Recurrent Disease

Surgery is curative for the majority of patients with endometrial carcinoma, so it is important to identify patients at high risk of recurrence who merit imaging follow-up; these factors include advanced stage at diagnosis, high-grade disease, and lymphovascular space invasion. Of recurrences, 87% occur within 3 years of the initial diagnosis, most commonly with recurrent disease to the vaginal vault (42%) and lymph node metastases (46%).[35] Computed tomography (CT) is commonly used to identify tumor recurrence; however, MR imaging is more sensitive in the identification of early vaginal vault recurrence. The use of DCE-MR imaging and DW-MR imaging aids recurrent tumor detection and allows differentiation from postradiotherapy changes.[36] Nakamura and colleagues[37] found that patients with a low minimum ADC of the primary tumor had a significantly lower disease-free survival than those with a high minimum ADC. Notably, the minimum ADC of the primary endometrial cancer was an independent predictive factor for disease recurrence in a multivariate analysis.

CERVICAL CANCER
Detection

Cervical cancer occurs in a younger population of women (peak age incidence is 30 years). Cytologic screening has resulted in earlier diagnosis and surgery is the mainstay of management in these cases. Accurate depiction of the presence and extent of tumor is critical, particularly if fertility-sparing procedures are being considered. The performance of DW-MR imaging for tumor detection is equivalent to DCE-MR imaging[38]; the lack of requirement of an extrinsic contrast agent makes it preferable. The derived ADC value of malignant cervical tissues is significantly lower than that of normal tissue. This was shown in a metaanalysis of 13 cohort studies (645 tumor tissues and 504 normal tissues) and held true, regardless of data from 6 different scanner types within the analysis[39] and of b-value combination.[40] This is not surprising given the large differences in ADC between benign and malignant tissue, which is greater than the variability in the ADC calculation.

Where cervical cancer is detected incidentally on LLETZ/knife cone to treat dysplasia, imaging is required to identify residual disease or extension up the endocervical canal beyond the superior extent of the surgical specimen. In these small lesions, signal return may be improved 4 to 10 times by the use of endovaginal coils placed in close proximity to the cervix. In a study of 45 patients with small tumors (0.2 cm³), one-third of whom had residual disease at fertility-sparing surgery, the sensitivity of detection using a 37-mm internal ring coil was 87% and specificity 80% and 90%, respectively, for 2 observers when DW-MR imaging was part of the evaluation (Fig. 5).[41] The use of DW sequences was particularly effective in improving sensitivity of tumor detection without loss of specificity after some form of local surgical excision (LLETZ or knife cone).[42] A 10% to 30% increase in sensitivity of detected stage Ia and Ib1 tumors was achieved without a loss of specificity when an ADC threshold was applied and used in combination with T2-W images for disease detection.[43] This technique, therefore, is helpful in selecting the appropriate operative procedure and in 1 study was shown to alter surgical management in 39% of cases.[44] In small volume disease, DCE-MR imaging techniques have no place, because they are neither more sensitive nor more specific than T2-W imaging, nor is the information they provide adjunctive to the T2-W imaging data. MRS has insufficient spatial resolution in vivo, even with the increased signal available with an endovaginal technique. The most striking biochemical changes in malignant voxels are not only the increase in choline signals,[45] but also the increased lipid resonances at 1.3 ppm (CH_2 – resonances), 0.9 ppm (CH_3 – resonances), and 2 ppm (NH-CH resonances). The technical issues with performing MRS in vivo, however, limit its translation into clinical practice.

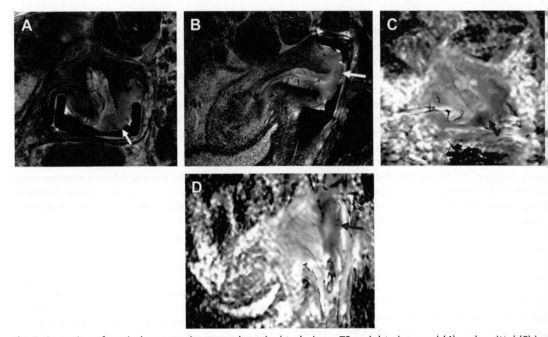

Fig. 5. Detection of cervical cancer using an endovaginal technique. T2-weighted coronal (*A*) and sagittal (*B*) images through the cervix showing a lobulated exophytic tumor on the left (*arrows*). The corresponding apparent diffusion coefficient (ADC) maps in coronal (*C*) and sagittal (*D*) planes show a restricted diffusion mass (*arrows*) but the heterogeneity of the ADC values within this adenocarcinoma are appreciated on these high spatial resolution images.

Staging

The use of DCE-MR imaging in distinguishing stage Ib1 from Ib2 tumors is equivalent to DW-MR imaging,[46] and the need for an extrinsic contrast agent adds additional complexity and cost. A retrospective analysis of 152 cases for distinguishing stage 2b disease (parametrial invasion) using a whole-body technique showed that fused T2-W + DW-MR imaging had a higher specificity but not sensitivity than T2-W imaging for 2 readers: reader 1, 99% versus 88.7%; and reader 2, 96.5% versus 85.2%. Sensitivity for each reader remained between 67% and 75%, regardless of whether DW-MR imaging was added or not.[47] The detection of parametrial extension may be boosted by the addition of tumor ADC data to the assessment of the parametrium itself (Fig. 6) and in 117 patients treated surgically, tumor ADC and parametrial invasion on T2-W MR imaging were shown to be independent predictors of parametrial invasion on pathology.[48] MRS has no role in this regard, because parametrial fat signals dominate and mask the recognition of smaller metabolites.

Early data investigating ADC for detecting malignant nodes did not support its use,[49] which is unsurprising because the parameter partly reflects the high cellular density present in lymphatic tissue. What is clear is that when nodes are enlarged the use of ADC is helpful; a significant difference in mean ADC has been shown in nodes greater than 5 mm (17 metastatic and 140 nonmetastatic).[5] Therefore, when considered generally and without regard to size, ADC does not improve diagnostic accuracy; a prospective study of 68 patients showed a low sensitivity (25%–33%) on both a patient and regional node level for 2 observers; specificity was 83% to 97%.[51] Of interest is the reproducibility of the detection of pelvic lymph nodes by DW-MR imaging, which has been shown to be equivalent to T2-W MR imaging, ranging between 42% and 65% for both methods.[52] When compared with the current imaging gold standard 18-fluorodeoxyglucose ([18]FDG) PET-CT, ADC has been shown to be significantly different in PET positive versus PET-negative nodes.[53] However the question remains as to whether the use of MR imaging is justified for delineating metastatic nodes if [18]FDG PET-CT can achieve a higher accuracy.

Characterization and Prognostication

Attempts have been made to derive imaging biomarkers that relate to histologic prognostic

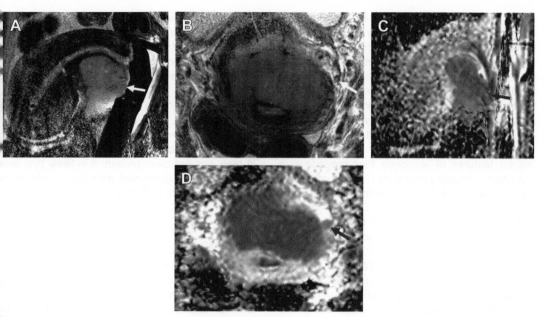

Fig. 6. Staging a bulky cervical tumor. T2-weighted sagittal (*A*) and transverse (*B*) images through the cervix showing a homogenous, solid tumor anteriorly (*arrows*). The corresponding apparent diffusion coefficient (ADC) maps in sagittal (*C*) and transverse (*D*) planes show a restricted diffusion mass. The extension into the parametrium on the left is appreciated on the transverse ADC maps, but is not easily identifiable on the T2-weighted image (*arrows*).

features. With DCE-MR imaging, the use of non-modelled parameters such as the normalized relative signal increase and normalized area under the gadolinium enhancement curve are intrinsically more robust to obtain than modeled parameters and are potentially more useful. A retrospective study of 50 patients demonstrated the utility of a very simple parameter, the enhancing fraction (which represents the proportion of enhancing voxels within the tumor region) for indicating disease-free survival.[54] Several pharmacokinetic parameters have also been associated positively both with locoregional control and progression-free survival; a prospectively collected cohort of 31 patients indicated that their prognostic impact was independent of tumor stage, volume, and lymph node status, was able to predict long-term locoregional control,[55] and may be used as indicators of treatment failure.[56]

More recently, the ADC has been shown to be an important prognostic indicator. Patients with lower mean or minimum ADC before hysterectomy had shorter disease-free survival than those with higher mean/minimum ADC values.[57] This is supported by the relationship between ADC and histology: higher grade tumors have lower ADC values than their low-grade counterparts.[58] Because the heterogeneity of tumors is increasingly recognized, histograms of voxel-wise analysis have proved more useful in distinguishing

poorly differentiated from well differentiated tumors as well as adeno from squamous cancers.[59,60] Intravoxel incoherent motion analyses in a small cohort of 16 patients distinguished well from poorly perfused tumors with good correlation between the intravoxel incoherent motion–derived perfusion parameter "f" (perfusion fraction) and K^{trans} derived from DCE-MR imaging studies.[61] More sophisticated analyses have attempted to combine ADC with total choline derived from MRS to classify tumors by type and grade, but the addition of the total choline measurement did not provide additional benefit.[62]

Assessment of Treatment Response

Functional MR imaging is increasingly exploited during treatment to monitor response. Significant increases in DCE-MR imaging parameters (K^{trans} and V_e) have been shown within tumor, but not in normal muscle, 4 weeks into treatment[63] or after 1 cycle of neoadjuvant chemotherapy that correlate with eventual tumor volume response rate.[64] ADC values after 4 weeks of treatment also correlate with volume response and clinical response.[65,66] Other studies have confirmed that the percentage ADC change after 1 month of chemoradiotherapy correlates positively with the percentage size reduction after 2 months of treatment.[67] A larger study of 75 patients imaged after 2 and 4 weeks of commencement of chemoradiotherapy and at completion indicated a higher percentage increase in those confirmed as complete responders on tumor size criteria at 6 months than in those classified as partial responders.[68] Similar early increases in ADC are evident in those treated with neoadjuvant chemotherapy.[69] ADC increases correlate negatively with proliferating cell nuclear antigen and with cell density in those who respond indicating their relationship to cellular features of response that precede size reduction.[70] Imaging very early (1 week) after initiation of chemoradiotherapy treatment with a combined DCE-MR imaging and DW-MR imaging approach in 16 patients showed that the changes in ADC correlated with size reduction on completion, although the changes in DCE did not, indicating a better sensitivity for DW-MR imaging as an early response biomarker[71] and its future potential for directing therapeutic interventions at much earlier time points. At the other end of the spectrum, ADC measured at the end of treatment in a metaanalysis of 9 studies with 231 patients also showed that responders had higher ADC values and a greater change in ADC than nonresponders.[72]

Follow-up and Detection of Disease Recurrence

The 4 factors most predictive of recurrence are size greater than 3 cm, adenocarcinoma, lymphovascular space invasion, and deep (outer third) stromal invasion.[73] Between one-quarter and one-half of recurrences are asymptomatic.[74,75] Because 64% to 87% of recurrences happen within 2 years and 89% to 98% within 5 years,[76] there is a strong argument for 5-year surveillance. Morphologic pelvic MR imaging with T2-W sequences forms the mainstay in defining recurrent pelvic disease, whereas [18]FDG PET-CT remains the imaging modality of choice for estimating lymph nodes and distant disease, with a sensitivity and specificity of 96% and 95%, respectively.[77] In patients with greater than 2 cm or node-positive disease treated surgically, a PET-CT at 3 months is recommended; in those treated with chemoradiotherapy, this should be delayed to 6 months to avoid false positives owing to postradiation effects on the images. MR imaging is reserved for symptomatic patients. However, in early cervical disease of less than 2 cm and node negative at the outset, follow-up imaging is warranted only if patients become symptomatic or if the physical examination is abnormal. T2-W MR imaging is the

modality of choice for detecting locally recurrent disease in these cases.

The use of ultra-small iron oxide particles as a lymph node contrast agent enjoyed some early excitement[78] and data from trials have affirmed its usefulness.[79,80] Normal nodes take up the ultra-small iron oxide particles and become dark on T2* imaging, whereas metastatic involved nodes do not. However, these agents remain unlicensed for clinical use as their efficacy in phase III trials has not been proven. It is likely that their utility will be superseded with the development and availability of PET-MR.

OVARIAN CANCER
Detection

MR imaging has been found to improve the specificity of characterizing adnexal masses using standard sequences including T1, T2, and T with fat saturation before and after intravenous contrast administration.[81–84] A recent systematic review has concluded that MR imaging with contrast enhancement provides the highest post test probability of ovarian cancer.[84] Thus, MR imaging offers the possibility of decreasing the number of patients undergoing inappropriate cancer operations for a benign lesion.

Early enhancement of solid components in a complex adnexal mass was initially thought to be an indicator of malignancy,[82] and a recent systematic review confirmed a high specificity.[84] A rapid wash-in of contrast has been found to have a high specificity for invasive malignancy.[85,86] Quantitative measures of perfusion as well as qualitative time–intensity curve of the enhancement is significantly associated with the risk of malignancy,[87,8] but requires a time resolution of at least 15 seconds with the adjacent myometrium acting as an internal reference (Fig. 7). A low-level gradual enhancement curve is associated with benign lesions, an intermediate enhancement curve with a "shoulder" is associated most frequently with borderline tumors, and a curve that has more rapid and higher level enhancement than the adjacent myometrium is predominantly seen in invasive ovarian masses.

Solid components of malignant adnexal masses typically retain high signal intensity on high b-value images, with low ADC, consistent with restricted diffusion (Fig. 8).[89–91] However significant overlap in diffusion characteristics has been identified with certain benign lesions including benign cystic teratomas, endometriotic cysts, some fibrothecomas, degenerating fibroids, or Brenner tumors.[92–94] Although ADC has been found to be lower generally in malignant

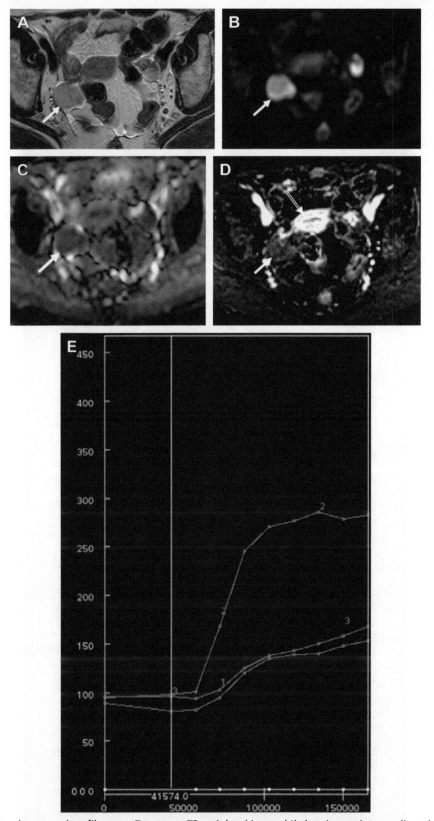

ig. 7. Bilateral serous adenofibromas. Transverse T2-weighted image (*A*) showing an intermediate signal inten-
ity mass (*arrow*) that is restricted in diffusion on diffusion-weighted imaging (b = 1000 s/mm²; *B, arrow*) and on
he apparent diffusion coefficient map (*C, arrow*). A corresponding dynamic contrast enhanced slice with a 15-
econd time resolution (*D, arrow*) demonstrates visibly lower level of enhancement in the mass than the adjacent
myometrium (*open arrow*). The time–intensity enhancement curve confirms low level gradual enhancement (*E,
rrow*) when compared with the myometrium (*open arrow*).

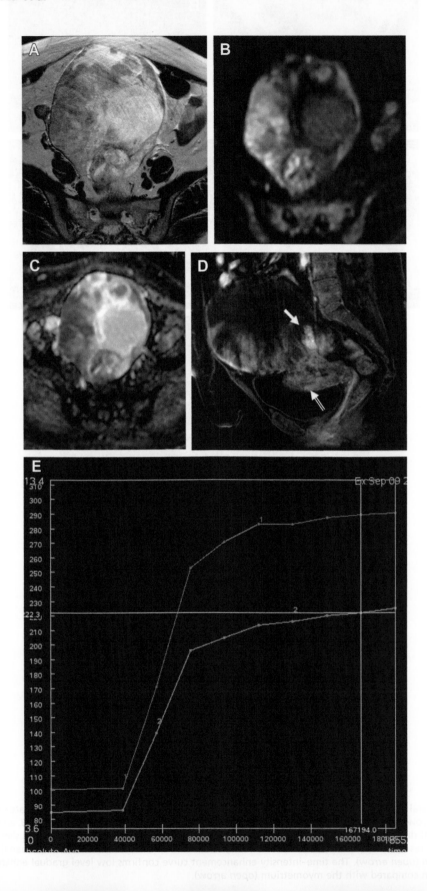

than in benign lesions,[94,95] there is marked over-ap.[96] However, if the signal intensity of a solid component is low on the high b-value image, the likelihood of malignancy is extremely low, particularly when the solid component also has low T2 signal intensity[87,94,97–99] so that DW-MR imaging can be used as a tool to "rule out" malignancy with a high negative predictive value. This is of particular importance in cases where intravenous gadolinium contrast medium is contraindicated, such as in a pregnant woman with a complex adnexal mass. More recent work has included DCE-MR imaging and DW-MR imaging together to offer a robust algorithmic approach. By considering morphology, T2-W and DW-MR imaging signal intensity and the enhancement curve analysis, a 5-point scoring system has been proposed which has very good discriminatory characteristics and reproducibility (Table 1).[87]

Staging Accuracy and Predicting Surgical Cytoreduction

The majority of women with suspected ovarian cancer present with disease that is disseminated into the peritoneal cavity. CT is used to determine the extent of disease and highlight likely inoperable disease, such as liver metastases. However, CT fails to adequately identify which patients are unlikely to undergo optimal or complete cytoreductive surgery (15%–51% of patients undergo suboptimal cytoreduction).[100–108] Conversely, 2 studies reported low positive predictive values on CT for suboptimal cytoreduction, suggesting that many patients who were predicted to have suboptimal cytoreduction would in fact have optimal cytoreduction.[106,109]

The use of DW-MR imaging increases the sensitivity and specificity for detecting peritoneal metastatic disease largely owing to the high contrast resolution (Fig. 9).[6,110,111] A prospective study of CT, [18]FDG PET-CT, and whole body DW-MR imaging in 32 patients found that DW-MR imaging could identify bowel serosal and mesenteric disease with an accuracy of 91% compared with 75% on CT and 71% on [18]FDG PET-CT.[112] Metastatic disease outside the abdomen was detected by DW-MR imaging with equal accuracy to [18]FDG

Table 1 Adnex MR score	
Adnex MR Score	**Positive Likelihood Ratio**
1. No adnexal mass	—
2. Benign mass	0
Purely cystic	—
Purely endometriotic	—
Purely fatty	—
Absence of wall enhancement	—
Low b1000 and low T2 Signal Intensity in solid component	—
3. Probably benign	<0.01
Curve type 1 within solid tissue	—
Masses without solid tissue (except purely cystic/endometriotic or fatty)	—
4. Indeterminate MR mass	0.1–10
Curve type 2 within solid tissue	—
5. Probably malignant mass	>10
Peritoneal implants	—
Curve type 3 within solid tissue	—

PET-CT. Thus, the use of DCE-MR imaging and DW-MR imaging is increasingly creeping into clinical practice in some cancer centers although a firm evidence base for its use yet needs to be established.

Three early studies in MR imaging, before the availability of DW-MR imaging, compared MR imaging with CT for predicting resectability and did not provide substantial evidence of an improvement.[102,105,113] More recently, the peritoneal cancer index scores in 35 patients (n = 8 ovarian primary) based on MR imaging with both DCE-MR imaging and DW-MR imaging[114] has been shown to match closely an overall sensitivity and specificity for all sites of disease of 88% and 74% and scoring peritoneal disease indicated a 91% diagnostic accuracy

Fig. 8. Characterization of a complex adnexal mass noted on ultrasound. Transverse T2-weighted imaging (A), diffusion-weighted imaging (b 1000 s/mm²: B), apparent diffusion coefficient map (C), sagittal dynamic-contrast enhanced MR imaging (D), and time–intensity curves (E) showing a mass of heterogenous intermediate signal intensity in A and heterogeneously restricted diffusion in B and C. In D and E, the straight arrow indicates early bright enhancement in the mass (type 3 curve) compared with the myometrium (open arrow). Histology confirmed stage 1C clear cell ovarian cancer.

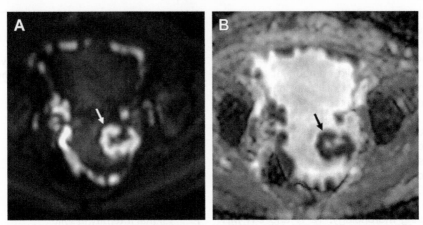

Fig. 9. Metastatic peritoneal disease in a primary peritoneal cancer. Transverse diffusion-weighted imaging through the pelvis (b = 1000 s/mm², A) and corresponding apparent diffusion coefficient map (B) showing extensive small volume tumor deposits lining the peritoneal cavity and the surface of the left ovary (arrows). The restricted diffusion tumor is readily identified owing to the high tumor to background signal intensity.

with 75% sensitivity for predicting suboptimal cytoreduction. No study has yet evaluated the impact of these measurements on treatment decisions and there has been no prospective evaluation of the impact on surgical outcomes.

Characterization

Differences in ADC between the primary ovarian tumor, omental deposits, and peritoneal deposits are recognized[115] owing to differences in underlying stroma.[116] The primary ovarian lesion seems to have a higher mean ADC and the peritoneal deposits a significantly lower mean ADC than the primary ovarian lesion or omental deposits. This site-specific heterogeneity is of potential interest in assessing disease aggressiveness and site-specific response.

Monitoring Treatment Response

Assessment of response to chemotherapy relies on a decrease in CA125 level and a reduction in tumor diameter using RECIST criteria on cross-sectional imaging, usually CT.[117] However, these criteria may take time and patients who are not responding to their chemotherapy regime cannot be identified after a single cycle of treatment using this traditional response assessment method. Early identification of nonresponders also has been reported using [18]FDG PET-CT, where the prediction of overall survival by [18]FDG uptake was superior to clinical response (P = .7), CA125 response (P = .5) and to histologic markers of response after delayed primary surgery (P = .09).[118]

More recently, DW-MR imaging has proven of interest in this regard: Kyriazi and colleagues[119] showed that, in patients classified clinically as

responders, the ADC increased after both the first and the third cycles of chemotherapy (P<.001), whereas in nonresponders no parameter changed significantly.[40] The DW-MR imaging parameter that best identified response was found to be the percentage change in the 25th percentile of the ADC histogram. Thus, an early increase in ADC could characterize the final chemotherapy response. In a multiparametric approach encompassing DCE-MR imaging, DW-MR imaging, and MRS, there was a greater increase in the ADC of the primary ovarian tumor in responders than in nonresponders in the primary ovarian tumor after 3 cycles of chemotherapy than at other disease sites. Significant changes also were also seen in the DCE-MR imaging characteristics of the primary tumor, but not at other sites. This imaging heterogeneity is an area of active future research, particularly for identifying phenotypic and genomic associations. A large, prospective, multicenter study in the UK (DISCOVAR, CCR 3694) is currently evaluating DW-MR imaging in chemotherapy response.

Detecting Disease Recurrence

Detecting recurrent disease relies primarily on an increase in the serum biomarker CA125. Increasingly, in patients with single-site recurrence, a surgical option may be available, so that detecting and defining the extent of recurrence is worthwhile. Remarkably, there are no reported studies formally evaluating DW-MR imaging or DCE-MR imaging for detecting recurrence in ovarian cancer, despite an early report of T2-W and conventional contrast enhanced MR imaging having a 90% accuracy in detecting recurrence in a

---

Box 2
What the referring physician needs to know

- MR imaging is the first choice for evaluating endometrial and cervical cancer at all stages of the clinical pathway—disease detection, staging, characterization, response monitoring, and identification of recurrence.

- CT remains the gold standard for assessing ovarian cancer, although the use of diffusion-weighted MR imaging in conjunction with T2-weighted imaging shows enormous potential for evaluating the extent of peritoneal metastatic disease. Its potential for predicting surgical outcomes needs to be established.

- MR imaging with diffusion-weighted imaging and dynamic-contrast enhanced are now well-established in the characterization of ultrasonographically indeterminate masses.

- Assessment of lymph nodes, even with the availability of functional MR imaging techniques, remains size related, and currently is best served by 18-fluorodeoxyglucose ([18]FDG) PET-CT.

- Quantification of functional MR imaging parameters for use as response biomarkers in clinical trials requires standardization of data acquisition and analysis methodology and rigorous quality control.

---

ongitudinal study in patients with a normal CA125.[120] This is largely because the treatment options for these patients are not aimed at cure. As therapeutic options improve, the impetus for detecting recurrence earlier with functional imaging techniques will increase.

SUMMARY

Functional MR imaging parameters derived from DCE-MR imaging and DW-MR imaging are now obtainable quickly and easily in a clinical setting on all modern MR imaging scanners. Their incorporation into the clinical workflow is becoming the norm. They have huge potential in improving the detection, staging, and characterization of gynecologic malignancies, as well as for monitoring response and identifying recurrence, thus profoundly impacting management (Box 2). The standardization of these quantitative parameters remains challenging and is essential before their successful incorporation into multicenter clinical trials.

REFERENCES

1. Colombo N, Carinelli S, Colombo A, et al. Endometrial cancer: ESMO clinical practice guidelines for diagnosis, treatment and follow-up. Ann Oncol 2011;22(Suppl 6):vi35–9.

2. Breijer MC, Timmermans A, van Doorn HC, et al. Diagnostic strategies for postmenopausal bleeding. Obstet Gynecol Int 2010;2010:850812.

3. Inada Y, Matsuki M, Nakai G, et al. Body diffusion-weighted MR imaging of uterine endometrial cancer: is it helpful in the detection of cancer in nonenhanced MR imaging? Eur J Radiol 2009;70(1):122–7.

4. Bharwani N, Miquel ME, Sahdev A, et al. Diffusion-weighted imaging in the assessment of tumour grade in endometrial cancer. Br J Radiol 2011; 84(1007):997–1004.

5. Fujii S, Matsusue E, Kigawa J, et al. Diagnostic accuracy of the apparent diffusion coefficient in differentiating benign from malignant uterine endometrial cavity lesions: initial results. Eur Radiol 2008;18(2):384–9.

6. Fujii S, Matsusue E, Kanasaki Y, et al. Detection of peritoneal dissemination in gynecological malignancy: evaluation by diffusion-weighted MR imaging. Eur Radiol 2008;18(1):18–23.

7. Zhang J, Cai S, Li C, et al. Can magnetic resonance spectroscopy differentiate endometrial cancer? Eur Radiol 2014;24(10):2552–60.

8. Celik O, Hascalik S, Sarac K, et al. Magnetic resonance spectroscopy of premalignant and malignant endometrial disorders: a feasibility of in vivo study. Eur J Obstet Gynecol Reprod Biol 2005; 118(2):241–5.

9. Kinkel K, Forstner R, Danza FM, et al. Staging of endometrial cancer with MRI: guidelines of the European Society of Urogenital Imaging. Eur Radiol 2009;19(7):1565–74.

10. Querleu D, Planchamp F, Narducci F, et al. Clinical practice guidelines for the management of patients with endometrial cancer in France: recommendations of the Institut National du Cancer and the Societe Francaise d'Oncologie Gynecologique. Int J Gynecol Cancer 2011;21(5):945–50.

11. Sironi S, Colombo E, Villa G, et al. Myometrial invasion by endometrial carcinoma: assessment with plain and gadolinium-enhanced MR imaging. Radiology 1992;185(1):207–12.

12. Ito K, Matsumoto T, Nakada T, et al. Assessing myometrial invasion by endometrial carcinoma with dynamic MRI. J Comput Assist Tomogr 1994; 18(1):77–86.

13. Manfredi R, Mirk P, Maresca G, et al. Local-regional staging of endometrial carcinoma: role of MR

imaging in surgical planning. Radiology 2004; 231(2):372–8.

14. Seki H, Kimura M, Sakai K. Myometrial invasion of endometrial carcinoma: assessment with dynamic MR and contrast-enhanced T1-weighted images. Clin Radiol 1997;52(1):18–23.

15. Yamashita Y, Harada M, Sawada T, et al. Normal uterus and FIGO stage I endometrial carcinoma: dynamic gadolinium-enhanced MR imaging. Radiology 1993;186(2):495–501.

16. Hricak H, Hamm B, Semelka RC, et al. Carcinoma of the uterus: use of gadopentetate dimeglumine in MR imaging. Radiology 1991;181(1):95–106.

17. Nakao Y, Yokoyama M, Hara K, et al. MR imaging in endometrial carcinoma as a diagnostic tool for the absence of myometrial invasion. Gynecol Oncol 2006;102(2):343–7.

18. Sala E, Crawford R, Senior E, et al. Added value of dynamic contrast-enhanced magnetic resonance imaging in predicting advanced stage disease in patients with endometrial carcinoma. Int J Gynecol Cancer 2009;19(1):141–6.

19. Wu LM, Xu JR, Gu HY, et al. Predictive value of T2-weighted imaging and contrast-enhanced MR imaging in assessing myometrial invasion in endometrial cancer: a pooled analysis of prospective studies. Eur Radiol 2013;23(2):435–49.

20. Utsunomiya D, Notsute S, Hayashida Y, et al. Endometrial carcinoma in adenomyosis: assessment of myometrial invasion on T2-weighted spin-echo and gadolinium-enhanced T1-weighted images. AJR Am J Roentgenol 2004;182(2):399–404.

21. Beddy P, Moyle P, Kataoka M, et al. Evaluation of depth of myometrial invasion and overall staging in endometrial cancer: comparison of diffusion-weighted and dynamic contrast-enhanced MR imaging. Radiology 2012;262(2):530–7.

22. Ascher SM, Reinhold C. Imaging of cancer of the endometrium. Radiol Clin North Am 2002;40(3): 563–76.

23. Shen SH, Chiou YY, Wang JH, et al. Diffusion-weighted single-shot echo-planar imaging with parallel technique in assessment of endometrial cancer. AJR Am J Roentgenol 2008;190(2): 481–8.

24. Rechichi G, Galimberti S, Signorelli M, et al. Myometrial invasion in endometrial cancer: diagnostic performance of diffusion-weighted MR imaging at 1.5-T. Eur Radiol 2010;20(3):754–62.

25. Whittaker CS, Coady A, Culver L, et al. Diffusion-weighted MR imaging of female pelvic tumors: a pictorial review. Radiographics 2009;29(3):759–74 [discussion: 774–8].

26. Lin G, Ho KC, Wang JJ, et al. Detection of lymph node metastasis in cervical and uterine cancers by diffusion-weighted magnetic resonance imaging at 3T. J Magn Reson Imaging 2008;28(1):128–35.

27. Rechichi G, Galimberti S, Signorelli M, et al. Endometrial cancer: correlation of apparent diffusion coefficient with tumor grade, depth of myometrial invasion, and presence of lymph node metastases. AJR Am J Roentgenol 2011;197(1):256–62.

28. Cao K, Gao M, Sun YS, et al. Apparent diffusion coefficient of diffusion weighted MRI in endometrial carcinoma-Relationship with local invasiveness. Eur J Radiol 2012;81(8):1926–30.

29. Woo S, Cho JY, Kim SY, et al. Histogram analysis of apparent diffusion coefficient map of diffusion weighted MRI in endometrial cancer: a preliminary correlation study with histological grade. Acta Radiol 2014;55(10):1270–7.

30. Sahdev A, Sohaib SA, Jacobs I, et al. MR imaging of uterine sarcomas. AJR Am J Roentgenol 2001; 177(6):1307–11.

31. Tamai K, Koyama T, Saga T, et al. The utility of diffusion-weighted MR imaging for differentiating uterine sarcomas from benign leiomyomas. Eur Radiol 2008;18(4):723–30.

32. Fujii S, Kaneda S, Tsukamoto K, et al. Diffusion-weighted imaging of uterine endometrial stromal sarcoma: a report of 2 cases. J Comput Assist Tomogr 2010;34(3):377–9.

33. Takeuchi M, Matsuzaki K, Harada M. Preliminary observations and clinical value of lipid peak in high-grade uterine sarcomas using in vivo proton MR spectroscopy. Eur Radiol 2013;23(9):2358–63.

34. Rijpkema M, Schuuring J, van der Meulen Y, et al. Characterization of oligodendrogliomas using short echo time 1H MR spectroscopic imaging. NMR Biomed 2003;16(1):12–8.

35. Sohaib SA, Houghton SL, Meroni R, et al. Recurrent endometrial cancer: patterns of recurrent disease and assessment of prognosis. Clin Radiol 2007; 62(1):28–34 [discussion: 35–6].

36. Kinkel K, Ariche M, Tardivon AA, et al. Differentiation between recurrent tumor and benign conditions after treatment of gynecologic pelvic carcinoma: value of dynamic contrast-enhanced subtraction MR imaging. Radiology 1997;204(1): 55–63.

37. Nakamura K, Imafuku N, Nishida T, et al. Measurement of the minimum apparent diffusion coefficient (ADCmin) of the primary tumor and CA125 are predictive of disease recurrence for patients with endometrial cancer. Gynecol Oncol 2012;124(2): 335–9.

38. Kuang F, Yan Z, Li H, et al. Diagnostic accuracy of diffusion-weighted MRI for differentiation of cervical cancer and benign cervical lesions at 3.0T: comparison with routine MRI and dynamic contrast-enhanced MRI. J Magn Reson Imaging 2015. [Epub ahead of print].

39. Hou B, Xiang SF, Yao GD, et al. Diagnostic significance of diffusion-weighted MRI in patients with

cervical cancer: a meta-analysis. Tumour Biol 2014;35(12):11761–9.

40. Hoogendam JP, Klerkx WM, de Kort GA, et al. The influence of the b-value combination on apparent diffusion coefficient based differentiation between malignant and benign tissue in cervical cancer. J Magn Reson Imaging 2010;32(2):376–82.

41. Downey K, Shepherd JH, Attygalle AD, et al. Pre-operative imaging in patients undergoing trache-lectomy for cervical cancer: validation of a combined T2- and diffusion-weighted endovaginal MRI technique at 3.0 T. Gynecol Oncol 2014; 133(2):326–32.

42. Charles-Edwards E, Morgan V, Attygalle AD, et al. Endovaginal magnetic resonance imaging of stage 1A/1B cervical cancer with A T2- and diffusion-weighted magnetic resonance technique: effect of lesion size and previous cone biopsy on tumor detectability. Gynecol Oncol 2011;120(3):368–73.

43. Charles-Edwards EM, Messiou C, Morgan VA, et al. Diffusion-weighted imaging in cervical cancer with an endovaginal technique: potential value for improving tumor detection in stage Ia and Ib1 dis-ease. Radiology 2008;249(2):541–50.

44. Downey K, Jafar M, Attygalle AD, et al. Influencing surgical management in patients with carcinoma of the cervix using a T2- and ZOOM-diffusion-weighted endovaginal MRI technique. Br J Cancer 2013;109(3):615–22.

45. De Silva SS, Payne GS, Thomas V, et al. Investiga-tion of metabolite changes in the transition from pre-invasive to invasive cervical cancer measured using (1)H and (31)P magic angle spinning MRS of intact tissue. NMR Biomed 2009;22(2):191–8.

46. Lin Y, Chen Z, Kuang F, et al. Evaluation of interna-tional federation of gynecology and obstetrics stage IB cervical cancer: comparison of diffusion-weighted and dynamic contrast-enhanced mag-netic resonance imaging at 3.0 T. J Comput Assist Tomogr 2013;37(6):989–94.

47. Park JJ, Kim CK, Park SY, et al. Parametrial inva-sion in cervical cancer: fused T2-weighted imaging and high-b-value diffusion-weighted imaging with background body signal suppression at 3 T. Radi-ology 2015;274(3):734–41.

48. Park JJ, Kim CK, Park SY, et al. Value of diffusion-weighted imaging in predicting parametrial inva-sion in stage IA2-IIA cervical cancer. Eur Radiol 2014;24(5):1081–8.

49. Nakai G, Matsuki M, Inada Y, et al. Detection and evaluation of pelvic lymph nodes in patients with gynecologic malignancies using body diffusion-weighted magnetic resonance imaging. J Comput Assist Tomogr 2008;32(5):764–8.

50. Yu SP, He L, Liu B, et al. Differential diagnosis of metastasis from non-metastatic lymph nodes in cervical cancers: pilot study of diffusion weighted

imaging with background suppression at 3T mag-netic resonance. Chin Med J (Engl) 2010;123(20): 2820–4.

51. Klerkx WM, Veldhuis WB, Spijkerboer AM, et al. The value of 3.0Tesla diffusion-weighted MRI for pelvic nodal staging in patients with early stage cervical cancer. Eur J Cancer 2012;48(18):3414–21.

52. Klerkx WM, Mali WM, Peter Heintz A, et al. Observer variation of magnetic resonance imaging and diffusion weighted imaging in pelvic lymph node detection. Eur J Radiol 2011;78(1):71–4.

53. Choi EK, Kim JK, Choi HJ, et al. Node-by-node cor-relation between MR and PET/CT in patients with uterine cervical cancer: diffusion-weighted imaging versus size-based criteria on T2WI. Eur Radiol 2009;19(8):2024–32.

54. Donaldson SB, Buckley DL, O'Connor JP, et al. Enhancing fraction measured using dynamic contrast-enhanced MRI predicts disease-free sur-vival in patients with carcinoma of the cervix. Br J Cancer 2010;102(1):23–6.

55. Andersen EK, Hole KH, Lund KV, et al. Dynamic contrast-enhanced MRI of cervical cancers: temp-oral percentile screening of contrast enhancement identifies parameters for prediction of chemora-dioresistance. Int J Radiat Oncol Biol Phys 2012; 82(3):e485–92.

56. Andersen EK, Hole KH, Lund KV, et al. Pharmaco-kinetic parameters derived from dynamic contrast enhanced MRI of cervical cancers predict chemo-radiotherapy outcome. Radiother Oncol 2013; 107(1):117–22.

57. Nakamura K, Joja I, Nagasaka T, et al. The mean apparent diffusion coefficient value (ADCmean) on primary cervical cancer is a predictive marker for disease recurrence. Gynecol Oncol 2012; 127(3):478–83.

58. Xue H, Ren C, Yang J, et al. Histogram analysis of apparent diffusion coefficient for the assessment of local aggressiveness of cervical cancer. Arch Gy-necol Obstet 2014;290(2):341–8.

59. Lin Y, Li H, Chen Z, et al. Correlation of histogram analysis of apparent diffusion coefficient with uter-ine cervical pathologic finding. AJR Am J Roent-genol 2015;204(5):1125–31.

60. Downey K, Riches SF, Morgan VA, et al. Relation-ship between imaging biomarkers of stage I cervi-cal cancer and poor-prognosis histologic features: quantitative histogram analysis of diffusion-weighted MR images. AJR Am J Roentgenol 2013;200(2):314–20.

61. Lee EY, Yu X, Chu MM, et al. Perfusion and diffu-sion characteristics of cervical cancer based on in-traxovel incoherent motion MR imaging-a pilot study. Eur Radiol 2014;24(7):1506–13.

62. Payne GS, Schmidt M, Morgan VA, et al. Evalua-tion of magnetic resonance diffusion and

spectroscopy measurements as predictive bio-markers in stage 1 cervical cancer. Gynecol Oncol 2010;116(2):246–52.

63. Kim JH, Kim CK, Park BK, et al. Dynamic contrast-enhanced 3-T MR imaging in cervical cancer before and after concurrent chemoradiotherapy. Eur Radiol 2012;22(11):2533–9.

64. Himoto Y, Fujimoto K, Kido A, et al. Assessment of the early predictive power of quantitative magnetic resonance imaging parameters during neoadjuvant chemotherapy for uterine cervical cancer. Int J Gynecol Cancer 2014;24(4):751–7.

65. Harry VN, Semple SI, Gilbert FJ, et al. Diffusion-weighted magnetic resonance imaging in the early detection of response to chemoradiation in cervical cancer. Gynecol Oncol 2008;111(2): 213–20.

66. Kim HS, Kim CK, Park BK, et al. Evaluation of therapeutic response to concurrent chemoradiotherapy in patients with cervical cancer using diffusion-weighted MR imaging. J Magn Reson Imaging 2013;37(1):187–93.

67. Liu Y, Bai R, Sun H, et al. Diffusion-weighted imaging in predicting and monitoring the response of uterine cervical cancer to combined chemoradiation. Clin Radiol 2009;64(11):1067–74.

68. Kuang F, Yan Z, Wang J, et al. The value of diffusion-weighted MRI to evaluate the response to radiochemotherapy for cervical cancer. Magn Reson Imaging 2014;32(4):342–9.

69. Fu C, Bian D, Liu F, et al. The value of diffusion-weighted magnetic resonance imaging in assessing the response of locally advanced cervical cancer to neoadjuvant chemotherapy. Int J Gynecol Cancer 2012;22(6):1037–43.

70. Fu C, Feng X, Bian D, et al. Simultaneous changes of magnetic resonance diffusion-weighted imaging and pathological microstructure in locally advanced cervical cancer caused by neoadjuvant chemotherapy. J Magn Reson Imaging 2015; 42(2):427–35.

71. Park JJ, Kim CK, Park SY, et al. Assessment of early response to concurrent chemoradiotherapy in cervical cancer: value of diffusion-weighted and dynamic contrast-enhanced MR imaging. Magn Reson Imaging 2014;32(8):993–1000.

72. Schreuder SM, Lensing R, Stoker J, et al. Monitoring treatment response in patients undergoing chemoradiotherapy for locally advanced uterine cervical cancer by additional diffusion-weighted imaging: a systematic review. J Magn Reson Imaging 2015;42(3):572–94.

73. Ryu SY, Kim MH, Nam BH, et al. Intermediate-risk grouping of cervical cancer patients treated with radical hysterectomy: a Korean Gynecologic Oncology Group study. Br J Cancer 2014;110(2): 278–85.

74. Ansink A, de Barros Lopes A, Naik R, et al. Recurrent stage IB cervical carcinoma: evaluation of the effectiveness of routine follow up surveillance. Br J Obstet Gynaecol 1996;103(11):1156–8.

75. Zola P, Fuso L, Mazzola S, et al. Could follow-up different modalities play a role in asymptomatic cervical cancer relapses diagnosis? An Italian multicenter retrospective analysis. Gynecol Oncol 2007;107(1 Suppl 1):S150–4.

76. Morice P, Deyrolle C, Rey A, et al. Value of routine follow-up procedures for patients with stage I/II cervical cancer treated with combined surgery-radiation therapy. Ann Oncol 2004;15(2):218–23.

77. Mittra E, El-Maghraby T, Rodriguez CA, et al. Efficacy of 18F-FDG PET/CT in the evaluation of patients with recurrent cervical carcinoma. Eur J Nucl Med Mol Imaging 2009;36(12):1952–9.

78. Keller TM, Michel SC, Fröhlich J, et al. USPIO enhanced MRI for preoperative staging of gynecological pelvic tumors: preliminary results. Eur Radiol 2004;14(6):937–44.

79. Vilarino-Varela MJ, Taylor A, Rockall AG, et al. A verification study of proposed pelvic lymph node localisation guidelines using nanoparticle-enhanced magnetic resonance imaging. Radiother Oncol 2008;89(2):192–6.

80. Rockall AG, Sohaib SA, Harisinghani MG, et al. Diagnostic performance of nanoparticle-enhanced magnetic resonance imaging in the diagnosis of lymph node metastases in patients with endometrial and cervical cancer. J Clin Oncol 2005; 23(12):2813–21.

81. Sohaib SA, Mills TD, Sahdev A, et al. The role of magnetic resonance imaging and ultrasound in patients with adnexal masses. Clin Radiol 2005;60(3): 340–8.

82. Sohaib SA, Sahdev A, Van Trappen P, et al. Characterization of adnexal mass lesions on MR imaging. AJR Am J Roentgenol 2003;180(5):1297–304.

83. Kaijser J, Vandecaveye V, Deroose CM, et al. Imaging techniques for the pre-surgical diagnosis of adnexal tumours. Best Pract Res Clin Obstet Gynaecol 2014;28(5):683–95.

84. Anthoulakis C, Nikoloudis N. Pelvic MRI as the "gold standard" in the subsequent evaluation of ultrasound-indeterminate adnexal lesions: a systematic review. Gynecol Oncol 2014;132(3):661–8.

85. Bernardin L, Dilks P, Liyanage S, et al. Effectiveness of semi-quantitative multiphase dynamic contrast-enhanced MRI as a predictor of malignancy in complex adnexal masses: radiological and pathological correlation. Eur Radiol 2012; 22(4):880–90.

86. Dilks P, Narayanan P, Reznek R, et al. Can quantitative dynamic contrast-enhanced MRI independently characterize an ovarian mass? Eur Radiol 2010;20(9):2176–83.

87. Thomassin-Naggara I, Aubert E, Rockall A, et al. Adnexal masses: development and preliminary validation of an MR imaging scoring system. Radiology 2013;267(2):432–43.

88. Thomassin-Naggara I, Balvay D, Aubert E, et al. Quantitative dynamic contrast-enhanced MR imaging analysis of complex adnexal masses: a preliminary study. Eur Radiol 2012;22(4):738–45.

89. Moteki T, Ishizaka H. Evaluation of cystic ovarian lesions using apparent diffusion coefficient calculated from turboFLASH MR images. Br J Radiol 1998;71(846):612–20.

90. Katayama M, Masui T, Kobayashi S, et al. Diffusion-weighted echo planar imaging of ovarian tumors: is it useful to measure apparent diffusion coefficients? J Comput Assist Tomogr 2002;26(2):250–6.

91. Sarty GE, Kendall EJ, Loewy J, et al. Magnetic resonance diffusion imaging of ovarian masses: a first experience with 12 cases. MAGMA 2004; 16(4):182–93.

92. Fujii S, Kakite S, Nishihara K, et al. Diagnostic accuracy of diffusion-weighted imaging in differentiating benign from malignant ovarian lesions. J Magn Reson Imaging 2008;28(5):1149–56.

93. Bakir B, Bakan S, Tunaci M, et al. Diffusion-weighted imaging of solid or predominantly solid gynaecological adnexal masses: is it useful in the differential diagnosis? Br J Radiol 2011;84(1003): 600–11.

94. Zhang P, Cui Y, Li W, et al. Diagnostic accuracy of diffusion-weighted imaging with conventional MR imaging for differentiating complex solid and cystic ovarian tumors at 1.5T. World J Surg Oncol 2012; 10:237.

95. Li W, Chu C, Cui Y, et al. Diffusion-weighted MRI: a useful technique to discriminate benign versus malignant ovarian surface epithelial tumors with solid and cystic components. Abdom Imaging 2012; 37(5):897–903.

96. Kierans AS, Bennett GL, Mussi TC, et al. Characterization of malignancy of adnexal lesions using ADC entropy: comparison with mean ADC and qualitative DWI assessment. J Magn Reson Imaging 2013;37(1):164–71.

97. Takeuchi M, Matsuzaki K, Harada M. Ovarian adenofibromas and cystadenofibromas: magnetic resonance imaging findings including diffusion-weighted imaging. Acta Radiol 2013;54(2):231–6.

98. Takeuchi M, Matsuzaki K, Nishitani H. Diffusion-weighted magnetic resonance imaging of ovarian tumors: differentiation of benign and malignant solid components of ovarian masses. J Comput Assist Tomogr 2010;34(2):173–6.

99. Cappabianca S, Iaselli F, Reginelli A, et al. Value of diffusion-weighted magnetic resonance imaging in the characterization of complex adnexal masses. Tumori 2013;99(2):210–7.

100. Dowdy SC, Mullany SA, Brandt KR, et al. The utility of computed tomography scans in predicting suboptimal cytoreductive surgery in women with advanced ovarian carcinoma. Cancer 2004; 101(2):346–52.

101. Bristow RE, Duska LR, Lambrou NC, et al. A model for predicting surgical outcome in patients with advanced ovarian carcinoma using computed tomography. Cancer 2000;89(7):1532–40.

102. Qayyum A, Coakley FV, Westphalen AC, et al. Role of CT and MR imaging in predicting optimal cytoreduction of newly diagnosed primary epithelial ovarian cancer. Gynecol Oncol 2005;96(2):301–6.

103. Meyer JI, Kennedy AW, Friedman R, et al. Ovarian carcinoma: value of CT in predicting success of debulking surgery. AJR Am J Roentgenol 1995; 165(4):875–8.

104. Ferrandina G, Sallustio G, Fagotti A, et al. Role of CT scan-based and clinical evaluation in the preoperative prediction of optimal cytoreduction in advanced ovarian cancer: a prospective trial. Br J Cancer 2009;101(7):1066–73.

105. Forstner R, Hricak H, Occhipinti KA, et al. Ovarian cancer: staging with CT and MR imaging. Radiology 1995;197(3):619–26.

106. Gemer O, Gdalevich M, Ravid M, et al. A multicenter validation of computerized tomography models as predictors of non- optimal primary cytoreduction of advanced epithelial ovarian cancer. Eur J Surg Oncol 2009;35(10):1109–12.

107. Kebapci M, Akca AK, Yalcin OT, et al. Prediction of suboptimal cytoreduction of epithelial ovarian carcinoma by preoperative computed tomography. Eur J Gynaecol Oncol 2010;31(1):44–9.

108. Nelson RC, Chezmar JL, Hoel MJ, et al. Peritoneal carcinomatosis: preoperative CT with intraperitoneal contrast material. Radiology 1992;182(1):133–8.

109. Axtell AE, Lee MH, Bristow RE, et al. Multi-institutional reciprocal validation study of computed tomography predictors of suboptimal primary cytoreduction in patients with advanced ovarian cancer. J Clin Oncol 2007;25(4):384–9.

110. Kyriazi S, Collins DJ, Morgan VA, et al. Diffusion-weighted imaging of peritoneal disease for non-invasive staging of advanced ovarian cancer. Radiographics 2010;30(5):1269–85.

111. Low RN, Sebrechts CP, Barone RM, et al. Diffusion-weighted MRI of peritoneal tumors: comparison with conventional MRI and surgical and histopathologic findings–a feasibility study. AJR Am J Roentgenol 2009;193(2):461–70.

112. Michielsen K, Vergote I, Op de Beeck K, et al. Whole-body MRI with diffusion-weighted sequence for staging of patients with suspected ovarian cancer: a clinical feasibility study in comparison to CT and FDG-PET/CT. Eur Radiol 2014; 24(4):889–901.

113. Tempany CM, Zou KH, Silverman SG, et al. Staging of advanced ovarian cancer: comparison of imaging modalities–report from the Radiological Diagnostic Oncology Group. Radiology 2000;215(3): 761–7.

114. Low RN, Barone RM. Combined diffusion-weighted and gadolinium-enhanced MRI can accurately predict the peritoneal cancer index preoperatively in patients being considered for cytoreductive surgical procedures. Ann Surg Oncol 2012;19(5): 1394–401.

115. Sala E, Priest AN, Kataoka M, et al. Apparent diffusion coefficient and vascular signal fraction measurements with magnetic resonance imaging: feasibility in metastatic ovarian cancer at 3 Tesla: technical development. Eur Radiol 2010;20(2):491–6.

116. Kyriazi S, Nye E, Stamp G, et al. Value of diffusion-weighted imaging for assessing site-specific response of advanced ovarian cancer to neoadjuvant chemotherapy: correlation of apparent diffusion coefficients with epithelial and stromal densities on histology. Cancer Biomark 2010;7(4):201–10.

117. Rustin GJ, Vergote I, Eisenhauer E, et al. Definitions for response and progression in ovarian cancer clinical trials incorporating RECIST 1.1 and CA 125 agreed by the Gynecological Cancer Intergroup (GCIG). Int J Gynecol Cancer 2011;21(2): 419–23.

118. Avril N, Sassen S, Schmalfeldt B, et al. Prediction of response to neoadjuvant chemotherapy by sequential F-18-fluorodeoxyglucose positron emission tomography in patients with advanced-stage ovarian cancer. J Clin Oncol 2005;23(30):7445–53.

119. Kyriazi S, Collins DJ, Messiou C, et al. Metastatic ovarian and primary peritoneal cancer: assessing chemotherapy response with diffusion-weighted MR imaging–value of histogram analysis of apparent diffusion coefficients. Radiology 2011; 261(1):182–92.

120. Low RN, Saleh F, Song SY, et al. Treated ovarian cancer: comparison of MR imaging with serum CA-125 level and physical examination–a longitudinal study. Radiology 1999;211(2):519–28.

Multiparametric MR Imaging of Breast Cancer

Habib Rahbar, MD, Savannah C. Partridge, PhD*

KEYWORDS

- Multiparametric breast MR imaging • Dynamic contrast enhanced • Diffusion-weighted imaging
- Magnetic resonance spectroscopy • Breast cancer

KEY POINTS

- Current clinical breast MR imaging approaches focus on high morphologic detail and semiquantitative kinetic information that allow high sensitivity and moderate specificity for breast cancer detection.
- Advanced functional MR imaging parameters can improve the ability to assess biology in vivo using imaging correlates of vascularity, cellularity, and chemical composition of breast lesions.
- Preliminary findings support the use of a functional, multiparametric breast approach to improve breast MR imaging specificity and the biological characterization of breast cancer.
- Currently, technical challenges and a lack of standardization in approach limit applicability of many functional breast MR imaging techniques, which should be addressed with future research.

INTRODUCTION

Breast cancer is extremely common, striking 1 in 8 American women, and is the second leading cause of cancer death among women in the United States.[1] Breast cancer mortality has decreased substantially over the past several decades, owing both to earlier-stage breast cancer detection through improved imaging techniques and improved therapeutics. Although breast MR imaging is a recent imaging technique, it was first proposed to aid early breast cancer detection in the 1970s,[2] which was supported by the discovery that abnormal breast tissue demonstrates differences in longitudinal (T1) and transverse (T2) relaxation times in vitro compared with normal tissue.[3] It was not until the elucidation, however, that most breast cancers demonstrate higher signal on T1-weighted images after the administration of gadolinium-based contrast material that breast MR imaging became a widely used tool for in vivo characterization of breast cancer.[4] Although optimal evidence-based uses continue to evolve, common clinical indications for conventional contrast-enhanced breast MR imaging currently include supplemental screening for high-risk women, preoperative evaluation of breast cancer extent of disease, assessment of equivocal findings on standard imaging and/or clinical examination, and evaluation of breast cancer response to neoadjuvant chemotherapy.

Perhaps the greatest driving force behind the increasingly wide adoption of breast MR imaging at many centers is its exquisite sensitivity

Drs H. Rahbar and S.C. Partridge have received support from the following grants: National Institutes of Health R01CA151326 and P50CA138293 and Radiological Society of North America Research Scholar Grant (Rahbar).
Breast Imaging Section, Department of Radiology, Seattle Cancer Care Alliance, University of Washington, 825 Eastlake Avenue East, PO Box 19023, Seattle, WA 98109–1023, USA
* Corresponding author.
E-mail address: scp3@uw.edu

Magn Reson Imaging Clin N Am 24 (2016) 223–238
http://dx.doi.org/10.1016/j.mric.2015.08.012
1064-9689/16/$ – see front matter © 2016 Elsevier Inc. All rights reserved.

(reported to approach 100%) for breast cancer detection. Multiple studies have shown that conventional contrast-enhanced breast MR imaging has the highest sensitivity of any imaging modality for breast cancer detection in asymptomatic high-risk women[5–8] and mammographically and clinically occult additional disease in the contralateral[6] and ipsilateral breast[9] in patients with recently diagnosed breast cancer. A major barrier to wider adoption of this technique for average and intermediate risk patients, however, is its modest specificity due to overlap in the imaging features of benign and malignant lesions, with wide variations in the positive predictive value of breast MR imaging reported in the literature (24%–89%).[10]

MR imaging also has been increasingly been studied as a tool to determine which newly diagnosed breast cancers are likely to respond to presurgical, or neoadjuvant, chemotherapy. Several early studies examining the use of MR imaging to assess early response to neoadjuvant chemotherapy found that changes in size or volume and enhancement kinetic profiles on MR imaging were associated with favorable responses to therapy, including pathologic complete response (pCR).[11,12] These findings suggested that MR imaging could be used to optimize medical therapy regimens for each individual. The general superiority of MR imaging over clinical examination and standard imaging techniques for predicting pCR was suggested in multiple single-center studies[13,14] and confirmed in a large multicenter trial.[15] Although standard contrast-enhanced MR imaging is the most accurate modality for predicting important neoadjuvant therapy outcomes, its clinical impact has been limited by its cost and modest overall performance in this setting.

Although MR imaging is commonly used at many centers to further evaluate equivocally suspicious clinical or imaging findings, several obstacles have limited application of MR imaging in this clinical setting. Barriers to cost-effective implementation of MR imaging to reduce unnecessary biopsies prompted by conventional imaging or clinical examination include the low cost associated with image-guided biopsies, which are highly accurate and safe compared with serial imaging,[16] and the high negative predictive value (NPV) (approximately 98%) needed to obviate the biopsy of a suspicious finding based on current American College of Radiology (ACR) Breast Imaging-Reporting and Data System (BI-RADS) guidelines.[17] Early studies have demonstrated that the NPV of MR imaging for this clinical indication ranges from 76% for further evaluation of suspicious mammographic calcifications[18] to

85% in the setting of any suspicious mammographic or clinical finding.[19] Studies from the authors' institution found that although breast MR imaging has high sensitivity and high NPV for this clinical indication, the added breast cancer yield was too low to routinely recommend breast MR imaging for problem solving.[20] More recently, Strobel and colleagues[21] found that the use of conventional breast MR imaging to evaluate suspicious (BI-RADS category 4) findings identified on screening mammography or ultrasound could help avoid up to 92% of unnecessary biopsies and was particularly accurate in evaluating lesions that were not comprised entirely of calcifications.

The basis for the strong clinical performance of conventional breast MR imaging has been through utilization of an imaging approach that emphasizes anatomic and morphologic detail through high spatial resolution and limited temporal resolution dynamic contrast-enhanced (DCE) technique (DCE–MR imaging). This approach provides limited insight on physiologic features of breast tissue and pathology through the measurement of semiquantitative kinetic features. Although these basic kinetic enhancement features, including peak initial-phase and delayed-phase curve descriptors, have shown some ability to distinguish between malignant and benign lesions,[22] they in general have provided a small incremental value to standard morphologic descriptions.[19] As a result, there is increasing interest in exploring whether multiparametric approaches to breast MR imaging that incorporate more highly quantitative pharmacokinetic DCE–MR imaging modeling and other functional MR imaging techniques such as diffusion-weighted imaging (DWI) and magnetic resonance spectroscopy (MRS), to probe specific biological properties, such as abnormal vessel permeability, cellularity, and chemical composition, can further advance the use of MR imaging for these specific clinical settings.

BREAST MR IMAGING PARAMETERS

There is no single way to achieve high-quality breast MR imaging, and this is particularly true when considering a multiparametric approach to MR imaging acquisition. Nonetheless, MR imaging should include an acquisition using a high-field (B_0) magnet ($\geq$1.5T) that is bilateral with complete breast and axilla coverage. Only dedicated breast surface coils are appropriate for breast MR imaging applications, because the built-in body coil cannot provide enough signal-to-noise (SNR) for high-quality breast imaging.

Dynamic Contrast-Enhanced MR Imaging

Currently, a DCE–MR imaging acquisition is central to breast MR imaging protocols, and the ACR Breast MRI Accreditation Program (BMRAP) mandates that a multiphase T1-weighted acquisition be performed for clinical breast MR imaging. Due to time and technical restraints, DCE–MR imaging protocols generally emphasize either high spatial resolution and full coverage or high temporal resolution in imaging of contrast uptake kinetics in breast. More sophisticated acquisition strategies, however, that undersample the periphery of k-space on subsequent dynamic acquisitions and more frequently sample the center of k-space can provide simultaneous high spatial, high temporal resolution acquisitions with full bilateral coverage[23–25] (**Fig. 1**). There is wide variation among centers on the number of postcontrast phases acquired. The ACR BMRAP requires acquisition of a minimum of 2 postcontrast T1-weighted images, with the first postcontrast sequence acquired within 4 minutes of contrast injection. DCE–MR imaging acquisition provides 2 primary imaging features that can be used to evaluate breast lesions: morphology and kinetic enhancement characteristics.

Morphology

There are 3 general morphologic descriptors of enhancing findings of the breast, which are

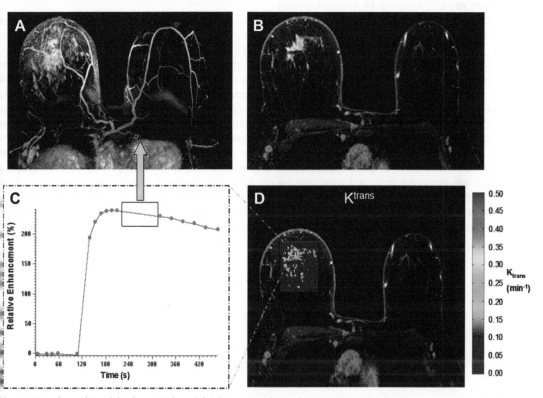

Fig. 1. Novel combined high spatial and high temporal resolution DCE–MR imaging scan approach, demonstrated in a subject with invasive ductal carcinoma. High spatial resolution phases (90-s scan; 0.6 × 0.6 × 2 mm resolution) are acquired before and 2 min and 6.5 min post–contrast injection, interleaved with high temporal resolution dynamic 4D THRIVE (Philips Healthcare, Best, Netherlands) acquisitions (15-s scan; 1 × 1 × 2 mm resolution). (*A*) Postcontrast subtraction maximum intensity projection generated from high spatial resolution images (*arrow*) acquired at 2 min post–contrast injection over the time frame indicated on the time-signal intensity curve (*c, box*). (*B*) Representative post–contrast high-resolution image through the lesion. (*C*) Time-signal intensity curve showing contrast enhancement dynamics for ROI in the invasive tumor. (*D*) Pharmacokinetic K^{trans} map calculated from the high temporal resolution images, overlaid on postcontrast image. Using this approach, 3-D extent of disease, along with lesion morphology can be accurately assessed on post–contrast high spatial resolution images, whereas more rigorous pharmacokinetic modeling can be performed using corresponding high temporal resolution data acquired during the same scan. (*Adapted from* Chen H, Olson ML, Partridge SC, et al, editors. Reducing the scan time in quantitative dynamic contrast enhanced MRI of the breast using the extended graphical model. Proceedings of the ISMRM Annual Meeting. Salt Lake City, UT, April 20–26 2013.)

defined by the ACR BI-RADS atlas: foci, masses, and nonmass enhancements (NMEs). Masses and NMEs also have additional descriptors that can further refine an interpreting radiologist's suspicion for malignancy. Prior studies have shown that morphologic features are perhaps the most important factor for initial assessment of likelihood of malignancy of a given lesion.[19] Suspicious morphologic features for masses include irregular shape, heterogeneous or rim internal enhancement, and irregular or spiculated margins. Suspicious NME morphologic features include segmental or linear distribution with heterogeneous or clustered ring enhancement. Breast cancers that present as NME are more likely to reflect in situ carcinoma than masses; however, significant overlap exists in morphologic presentation on MR imaging of invasive breast cancer, ductal carcinoma in situ, and atypical/high-risk lesions.

Dynamic contrast-enhanced kinetic enhancement features

Differential enhancement of malignancies relative to normal breast tissue is based on the fact that malignancies typically recruit abnormal new blood vessels to support their growth (ie, angiogenesis). The rate at which these abnormal vessels allow nutrients to spill into a tumor and the rate cell cycle byproducts are removed from a tumor can be characterized through assessing kinetic enhancement curves obtained from DCE–MR imaging. Most commonly, breast kinetic enhancement

features are measured semiquantitatively using modest temporal resolution with at least 2 to 3 postcontrast T1-weighted acquisitions, with k-space centered at approximately 90 to 120 seconds after contrast injection for the first postcontrast images. Using the data obtained at each of these time points, a time-signal intensity curve can be determined for a given lesion or region of interest (ROI), allowing assessment of 2 phases of enhancement: initial phase, within approximately 2 minutes of contrast injection, and late (or delayed) phase, after 2 minutes or after peak enhancement (Fig. 2). In the initial phase, enhancement classifications of slow, medium, and fast are determined by signal intensity increase ($SI_{\%increase}$) defined by the equation:

$$SI_{\%increase} = [(SI_{post} - SI_{pre})/SI_{pre}] \times 100\%$$

where SI_{pre} is the baseline signal intensity of an ROI and SI_{post} is the signal intensity of the same ROI after contrast injection.

In the delayed phase, enhancement curves can be classified by 3 basic curve types: persistent, plateau, and washout. Persistent delayed enhancement is generally considered a benign enhancement curve type, whereas plateau delayed enhancement is of intermediate suspicion for malignancy, and washout delayed enhancement is the most suggestive of malignancy. Although the most classic combined curve type for malignant breast lesions is fast initial enhancement followed by early washout (sometimes referred to as a type III curve[26]), there is significant

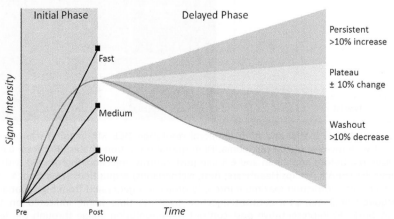

Fig. 2. Semiquantitative breast DCE kinetics analysis approach, as defined in the ACR BI-RADS atlas. The initial phase is classified based on the percent increase in signal intensity from precontrast levels, with increases of less than 50%, 50% to 100%, and greater than 100% classified as slow, medium, and fast, respectively. The delayed phase is classified by the curve type after initial peak enhancement as persistent (defined as a continuous increase in enhancement of >10% initial enhancement), plateau (constant signal intensity once peak is reached ± 10% initial enhancement), or washout (decreasing signal intensity after peak enhancement >10% initial enhancement).

overlap of semiquantitative kinetic curve types among benign and malignant lesions.

MR imaging techniques that acquire postcontrast images with high temporal resolution can allow for more elegant assessment of contrast kinetics through pharmacokinetic modeling techniques. Pharmacokinetic models enable quantitative assessments of contrast agent exchange between the intravascular and the interstitial space, providing measures related to tumor blood flow, microvasculature, and capillary permeability. A 2-compartment model is the most commonly used approach, measuring the exchange of contrast between tissue (in this case breast tissue) and the plasma space and was first proposed in an MR imaging context by Tofts and Kermode.[27] The concentrations of the gadolinium tracer for each compartment vary with time after the bolus injection of the contrast agent, and quantitative metrics can be measured by this model using the following relationship:

$$k_{ep} = K^{trans}/v_e \qquad (2)$$

where the volume transfer constant K^{trans} reflects the rate of transfer of gadolinium from plasma to the tissue (unit: min^{-1}) (see Fig. 1D); the transfer rate constant k_{ep} (min^{-1}) reflects the reflux of contrast agent from the extravascular extracellular space to the plasma compartment; and v_e (%) reflects the leakage of fractional volume from the extravascular extracellular space into the plasma compartment.

Promising clinical applications of quantitative dynamic contrast-enhanced MR imaging

Several investigators have demonstrated that some of these pharmacokinetic parameters, in particular K^{trans} and k_{ep}, hold value for improved discrimination of malignant from benign breast pathologies and may even be used as biomarkers of disease subtypes. Li and colleagues[28] demonstrated that K^{trans} and k_{ep} values progressively increased when measuring normal glands, benign lesions, and malignant lesions, noting that invasive ductal carcinomas and ductal carcinoma in situ lesions exhibited significantly higher K^{trans} and k_{ep} values than ductal dysplasias. Huang and colleagues[29] demonstrated that using K^{trans} values of lesions found suspicious on standard clinical breast MR imaging, a potential cutoff value could be used such that lesions with lower K^{trans} values could avoid biopsy and thereby decrease false-positive MR examinations. Finally, DCE–MR imaging holds potential for assessing alterations in tumor perfusion in response to preoperative therapies (Fig. 3). K^{trans} values have been shown in a recent meta-analysis to be among the most promising MR imaging parameters for prediction of near-pCR to neoadjuvant chemotherapy, outperforming standard tumor size measurements.[30]

Technical challenges and considerations of quantitative dynamic contrast-enhanced MR imaging

To perform DCE–MR imaging pharmacokinetic modeling and calculate quantitative parameters, knowledge of both the precontrast T1 relaxation times of the tumor or tissue being imaged and the arterial input function (AIF), or the concentration of contrast agent as it changes over time within the arterial blood, is required. Measuring each of these parameters introduces unique challenges and potential for error. Precontrast T1 mapping is an essential step to convert DCE–MR imaging signal intensity into contrast agent concentration. T1 mapping requires acquisition of an additional series of images prior to DCE–MR imaging, most commonly using varying flip angle or inversion recovery approaches, and thus adds to the overall examination times. Moreover, variable flip angle approaches are prone to inaccuracies due to B1 inhomogeneity, a common issue for breast imaging, particularly at higher field strengths.[31] Most models require that the AIF be measured directly for each subject,[32] which is often challenging to perform and necessitates acquisition tradeoffs (in coverage and/or spatial resolution) to achieve the very high temporal resolution required to accurately sample the rapidly changing AIF. Furthermore, AIF measures can be sensitive to patient motion between dynamic acquisitions. One common approach to avoid the challenge of directly calculating the AIF is to use an average AIF calculated from a larger population for whom the injection site, dose, and rate were kept constant.[29] Yankeelov and colleagues[33] have proposed another method to circumvent this problem by estimating the AIF using a reference region model and found that such an approach correlated well with direct AIF measurement. Novel high spatiotemporal DCE–MR imaging acquisition strategies, as described previously, hold potential to provide high temporal resolution sampling of contrast enhancement curves without undesirable tradeoffs in spatial resolution and coverage, which may improve feasibility for utilization of pharmacokinetic analysis in clinical breast applications.[25]

Theoretically, model-based pharmacokinetic parameters have the advantage over semiquantitative enhancement curve assessments of being objective measures of underlying physiology that are not affected by variability in scan parameters. Given the different modeling algorithms, multiple challenges, and varying potential solutions, however, each of which can create significant differences

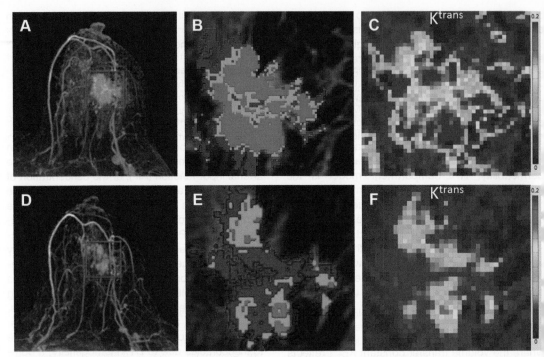

Fig. 3. DCE–MR imaging in a 51-year-old woman undergoing neoadjuvant chemotherapy for invasive ductal car cinoma (grade 3, estrogen receptor [ER]+/progesterone receptor [PR]+/human epidermal growth factor recepto 2 [HER2]+). The subject was imaged prior to therapy and 14 days after starting treatment with paclitaxel and tras tuzumab. Shown are pretreatment images of (A) post-contrast subtraction maximum intensity projection; (B) co lor-coded lesion curve type map ([blue] persistent enhancement, [green] plateau enhancement, and [red washout); (C) lesion Ktrans map, and corresponding post-14 days treatment images of (D) post-contrast subtrac tion maximum intensity projection; (E) color-coded curve type map; (F) Ktrans map. Changes in both lesion size and enhancement profile are evident at the early 14 day treatment time point.

in quantitative measurements, the generalizability of individual studies of advanced pharmacokinetic parameters will require standardization of the technical approach and multicenter testing.[34]

Diffusion-Weighted MR Imaging

DWI is a noncontrast MR imaging technique that measures the mobility of water molecules in vivo and probes tissue organization at the microscopic level. This water movement due to molecular diffusion, called brownian motion, is random in pure water. The motion of water molecules in vivo, however, is restricted by hindrances within intracellular and extracellular compartments. As a result, DWI reflects the microscopic cellular environment and is sensitive to biophysical characteristics, such as cell density, membrane integrity, and microstructure.

DWI has shown promise for the detection and characterization of breast cancer.[35] Numerous studies have shown that malignant breast lesions exhibit decreased water diffusion, attributed primarily to the increased cell density associated with breast tumors.[36] DWI is a short scan available on most commercial MR scanners that does not

require any exogenous contrast and can be added to breast MR imaging examinations to provide additional unique information on tissue micro structural properties.

Apparent diffusion coefficient calculation

DWI uses motion-sensitizing gradients during MR image acquisition to probe local diffusion characteristics. The diffusion-weighted MR imaging signal is reduced in intensity proportional to the water mobility and is commonly described by the monoexponential equation:

$$S_D = S_0\, e^{-b*ADC} \tag{3}$$

where S_0 is the signal intensity without diffusion weighting, S_D is the signal intensity with diffusion weighting, b is the applied diffusion sensitization (s/mm^2), and ADC is the apparent diffusion coefficient, defined as the average area a water molecule occupies per unit time (mm^2/s).[37] In general ADC can be calculated directly from a minimum of 2 acquisitions with different diffusion sensitizations (b-values) using:

$$ADC = \ln(S_1/S_2)/(b_2 - b_1) \tag{4}$$

where b_1 is the minimum b-value (eg, 0 s/mm^2) and b_2 is the maximum b-value (eg, 800 s/mm^2); S_1 is the signal intensity at $b = b_1$, S_2 is the signal intensity at $b = b_2$, and repetition time and echo time remain constant.[38] Due to restricted diffusion, breast malignancies commonly exhibit hyperintensity on DWI and lower ADC relative to normal breast parenchyma (Fig. 4).

Promising clinical applications of breast diffusion-weighted imaging

DWI holds strong potential as an adjunct MR imaging technique to reduce false-positive results and unnecessary biopsies. This has been the most widely explored application of DWI for breast imaging, and numerous groups have demonstrated restricted water diffusion in breast malignancies and significant differences in ADC values of benign and malignant lesions[36,39-41] (Figs. 5-7). A meta-analysis of 13 studies evaluating the diagnostic performance of DWI in 964 breast lesions (615 malignant and 349 benign) reported a pooled sensitivity of 84% (95% CI, 82%-87%) and specificity of 79% (95% CI, 75%-82%). ADC values for malignancies ranged from 0.87 to 1.36 $\times$ 10^{-3} mm^2/s, and recommended threshold ADC cutoffs to discriminate benign and malignant lesions varied from 0.90 to 1.76 $\times$ 10^{-3} mm^2/s (with 10/13 studies using a maximum b-value of 1000 s/mm^2).[42] Furthermore, multiple studies across a variety of field strengths have found that ADC measures are complementary to DCE-MR imaging parameters for discriminating benign and malignant breast lesions and can increase the accuracy of conventional breast MR imaging assessment.[43-46]

Another promising application for DWI is in monitoring breast cancer treatment. Alterations in cell membrane integrity and reduced tumor cellularity due to cytotoxic effects of chemotherapy result in increased water mobility within the damaged tumor tissue. A corresponding increase in tumor ADC in response to treatment may be detectable earlier than changes in tumor size or vascularity as measured by DCE-MR imaging, suggesting DWI may provide valuable early indication of treatment efficacy.[47,48] In a recent study of 118 women undergoing neoadjuvant chemotherapy for locally advanced breast cancer, Richard and colleagues[49] found that pretreatment tumor ADC values differed between intrinsic subtypes and were predictive of pathologic response in triple-negative tumors.

DWI may also offer a viable noncontrast method of breast MR screening. Many mammographically and clinically occult breast cancers detected by DCE-MR imaging are also visible on DWI and can be differentiated from benign breast lesions based on ADC.[50] In 1 study of asymptomatic women, DWI provided higher accuracy than screening mammography for the detection of breast malignancies.[51] The potential of DWI as a noncontrast alternative for breast MR screening has only been explored in a handful of studies and requires further investigation.

Technical challenges of breast diffusion-weighted imaging

Although a growing number of imaging centers are incorporating DWI into the clinical breast MR examination, several factors currently limit widespread clinical implementation.[35] The techniques used to acquire DW images of the breast, including the choice of b-values, vary considerably across studies in the literature. There is also wide variation in image quality of breast DWI due to the particular challenges of off-isocenter imaging, air-tissue interfaces, and significant fat content in the breast. Complete fat suppression is necessary to avoid detrimental chemical shift artifacts in

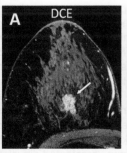 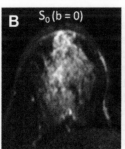 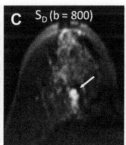 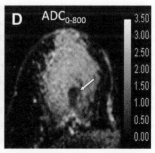

Fig. 4. Example DWI images obtained in a 52-year-old woman with an invasive lobular breast cancer. (A) DCE-MR imaging postcontrast slice as reference. Shown are corresponding slices from DWI of (B) S_0 with $b = 0$ s/mm^2 (primarily T2 weighted), (C) S_D with $b = 800$ s/mm^2, and (D) ADC map. The tumor (arrows) exhibits reduced diffusivity on DWI, appearing hyperintense on the S_D ($b = 800$ s/mm^2) image (C) and hypointense (mean ADC = 0.89 $\times$ 10^{-3} mm^2/s) on the ADC map (D).

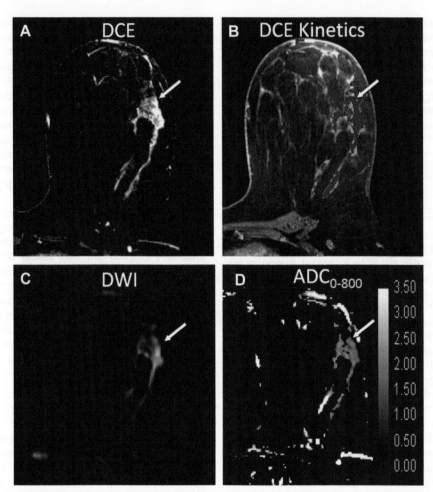

Fig. 5. Benign adenosis breast lesion in a 34-year-old woman with a BRCA1 gene mutation who underwent 1.5 breast MR imaging high-risk screening. (*A*) Postcontrast T1-weighted subtraction image shows an 84 mm segmental area of NME in the left breast (*arrow*). (*B*) DCE: the lesion shows mixed kinetics ([*blue*] 96% delayed persistent enhancement and [*green*] 4% delayed plateau enhancement). (*C*) DWI (b = 600 s/mm^2): the lesion demonstrates hyperintensity. (*D*) ADC map: the lesion exhibits moderately high diffusivity, with a mean ADC of 1.68 × 10^{-3} mm^2/s. (*Adapted from* Parsian S, Rahbar H, Allison KH, et al. Nonmalignant breast lesions: ADC of benign and high-risk subtypes assessed as false-positive at dynamic enhanced MR imaging. Radiology 2012;265(3):696–706; with permission.)

echo-planar DWI and confounding effects of residual intravoxel fat signal on breast tissue ADC measures.[52] Furthermore, differences in data analysis approaches, including postprocessing, ADC calculation, and ROI methods, result in considerable differences in the reported ADC values of similar breast pathologies. This lack of standardization in image acquisition and postprocessing methods makes it difficult to define generalizable interpretation strategies for breast DWI and to reliably assess the clinical utility of the technique.

Advanced methods of breast diffusion-weighted imaging

Several compelling advancements in DWI acquisition strategies are under development to overcome

the technical issues of spatial distortion and low resolution that currently prevent direct correlation and one-to-one mapping of DCE–MR imaging and DWI features and limit clinical implementation of breast DWI.[53–56] Furthermore, advanced modeling approaches are also being investigated to extract more valuable biological information from breast DWI scans. These include intravoxel incoherent motion (IVIM) modeling, which provides characterization of tissue perfusion in addition to diffusion[57–60]; diffusion kurtosis modeling, which characterizes deviation from unrestricted diffusion behavior (evident in vivo at high *b*-values >1500 s/ mm^2) and accounts for tissue complexity or physical barriers to diffusion within tissue (cell membranes, organelles, stromal desmoplasia, and so

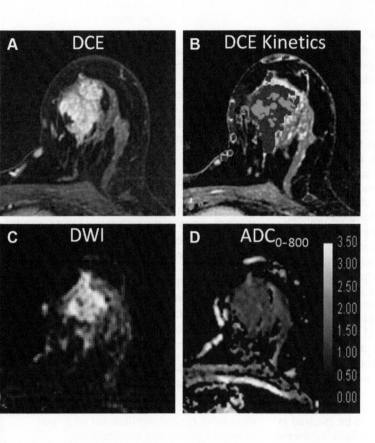

Fig. 6. High-grade ductal carcinoma in situ in 37-year-old woman who underwent 1.5T breast MR imaging. (A) Postcontrast T1-weighted fat-suppressed image shows a 51-mm enhancing lobular mass with irregular margins and heterogeneous internal and rapid enhancement in the left breast. (B) DCE–MR imaging: the mass demonstrates 146% peak initial enhancement with predominantly delayed persistent (blue) and plateau (green) enhancement kinetic features. (C) DWI (b = 600 s/mm^2): the lesion demonstrates high signal intensity. (D) ADC map: the lesion demonstrates low diffusivity, with a mean ADC of 1.45×10^{-3} mm^2/s. (Adapted from Rahbar H, Partridge SC, DeMartini WB, et al. In vivo assessment of ductal carcinoma in situ grade: a model incorporating dynamic contrast-enhanced and diffusion-weighted breast MR imaging parameters. Radiology 2012;263(2): 374–82; with permission.)

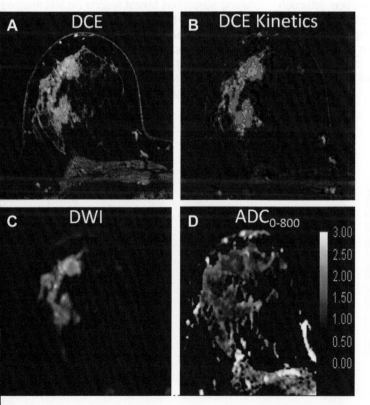

Fig. 7. High-grade invasive ductal carcinoma in a 35-year-old woman who underwent 3T breast MR imaging. (A) Postcontrast T1-weighted fat-suppressed image shows a large 47-mm enhancing irregular mass with heterogeneous internal and rapid enhancement in the right breast. (B) DCE–MR imaging: the mass demonstrates 489% peak initial enhancement with 66% delayed washout (red). (C) DWI (b = 800 s/mm^2): the lesion demonstrates high signal intensity. (D) ADC map: the lesion demonstrates low diffusivity, with a mean ADC of 0.94×10^{-3} mm^2/s.

forth)[58,61]; and diffusion tensor imaging, which characterizes the directionality of water diffusion in addition to the rate and may provide further insights on glandular organization (ducts and lobules) and microarchitecture.[62–64]

Magnetic Resonance Spectroscopy

MRS is a noninvasive technique that reflects the chemical composition of tissue. Rather than images, MRS techniques produce spatially localized signal spectra, with spectral peaks representing the structure and concentration of different chemical compounds in that region. MRS can differentiate tissue states, such as normal, malignant, necrotic, or hypoxic, based on varying levels of associated detectable metabolites. Proton MRS studies of the breast have demonstrated highly elevated levels of the metabolite choline in malignant lesions compared with benign lesions and normal breast tissue.[65–68] The choline peak observed in vivo, located at approximately 3.2 ppm, actually represents a composite of several different choline-containing compounds (including free choline, phosphocoline, and glycerophosphocholine, resolvable using ex vivo methods[69]) and is typically referred to as total choline (tCho). Choline is known to be involved in cell membrane turnover (phospholipid synthesis and degradation) and is, therefore, generally considered a marker of cell proliferation. Although the underlying biochemical process is not yet well understood, elevated choline signal in malignancies is thought to result from a combination of both increased intracellular phosphocholine concentration and increased cell density in the lesion.[69,70]

Techniques for acquisition and analysis of breast MRS have been reviewed extensively in a recent article by Bolan.[71] In general, single-voxel MRS is the most widely used acquisition approach, which produces a single spatially localized spectrum representing the average chemical signal from a 3-D cuboid volume (voxel) centered within a lesion identified on contrast-enhanced MR imaging (**Fig. 8**). Some manufacturers currently offer single-voxel protocols specifically optimized for breast MRS. An alternative localization technique is chemical shift imaging, or MRS imaging (MRSI), in which a larger volume is excited and 2-D or 3-D phase encoding is used to produce a spatially resolved grid of spectra. Breast MRS analysis centers on evaluation of the tCho signal and has been performed using a variety of approaches that can be generally categorized as (1) qualitative—detection of the presence of a tCho peak, (2) semiquantitative—measurement of tCho SNR, peak height, or peak integral, or (3) absolute quantification—calculation of tCho concentration (using internal referencing to unsuppressed water signal or external referencing to a phantom with a known chemical concentration).[71]

Promising clinical applications of breast magnetic resonance spectroscopy

MRS may help improve the accuracy of diagnosing suspicious breast lesions on MR imaging. Hydrogen (^{1}H)-MRS measures of choline levels in suspicious breast lesions have been shown to provide high specificity for distinguishing benign from malignant lesions.[72–74] A majority of breast MRS studies to date have been performed at 1.5T using single-voxel approaches. In a recent

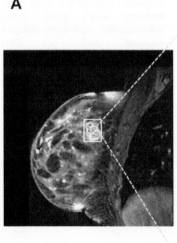

A

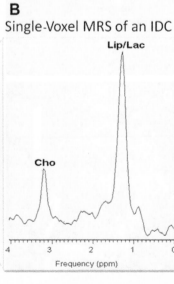

B

Single-Voxel MRS of an IDC

Fig. 8. Example of single-voxel breast ^{1}H-MRS acquired at 1.5T in a patient with invasive ductal carcinoma (2.1 cm, grade 2). (A) The voxel was positioned encompassing the enhancing lesion as indicated on the sagittal postcontrast T1-weighted image. (B) The resulting spectra demonstrated choline (Cho) peak at 3.2 ppm. A peak representing lipid (Lip) and lactate (Lac) is also present. (Courtesy of Wei Huang, PhD, Advanced Imaging Research Center, Oregon Health & Science University, Portland, Oregon.)

meta-analysis of 19 breast MRS studies, including 1198 lesions (773 malignant and 452 benign), Baltzer and Dietzel[75] found a pooled sensitivity of 73% (95% CI, 85%–91%) and specificity of 88% (95% CI, 64%–82%) for lesion diagnosis. Their analysis did not show any significant performance advantages of 3T over 1.5T field strength or MRSI over single-voxel techniques, or qualitative over quantitative tCho assessments, although the numbers of studies using 3T (n = 2/19) and MRSI (n = 3/19) were small. More recently, Pinker and colleagues[76] reported a high diagnostic accuracy for assessing suspicious breast lesions using a multiparametric MR imaging breast examination incorporating MRSI.

Whereas simple qualitative detection of the presence of a tCho peak was a reliable marker of malignancy in earlier investigations,[77] newer approaches using higher field strengths and higher sensitivity breast coil designs require more quantitative diagnostic methods because choline also becomes detectable even in normal breast tissue at higher SNR levels.[71,78] A threshold of tCho SNR greater than 2 is a commonly used threshold for malignancy in prior studies.

Breast MRS may play a valuable role in assessing response to neoadjuvant therapy. Breast tumor choline levels may reflect treatment-induced alterations in cell proliferation prior to any changes in tumor size and thus provide an early predictive marker of treatment response. In support of this, Haddadin and colleagues[70,79] found acute decreases in tumor tCho concentration were measurable at 4T as early as 24 hours after the first dose of chemotherapy and correlated with final changes in tumor size. In a large study of 184 patients with breast cancer, Shin and colleagues[80] further showed that tumor tCho measures were higher in invasive versus in situ cancers and correlated with several prognostic factors, including nuclear grade, histologic grade, and estrogen receptor (ER) status.

Technical challenges of breast magnetic resonance spectroscopy

There are several challenges to routine clinical use of MRS of the breast. As with breast DWI, high-quality shimming and lipid suppression are critical for successful breast MRS. Poor shimming results in B0 field inhomogeneities that broaden spectral line widths, causing reduced SNR and a reduced ability to separate different chemical resonances, and may also compromise the performance of chemically selective fat and water suppression in localized MRS. Shimming n be especially challenging in the breast with egions of mixed fibroglandular and adipose

tissues and in the presence of metallic biopsy clips. Without adequate fat suppression, lipid sidebands can obscure choline peaks in the spectra. A variety of fat-suppression strategies have been used across prior breast MRS studies and there is no clear consensus on the optimal method.[71,75]

A major limitation of breast MRS with current approaches is low sensitivity for detecting choline levels in smaller lesions (<10 mm),[71] which limits the applicability of the technique as an adjunct to clinical breast MR imaging to reduce false-positive results. Although breast tumor choline levels can be successfully measured using 1.5T magnetic resonance scanners, increases in both SNR and spectral resolution at higher field strength can improve choline detectability, decrease measurement errors, and enable the assessment of smaller lesions.[70] Another factor limiting clinical implementation is that single-voxel MRS requires voxel placement to be performed at the time of acquisition, which can be disruptive to clinical workflow because it requires real-time review by experienced radiologists specializing in breast MR imaging and some level of operator expertise. Furthermore, a single-voxel MRS technique is not helpful for breast cancer screening because of the limitations in breast coverage and voxel localization. Alternatively, multivoxel MRS approaches are under investigation and hold strong potential for improving the clinical utility of MRS for lesion detection and local staging of disease, as described later.

Advanced methods of breast magnetic resonance spectroscopy

MRSI, or chemical shift imaging, is a multivoxel approach that enables more extensive spatial sampling of the breast, providing several potential advantages over single-voxel methods. These include the ability to evaluate multiple lesions simultaneously, to characterize tumor heterogeneity, and to assess the extent of disease infiltration into surrounding tissue.[81] By providing wider coverage, MRSI reduces the need for a priori knowledge of lesion location and real-time expertise during the MR scan and may increase the feasibility of performing MRS in screening examinations. Furthermore, MRSI also allows for internal referencing for signal normalization. MRSI is more technically challenging, however, than single-voxel MRS with regard to shimming and fat suppression and requires longer scan times to achieve the extended breast coverage and as a result has not been widely implemented. With advancements in MR imaging hardware and software, a growing number of groups are implementing breast MRSI research protocols.[78,82–86]

Phosphorus (^{31}P)-MRS, a compelling alternative to conventional ^{1}H-MRS, holds promise to overcome some of the current challenges of breast MRS. ^{31}P-MRS enables direct measurement of phosphocholine and other key metabolites without the issues of lipid contamination present in ^{1}H MRS signal. Due to the inherently low SNR of ^{31}P-MRS caused by low abundance of phosphorus in the body, this approach becomes more feasible at high field strengths.[87] A recent study at 7T demonstrated associations between relative levels of ^{31}P-MRS phosphodiester and phosphomonoester peaks and metabolic activity as assessed by mitotic count in breast cancers.[88]

Emerging Functional Breast MR imaging Approaches

There are several other functional MR imaging approaches at early stages of development that are showing promise for advancing breast cancer characterization in preliminary investigations. These include ^{23}Na (sodium)-MR imaging and blood oxygen level–dependent (BOLD) MR imaging, described briefly later, as well as other techniques, such as MR elastography,[89] chemical exchange saturation transfer,[90,91] and high spectral spatial resolution imaging,[92] which are beyond the scope of this article.

Sodium MR imaging

Although MR imaging is typically performed to image the ^{1}H nucleus, it can also image other nuclei, such as ^{23}Na (sodium). Sodium is present at abundant levels in the body and has important biologic implications. Physiologic and biochemical changes associated with proliferating malignant tumors lead to an increase in tissue sodium. Sodium MR imaging may provide valuable insights to breast tumor metabolism and response to therapy. ^{23}Na-MR imaging studies have demonstrated elevated sodium levels in breast malignancies[93] and have shown that decreases in tumor sodium concentrations may reflect changes in cellular metabolism and membrane integrity with effective treatment.[94]

Blood oxygen level–dependent MR imaging

BOLD MR imaging, also known as intrinsic susceptibility-weighted imaging, can provide a noninvasive method of indirectly measuring tumor perfusion and hypoxia. Tumor hypoxia, a condition of low oxygenation, is a common feature of many solid tumors because rapidly proliferating cells outgrow the existing vasculature. Increased levels of paramagnetic deoxyhemoglobin concentration provide an endogenous contrast agent for imaging tissue hypoxia using BOLD MR imaging.[95,96] Tumor hypoxia is associated with tumor progression, angiogenesis, treatment resistance, local recurrence, and metastasis[97] and may be a useful biomarker of breast cancer prognosis and response to chemotherapy. BOLD for breast cancer is at an early stage of implementation and optimization, with only a few published studies to date.[95,96,98,99]

SUMMARY

Perhaps more than any other organ system, the breast holds great potential for clinical benefit from the use of a multiparametric MR imaging approach. This is due in part to the already broad use of breast MR imaging in clinical practice, which allows for relatively rapid translation of novel imaging techniques. Several groups have implemented sophisticated multiparametric functional MR imaging examinations to characterize breast lesions and have demonstrated dramatic ability to improve the diagnostic accuracy of conventional contrast-enhanced breast MR imaging,[7] to predict and monitor response to medical therapies,[94,100,101] and to discriminate biological subtypes of cancer.[88] There are obstacles to routine clinical application of advanced multiparametric breast MR imaging, however. Future work to address the many technical challenges unique to each of the individual functional MR imaging parameters and the lack of standardization of imaging approaches across institutions is needed. Ultimately, multicenter trials must be conducted (several of which are currently underway through ACRIN[102–104]) to validate single-institution findings prior to widespread implementation of these advanced functional breast MR imaging techniques.

REFERENCES

1. American Cancer Society. Cancer Facts and Figures. Atlanta (GA): American Cancer Society. 2015
2. Damadian R. Tumor detection by nuclear magnetic resonance. Science 1971;171(3976):1151–3.
3. Bovee WM, Getreuer KW, Smidt J, et al. Nuclear magnetic resonance and detection of human breast tumor. J Natl Cancer Inst 1978;61(1):53–5.
4. Kaiser WA, Zeitler E. MR imaging of the breast: fast imaging sequences with and without Gd-DTPA. Preliminary observations. Radiology 1989;170(Pt 1):681–6.
5. Kriege M, Brekelmans CT, Boetes C, et al. Efficacy of MRI and mammography for breast-cancer

screening in women with a familial or genetic pre-disposition. N Engl J Med 2004;351(5):427–37.

6. Lehman CD, Isaacs C, Schnall MD, et al. Cancer yield of mammography, MR, and US in high-risk women: prospective multi-institution breast cancer screening study. Radiology 2007;244(2):381–8.

7. Saslow D, Boetes C, Burke W, et al. American Cancer Society guidelines for breast screening with MRI as an adjunct to mammography. CA Cancer J Clin 2007;57(2):75–89.

8. Warner E, Plewes DB, Hill KA, et al. Surveillance of BRCA1 and BRCA2 mutation carriers with magnetic resonance imaging, ultrasound, mammography, and clinical breast examination. JAMA 2004;292(11):1317–25.

9. Schnall MD, Blume J, Bluemke DA, et al. MRI detection of distinct incidental cancer in women with primary breast cancer studied in IBMC 6883. J Surg Oncol 2005;92(1):32–8.

10. Elmore JG, Armstrong K, Lehman CD, et al. Screening for breast cancer. JAMA 2005;293(10): 1245–56.

11. Martincich L, Montemurro F, De Rosa G, et al. Monitoring response to primary chemotherapy in breast cancer using dynamic contrast-enhanced magnetic resonance imaging. Breast Cancer Res Treat 2004;83(1):67–76.

12. Pickles MD, Lowry M, Manton DJ, et al. Role of dynamic contrast enhanced MRI in monitoring early response of locally advanced breast cancer to neoadjuvant chemotherapy. Breast Cancer Res Treat 2005;91(1):1–10.

13. Rosen EL, Blackwell KL, Baker JA, et al. Accuracy of MRI in the detection of residual breast cancer after neoadjuvant chemotherapy. AJR Am J Roentgenol 2003;181(5):1275–82.

14. Weatherall PT, Evans GF, Metzger GJ, et al. MRI vs. histologic measurement of breast cancer following chemotherapy: comparison with x-ray mammography and palpation. J Magn Reson Imaging 2001;13(6):868–75.

15. Hylton NM, Blume JD, Bernreuter WK, et al. Locally advanced breast cancer: MR imaging for prediction of response to neoadjuvant chemotherapy–results from ACRIN 6657/I-SPY TRIAL. Radiology 2012;263(3):663–72.

16. Lee CI, Bensink ME, Berry K, et al. Performance goals for an adjunct diagnostic test to reduce unnecessary biopsies after screening mammography: analysis of costs, benefits, and consequences. J Am Coll Radiol 2013;10(12):924–30.

17. DeMartini W, Lehman C. A review of current evidence-based clinical applications for breast magnetic resonance imaging. Top Magn Reson Imaging 2008;19(3):143–50.

18. Cilotti A, Iacconi C, Marini C, et al. Contrast-enhanced MR imaging in patients with BI-RADS 3-5 microcalcifications. Radiol Med 2007;112(2): 272–86.

19. Bluemke DA, Gatsonis CA, Chen MH, et al. Magnetic resonance imaging of the breast prior to biopsy. JAMA 2004;292(22):2735–42.

20. Yau EJ, Gutierrez RL, DeMartini WB, et al. The utility of breast MRI as a problem-solving tool. Breast J 2011;17(3):273–80.

21. Strobel K, Schrading S, Hansen NL, et al. Assessment of BI-RADS category 4 lesions detected with screening mammography and screening US: utility of MR imaging. Radiology 2015;274(2):343–51.

22. Wang LC, DeMartini WB, Partridge SC, et al. MRI-detected suspicious breast lesions: predictive values of kinetic features measured by computer-aided evaluation. AJR Am J Roentgenol 2009; 193(3):826–31.

23. Chen H, Olson ML, Partridge SC, et al. Reducing the scan time in quantitative dynamic contrast enhanced MRI of the breast using the extended graphical model. Proceedings of the ISMRM Annual Meeting. Salt Lake City, UT, April 20–26 2013.

24. Pinker K, Bogner W, Baltzer P, et al. Clinical application of bilateral high temporal and spatial resolution dynamic contrast-enhanced magnetic resonance imaging of the breast at 7 T. Eur Radiol 2014;24(4):913–20.

25. Tudorica LA, Oh KY, Roy N, et al. A feasible high spatiotemporal resolution breast DCE-MRI protocol for clinical settings. Magn Reson Imaging 2012; 30(9):1257–67.

26. Kuhl CK, Mielcareck P, Klaschik S, et al. Dynamic breast MR imaging: are signal intensity time course data useful for differential diagnosis of enhancing lesions? Radiology 1999;211(1):101–10.

27. Tofts PS, Kermode AG. Measurement of the blood-brain barrier permeability and leakage space using dynamic MR imaging. 1. Fundamental concepts. Magn Reson Med 1991;17(2):357–67.

28. Li L, Wang K, Sun X, et al. Parameters of dynamic contrast-enhanced MRI as imaging markers for angiogenesis and proliferation in human breast cancer. Med Sci Monit 2015;21:376–82.

29. Huang W, Tudorica LA, Li X, et al. Discrimination of benign and malignant breast lesions by using shutter-speed dynamic contrast-enhanced MR imaging. Radiology 2011;261(2):394–403.

30. Marinovich ML, Sardanelli F, Ciatto S, et al. Early prediction of pathologic response to neoadjuvant therapy in breast cancer: systematic review of the accuracy of MRI. Breast 2012;21(5):669–77.

31. Kuhl CK, Kooijman H, Gieseke J, et al. Effect of B1 inhomogeneity on breast MR imaging at 3.0 T. Radiology 2007;244(3):929–30.

32. Tofts PS, Brix G, Buckley DL, et al. Estimating kinetic parameters from dynamic contrast-enhanced

T(1)-weighted MRI of a diffusable tracer: standard-ized quantities and symbols. J Magn Reson Imaging 1999;10(3):223–32.

33. Yankeelov TE, Luci JJ, Lepage M, et al. Quantita-tive pharmacokinetic analysis of DCE-MRI data without an arterial input function: a reference region model. Magn Reson Imaging 2005;23(4):519–29.

34. Huang W, Li X, Chen Y, et al. Variations of dynamic contrast-enhanced magnetic resonance imaging in evaluation of breast cancer therapy response: a multicenter data analysis challenge. Transl Oncol 2014;7(1):153–66.

35. Partridge SC, McDonald ES. Diffusion weighted magnetic resonance imaging of the breast: proto-col optimization, interpretation, and clinical appli-cations. Magn Reson Imaging Clin N Am 2013; 21(3):601–24.

36. Guo Y, Cai YQ, Cai ZL, et al. Differentiation of clin-ically benign and malignant breast lesions using diffusion-weighted imaging. J Magn Reson Imag-ing 2002;16(2):172–8.

37. Le Bihan D, Breton E, Lallemand D, et al. MR imag-ing of intravoxel incoherent motions: application to diffusion and perfusion in neurologic disorders. Radiology 1986;161(2):401–7.

38. Le Bihan D, Breton E, Lallemand D, et al. Separa-tion of diffusion and perfusion in intravoxel inco-herent motion MR imaging. Radiology 1988; 168(2):497–505.

39. Rubesova E, Grell AS, De Maertelaer V, et al. Quan-titative diffusion imaging in breast cancer: a clinical prospective study. J Magn Reson Imaging 2006; 24(2):319–24.

40. Sinha S, Lucas-Quesada FA, Sinha U, et al. In vivo diffusion-weighted MRI of the breast: potential for lesion characterization. J Magn Reson Imaging 2002;15(6):693–704.

41. Woodhams R, Matsunaga K, Kan S, et al. ADC mapping of benign and malignant breast tumors. Magn Reson Med Sci 2005;4(1):35–42.

42. Chen X, Li WL, Zhang YL, et al. Meta-analysis of quantitative diffusion-weighted MR imaging in the differential diagnosis of breast lesions. BMC Can-cer 2010;10:693.

43. Ei Khouli RH, Jacobs MA, Mezban SD, et al. Diffu-sion-weighted imaging improves the diagnostic ac-curacy of conventional 3.0-T breast MR imaging. Radiology 2010;256(1):64–73.

44. Partridge SC, DeMartini WB, Kurland BF, et al. Quantitative diffusion-weighted imaging as an adjunct to conventional breast MRI for improved positive predictive value. AJR Am J Roentgenol 2009;193(6):1716–22.

45. Pinker K, Baltzer P, Bogner W, et al. Multiparamet-ric MR Imaging with High-Resolution Dynamic Contrast-enhanced and Diffusion-weighted Imag-ing at 7 T Improves the Assessment of Breast

Tumors: A Feasibility Study. Radiology 201! 276(2):360–70.

46. Rahbar H, Partridge SC, Demartini WB, et al In vivo assessment of ductal carcinoma in sit grade: a model incorporating dynamic contras enhanced and diffusion-weighted breast MR imac ing parameters. Radiology 2012;263(2):374–82.

47. Pickles MD, Gibbs P, Lowry M, et al. Diffusic changes precede size reduction in neoadjuvar treatment of breast cancer. Magn Reson Imagin 2006;24(7):843–7.

48. Sharma U, Danishad KK, Seenu V, et al. Longitud nal study of the assessment by MRI and diffusior weighted imaging of tumor response in patient with locally advanced breast cancer undergoin neoadjuvant chemotherapy. NMR Biomed 2009 22(1):104–13.

49. Richard R, Thomassin I, Chapellier M, et al. Diffu sion-weighted MRI in pretreatment prediction c response to neoadjuvant chemotherapy in patient with breast cancer. Eur Radiol 2013;23(9):2420–3`

50. Partridge SC, Demartini WB, Kurland BF, et al. Di ferential diagnosis of mammographically and clin cally occult breast lesions on diffusion-weighte MRI. J Magn Reson Imaging 2010;31(3):562–70.

51. Yabuuchi H, Matsuo Y, Sunami S, et al. Detection c non-palpable breast cancer in asymptomat women by using unenhanced diffusion-weighte and T2-weighted MR imaging: comparison wit mammography and dynamic contrast-enhance MR imaging. Eur Radiol 2011;21(1):11–7.

52. Partridge SC, Singer L, Sun R, et al. Diffusior weighted MRI: influence of intravoxel fat signa and breast density on breast tumor conspicuit and apparent diffusion coefficient measurement Magn Reson Imaging 2011;29(9):1215–21.

53. Bogner W, Pinker K, Zaric O, et al. Bilater diffusion-weighted MR imaging of breast tumor with submillimeter resolution using readou segmented echo-planar imaging at 7 T. Radiolog 2015;274(1):74–84.

54. Lee SK, Tan ET, Govenkar A, et al. Dynamic slice dependent shim and center frequency update i 3 T breast diffusion weighted imaging. Magn Re son Med 2014;71(5):1813–8.

55. Singer L, Wilmes LJ, Saritas EU, et al. High-resolu tion diffusion-weighted magnetic resonance imag ing in patients with locally advanced breas cancer. Acad Radiol 2012;19(5):526–34.

56. Teruel JR, Fjosne HE, Ostlie A, et al. Inhomoge neous static magnetic field-induced distortic correction applied to diffusion weighted MRI c the breast at 3T. Magn Reson Med 2014. http: dx.doi.org/10.1002/mrm.25489.

57. Bokacheva L, Kaplan JB, Giri DD, et al. Intravox(incoherent motion diffusion-weighted MRI at 3.0 differentiates malignant breast lesions from benig

lesions and breast parenchyma. J Magn Reson Imaging 2014;40(4):813–23.

58. Iima M, Yano K, Kataoka M, et al. Quantitative non-Gaussian diffusion and intravoxel incoherent motion magnetic resonance imaging: differentiation of malignant and benign breast lesions. Invest Radiol 2015;50(4):205–11.

59. Liu C, Liang C, Liu Z, et al. Intravoxel incoherent motion (IVIM) in evaluation of breast lesions: comparison with conventional DWI. Eur J Radiol 2013; 82(12):e782–9.

60. Sigmund EE, Cho GY, Kim S, et al. Intravoxel incoherent motion imaging of tumor microenvironment in locally advanced breast cancer. Magn Reson Med 2011;65(5):1437–47.

61. Jensen JH, Helpern JA. MRI quantification of non-Gaussian water diffusion by kurtosis analysis. NMR Biomed 2010;23(7):698–710.

62. Partridge SC, Ziadloo A, Murthy R, et al. Diffusion tensor MRI: preliminary anisotropy measures and mapping of breast tumors. J Magn Reson Imaging 2010;31(2):339–47.

63. Baltzer PA, Schafer A, Dietzel M, et al. Diffusion tensor magnetic resonance imaging of the breast: a pilot study. Eur Radiol 2011;21(1):1–10.

64. Eyal E, Shapiro-Feinberg M, Furman-Haran E, et al. Parametric diffusion tensor imaging of the breast. Invest Radiol 2012;47(5):284–91.

65. Roebuck JR, Cecil KM, Schnall MD, et al. Human breast lesions: characterization with proton MR spectroscopy. Radiology 1998;209(1):269–75.

66. Gribbestad IS, Singstad TE, Nilsen G, et al. In vivo 1H MRS of normal breast and breast tumors using a dedicated double breast coil. J Magn Reson Imaging 1998;8(6):1191–7.

67. Cecil KM, Schnall MD, Siegelman ES, et al. The evaluation of human breast lesions with magnetic resonance imaging and proton magnetic resonance spectroscopy. Breast Cancer Res Treat 2001;68(1):45–54.

68. Yeung DK, Cheung HS, Tse GM. Human breast lesions: characterization with contrast-enhanced in vivo proton MR spectroscopy–initial results. Radiology 2001;220(1):40–6.

69. Sitter B, Sonnewald U, Spraul M, et al. High-resolution magic angle spinning MRS of breast cancer tissue. NMR Biomed 2002;15(5):327–37.

70. Haddadin IS, McIntosh A, Meisamy S, et al. Metabolite quantification and high-field MRS in breast cancer. NMR Biomed 2009;22(1):65–76.

71. Bolan PJ. Magnetic resonance spectroscopy of the breast: current status. Magn Reson Imaging Clin N Am 2013;21(3):625–39.

72. Bartella L, Morris EA, Dershaw DD, et al. Proton MR spectroscopy with choline peak as malignancy marker improves positive predictive value for breast cancer diagnosis: preliminary study. Radiology 2006;239(3):686–92.

73. Meisamy S, Bolan PJ, Baker EH, et al. Adding in vivo quantitative 1H MR spectroscopy to improve diagnostic accuracy of breast MR imaging: preliminary results of observer performance study at 4.0 T. Radiology 2005;236(2):465–75.

74. Bartella L, Thakur SB, Morris EA, et al. Enhancing nonmass lesions in the breast: evaluation with proton (1H) MR spectroscopy. Radiology 2007;245(1): 80–7.

75. Baltzer PA, Dietzel M. Breast lesions: diagnosis by using proton MR spectroscopy at 1.5 and 3.0 T–systematic review and meta-analysis. Radiology 2013;267(3):735–46.

76. Pinker K, Bogner W, Baltzer P, et al. Improved diagnostic accuracy with multiparametric magnetic resonance imaging of the breast using dynamic contrast-enhanced magnetic resonance imaging, diffusion-weighted imaging, and 3-dimensional proton magnetic resonance spectroscopic imaging. Invest Radiol 2014;49(6):421–30.

77. Katz-Brull R, Lavin PT, Lenkinski RE. Clinical utility of proton magnetic resonance spectroscopy in characterizing breast lesions. J Natl Cancer Inst 2002;94(16):1197–203.

78. Zhao C, Bolan PJ, Royce M, et al. Quantitative mapping of total choline in healthy human breast using proton echo planar spectroscopic imaging (PEPSI) at 3 Tesla. J Magn Reson Imaging 2012; 36(5):1113–23.

79. Meisamy S, Bolan PJ, Baker EH, et al. Neoadjuvant chemotherapy of locally advanced breast cancer: predicting response with in vivo (1)H MR spectroscopy–a pilot study at 4 T. Radiology 2004;233(2): 424–31.

80. Shin HJ, Baek HM, Cha JH, et al. Evaluation of breast cancer using proton MR spectroscopy: total choline peak integral and signal-to-noise ratio as prognostic indicators. AJR Am J Roentgenol 2012;198(5):W488–97.

81. Jacobs MA, Barker PB, Argani P, et al. Combined dynamic contrast enhanced breast MR and proton spectroscopic imaging: a feasibility study. J Magn Reson Imaging 2005;21(1):23–8.

82. Danishad KK, Sharma U, Sah RG, et al. Assessment of therapeutic response of locally advanced breast cancer (LABC) patients undergoing neoadjuvant chemotherapy (NACT) monitored using sequential magnetic resonance spectroscopic imaging (MRSI). NMR Biomed 2010;23(3):233–41.

83. Dorrius MD, Pijnappel RM, van der Weide Jansen MC, et al. The added value of quantitative multi-voxel MR spectroscopy in breast magnetic resonance imaging. Eur Radiol 2012;22(4):915–22.

84. Gruber S, Debski BK, Pinker K, et al. Three-dimensional proton MR spectroscopic imaging at 3 T for the differentiation of benign and malignant breast lesions. Radiology 2011;261(3):752–61.

85. Hu J, Yu Y, Kou Z, et al. A high spatial resolution 1H magnetic resonance spectroscopic imaging technique for breast cancer with a short echo time. Magn Reson Imaging 2008;26(3):360–6.

86. Jacobs MA, Barker PB, Bottomley PA, et al. Proton magnetic resonance spectroscopic imaging of human breast cancer: a preliminary study. J Magn Reson Imaging 2004;19(1):68–75.

87. Klomp DW, van de Bank BL, Raaijmakers A, et al. 31P MRSI and 1H MRS at 7 T: initial results in human breast cancer. NMR Biomed 2011;24(10):1337–42.

88. Schmitz AM, Veldhuis WB, Menke-Pluijmers MB, et al. Multiparametric MRI With Dynamic Contrast Enhancement, Diffusion-Weighted Imaging, and 31-Phosphorus Spectroscopy at 7 T for Characterization of Breast Cancer. Invest Radiol 2015. http://dx.doi.org/10.1097/RLI.0000000000000183.

89. Sinkus R, Tanter M, Xydeas T, et al. Viscoelastic shear properties of in vivo breast lesions measured by MR elastography. Magn Reson Imaging 2005;23(2):159–65.

90. Klomp DW, Dula AN, Arlinghaus LR, et al. Amide proton transfer imaging of the human breast at 7T: development and reproducibility. NMR Biomed 2013;26(10):1271–7.

91. Dula AN, Arlinghaus LR, Dortch RD, et al. Amide proton transfer imaging of the breast at 3 T: establishing reproducibility and possible feasibility assessing chemotherapy response. Magn Reson Med 2013;70(1):216–24.

92. Medved M, Newstead GM, Fan X, et al. Fourier component imaging of water resonance in the human breast provides markers for malignancy. Phys Med Biol 2009;54(19):5767–79.

93. Ouwerkerk R, Jacobs MA, Macura KJ, et al. Elevated tissue sodium concentration in malignant breast lesions detected with non-invasive 23Na MRI. Breast Cancer Res Treat 2007;106(2):151–60.

94. Jacobs MA, Ouwerkerk R, Wolff AC, et al. Monitoring of neoadjuvant chemotherapy using multiparametric, (2)(3)Na sodium MR, and multimodality (PET/CT/MRI) imaging in locally advanced breast cancer. Breast Cancer Res Treat 2011;128(1):119–26.

95. Rakow-Penner R, Daniel B, Glover GH. Detecting blood oxygen level-dependent (BOLD) contrast in the breast. J Magn Reson Imaging 2010;32(1):120–9.

96. Li SP, Taylor NJ, Makris A, et al. Primary human breast adenocarcinoma: imaging and histologic correlates of intrinsic susceptibility-weighted MR imaging before and during chemotherapy. Radiology 2010;257(3):643–52.

97. Tatum JL, Kelloff GJ, Gillies RJ, et al. Hypoxia importance in tumor biology, noninvasive measurement by imaging, and value of its measurement in the management of cancer therapy. Int J Radiat Biol 2006;82(10):699–757.

98. Jiang L, Weatherall PT, McColl RW, et al. Blood oxygenation level-dependent (BOLD) contrast magnetic resonance imaging (MRI) for prediction of breast cancer chemotherapy response: a pilot study. J Magn Reson Imaging 2013;37(5):1083–92.

99. Liu M, Guo X, Wang S, et al. BOLD-MRI of breast invasive ductal carcinoma: correlation of R2* value and the expression of HIF-1alpha. Eur Radiol 2013;23(12):3221–7.

100. Jacobs MA, Stearns V, Wolff AC, et al. Multiparametric magnetic resonance imaging, spectroscopy and multinuclear ((2)(3)Na) imaging monitoring of preoperative chemotherapy for locally advanced breast cancer. Acad Radiol 2010;17(12):1477–85.

101. Li X, Abramson RG, Arlinghaus LR, et al. Multiparametric magnetic resonance imaging for predicting pathological response after the first cycle of neoadjuvant chemotherapy in breast cancer. Invest Radiol 2015;50(4):195–204.

102. American College of Radiology Imaging Network (ACRIN) 6657: Contrast-Enhanced Breast MR (and 1H-MRS) for Evaluation of Patients Undergoing Neoadjuvant Treatment for Locally Advanced Breast Cancer. Available at: https://www.acrin.org 6657_protocol.aspx. Accessed September 21, 2015.

103. American College of Radiology Imaging Network (ACRIN) 6702: A Multi-Center Study Evaluating the Utility of Diffusion Weighted Imaging for Detection and Diagnosis of Breast Cancer. Available at https://www.acrin.org/TabID/879/Default.aspx. Accessed September 21, 2015.

104. American College of Radiology Imaging Network (ACRIN) 6698: Diffusion Weighted MR Imaging Biomarkers for Assessment of Breast Cancer Response to Neoadjuvant Treatment: A sub-study of the I-SPY 2 TRIAL (Investigation of Serial Studies to Predict Your Therapeutic Response with Imaging And moLecular Analysis). Available at: https://www.acrin.org/TabID/825/Default.aspx. Accessed September 21, 2015.

Assessment of Musculoskeletal Malignancies with Functional MR Imaging

CrossMark

Joan C. Vilanova, MD, PhD[a],*,
Sandra Baleato-Gonzalez, MD, PhD[b],
Maria José Romero, MD[c], Javier Carrascoso-Arranz, MD[d],
Antonio Luna, MD[e,f]

KEYWORDS

- MR imaging • Malignant skeletal neoplasms • Diffusion-weighted image
- Magnetic resonance spectroscopy imaging • Dynamic contrast-enhanced perfusion imaging
- Soft tissue tumors • Bone tumors

KEY POINTS

- Functional MR imaging sequences include chemical shift (in-phase and opposed-phase) MR imaging, diffusion-weighted imaging (DWI) with apparent diffusion coefficient mapping, MR spectroscopy imaging, and dynamic contrast-enhanced imaging.
- Advanced MR imaging techniques can provide improved tools to characterize skeletal lesions and differentiate benign from malignant lesions.
- Whole-body MR imaging with DWI may become a widespread first-line tool for detection and therapy monitoring of malignancy on bone.
- Multiparametric MR imaging is an accurate and reliable imaging modality in local tumor staging in patients with soft tissue sarcoma.
- Posttreatment evaluation using functional MR imaging sequences adds value after chemotherapy and/or radiation therapy to help determine treatment response and distinguish postoperative fibrosis and inflammation.

INTRODUCTION

MR imaging is the technique of choice to manage malignant musculoskeletal masses.[1–3] The radiologic evaluation of musculoskeletal malignancies has changed within recent years, mainly because of the introduction of evolving new MR imaging sequences. The new advances in MR imaging have made the imaging of musculoskeletal masses more complex. MR imaging can be used for detection, characterization, staging, and assessment of tumor after treatment.[4]

Disclosure: The authors have nothing to disclose.
[a] Department of Radiology, Clínica Girona, IDI, Catalan Health Institute, University of Girona, Lorenzana 36, Girona 17002, Spain; [b] Department of Radiology, Complexo Hospitalario de Santiago de Compostela (CHUS), Choupana s/n, Santiago de Compostela 15706, Spain; [c] Musculoskeletal Imaging, DADISA, Health Time, Zona Franca, Avenida Consejo de Europa, Nave 1, Cadiz 11011, Spain; [d] Department of Diagnostic Imaging, Hospital Universitario Quirón, Diego de Velázquez 1, Pozuelo de Alarcón, Madrid 28223, Spain; [e] Department of Radiology, Health Time, Carmelo Torres 2, Jaén 23006, Spain; [f] Department of Radiology, University Hospitals of Cleveland, Case Western Reserve University, 11100 Euclid Ave, 44106 Cleveland, Ohio
* Corresponding author.
E-mail address: kvilanova@comg.cat

Magn Reson Imaging Clin N Am 24 (2016) 239–259
http://dx.doi.org/10.1016/j.mric.2015.08.006

mri.theclinics.com

Different combinations of pulse sequences might be necessary to provide additional value for the assessment of a musculoskeletal mass.[5] Each sequence, either conventional (anatomic) or advanced (functional), provides specific information through the analysis of anatomy, physiology (cellularity and vascular function), metabolism, or molecular biology of the tumor tissue.[6]

Functional MR imaging combines information on tumor morphology with quantitative information on underlying tissue characteristics using different imaging biomarkers. Advanced MR imaging sequences include chemical shift (in-phase and opposed-phase) MR imaging, diffusion-weighted imaging (DWI) with apparent diffusion coefficient (ADC) mapping, MR spectroscopy imaging (MRSI), and dynamic contrast-enhanced (DCE) MR imaging.[7] Table 1 lists the biological-pathogenic process studied by each functional MR imaging sequence.

In this article, the role of functional MR imaging in the evaluation of malignant musculoskeletal malignancies is discussed, with a focus on detection, characterization, staging, and tumor assessment after treatment. It also reviews the technical adjustments necessary in each sequence for the enhancement of their clinical applications in the musculoskeletal system in order to allow more confident decisions to be made when dealing with malignancies. Note the importance of performing a combined analysis of the information provided by conventional sequences (T1-weighted and fluid-sensitive sequences) together with the functional sequences, because each may provide some additional value for the assessment of a musculoskeletal lesion, in its characterization, determination of extent, or posttreatment evaluation.

FUNCTIONAL MR IMAGING TECHNIQUES
Chemical Shift Imaging

Chemical shift imaging is based on the principle of separately detecting protons that precess with very similar but slightly different frequencies (such as fat and water), to identify potential neoplastic lesions in bone marrow using 2 different echo times (TEs). When the protons of fat and water are located within the same voxel and are imaged while in phase, they are responsible for additive signal intensity on the image because the protons are in sync with each other; but when they are imaged in opposed phase they are responsible for a decrease in signal intensity on the image because the protons are out of sync with one another.[8] This condition occurs most prominently when the amounts of fat and water are similar. At 1.5 T, the most commonly used TEs are 2.3 milliseconds and ~4.7 milliseconds for opposed-phase and in-phase imaging, respectively. With current software, images at both TE can be obtained in the course of a signal dual echo acquisition.

Chemical shift imaging has the ability to reveal microscopic fat, which makes it especially useful in distinguishing normal bone marrow with abundant fat from a pathologic condition that may replace fatty marrow (Fig. 1). In contrast, in a process in which fatty marrow is not replaced (such as edema or red marrow mixed with yellow marrow) there is a decrease in signal intensity on the opposed-phase image compared with the in-phase image. The signal intensity ratio (SIR) of the marrow on the opposed-phase image to the in phase can be calculated, creating a region of interest (ROI). It has been shown that using an SIR greater than 0.8 is suggestive of malignant process and an SIR less than 0.8 is typical of nonmalignant processes.[9] The utility of the technique is likely greater for distinguishing a true marrow replacing tumor from other processes such as edema or hematopoietic marrow than for strictly distinguishing benign and malignant bone tumor.

It is important to remember that the voxel of interest must contain both lipid and water; hence, a benign tumor such as a lipoma may show no decrease in signal intensity on opposed-phase images compared with in-phase images, even though the neoplasm is benign. Modern MR magnets can combine the in-phase and out-of-phase images with water-only (fat-suppressed image) and fat-only images, resulting in the Dixon method. The current Dixon-type sequences produce 4 sets of images: water only, fat only, in phase, and out of phase. The fat-only images offer the potential for fat quantification.[10]

Diffusion-weighted MR Imaging

Only specific aspects of DWI relevant to the assessment of musculoskeletal malignancies are

---

Table 1
Functional MR imaging sequences and biological processes involved

Sequence	Biological Significance
Chemical shift imaging	Presence of microscopic fat
Perfusion, DCE, MR imaging	Vascularization (angiogenesis)
Diffusion (DWI)	Cellularity (viable tumor)
Spectroscopy (MRSI)	Metabolism (choline: cellular membrane turnover)

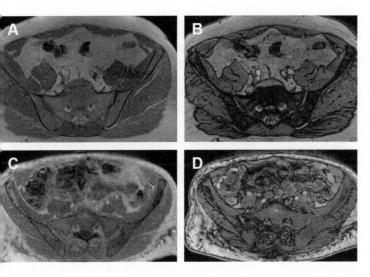

Fig. 1. Chemical shift imaging. (*A*) Axial gradient-recalled-echo in-phase image (10/4.4) and (*B*) the corresponding opposed-phase MR image (10/2.2) showing the decrease signal on opposed phase (*B*) caused by normal fatty bone marrow on a healthy patient. (*C, D*) Bone metastases in a 59-year-old woman with breast cancer. (*C*) Axial gradient-recalled-echo in-phase image (10/4.4) and (*D*) the corresponding opposed-phase MR image (10/2.2) showing the diffuse infiltration of the bone marrow because there is no decrease signal, caused by the replacement of fat by the metastases.

discussed here. However, a detailed explanation of the physics of DWI is presented elsewhere in this issue.[11] DWI complements the morphologic information obtained with conventional MR imaging. DWI measures the random motion of water at a microscopic level in the body, and is sensitive to changes in the microdiffusion of water within the intracellular and extracellular spaces, as well as transcellular and intravascular spaces (microcirculation-perfusion fraction).[12]

DWI is commonly performed using a single-shot or multishot echo-planar imaging (EPI). This sequence is faster and less sensitive to patient motion, and allows large volume coverage. However, EPI DWI images are prone to artifacts, particularly magnetic susceptibility artifacts, especially at tissue interfaces such as between air and soft tissue or bone and soft tissue. The EPI DWI images are also prone to geometric distortions, particularly in large fields of view.

To detect the characteristic differences in water movement, diffusion-probing gradients are applied during the scan period. The strength of these gradients determines the degree of diffusion weighting and is expressed by the b value. The typical DWI acquisition produces image sets at 2 or more b values. The signal intensity change over these different b values is quantified through calculation of the ADC, which is performed automatically for each voxel at the time of imaging, creating the ADC map, which is a visual representation of the calculated ADC values. It is possible to calculate the specific ADC value by drawing ROIs. Areas of restricted diffusion have low ADC values and high signal intensity on high–b-value diffusion-weighted images, with the reverse occurring for areas with unrestricted diffusion.

In addition to diffusion of water molecules in the extracellular space contributing to ADC values, the ADC values of tumors are increased by the degree of tumor perfusion. The perfusion fraction (microcirculation) tends to be higher in malignant than in benign tumors, and therefore contributes more to increasing ADC values in malignant tumors than it does in benign tumors. Hence, perfusion could increase the ADC value more in malignant tumors than in benign tumors, resulting in an overlap in ADC values between benign and malignant tumors. To overcome this analysis, it has been proposed to use a biexponential model of diffusion signal analysis, also known as intravoxel incoherent motion (IVIM), to separate tissue microcapillary perfusion from the true tissue diffusivity using quantitative parameters.[13] This model separates the diffusion signal decay in 2 different diffusion compartments. For low b values, between 0 and 100 s/mm^2, the diffusion signal experiences a fast decay because of the blood flow along the microvasculature, whereas for higher b values, more than 100 s/mm^2, the signal decay corresponds with the conventional diffusion of the tissue. This DWI sequence with the IVIM model obtains 2 diffusion coefficients, one related to molecular diffusion restriction (higher b values), D, and another related to the tissue perfusion, called D* (lower b values). Calculation and quantification of D* (perfusion contribution to signal decay), D (real diffusion of H$_2$0 molecules), and f (perfusion contribution to the diffusion signal) are possible with this approach, and they are more reliable markers of tissue diffusion than the previously used ADC. IVIM analysis can provide an independent measure of tissue perfusion, because malignant tumors show lower diffusion (D) and higher perfusion (D*) compared with benign tumors (Fig. 2). A easier way to moderate the effect of perfusion on ADC calculation is to avoid b values less than 100 s/mm² in ADC quantification in order to minimize perfusion effects; this parameter has been called perfusion-insensitive ADC by some investigators.[8]

Another important consideration to interpret DWI sequence is known as the T2 shine-through effect. Any tissue with sufficiently long T2 relaxivity (eg, fluid within a simple cyst) can show high signal intensity on the high–b-value image, even though diffusion may not be impeded in such tissues. However, T2 shine-through can be distinguished from true impeded diffusion by corroborating the signal intensity on the ADC map. A lesion with T2 shine-through shows high ADC value (Fig. 3).

It should be considered together the content of the tumor, with the interpretation of DWI (at low and high b value) and ADC images (Table 2), when analyzing skeletal tumors.[14] The ROI should be placed independently on different locations within the lesion according to solid, cystic, or necrotic tissues, instead of performing an average or a total placement of the ROI within the lesion, to minimize overlaps between ADC values of malignant and benign tumors (Fig. 4). Some investigators prefer the use of the minimum ADC value to mean ADC, because it reflects the area of the highest tumor cellularity.[15]

Magnetic Resonance Spectroscopic Imaging

MR spectroscopy (MRS) is a noninvasive metabolic imaging technique that has shown value in identifying malignant tumors. In clinical practice, MRS produces spectra from the patient with an anatomic/spatial reference. MRS is mainly based on ¹H, because hydrogen is one of the main elements in the human body. In vivo MRS allows the analysis and quantification of metabolites present in a tissue in a noninvasive way. MRS is based on the fact that protons in different molecules resonate at slightly different frequencies. This feature is secondary to the differences in the local electron cloud, which may shield the nucleus from the main

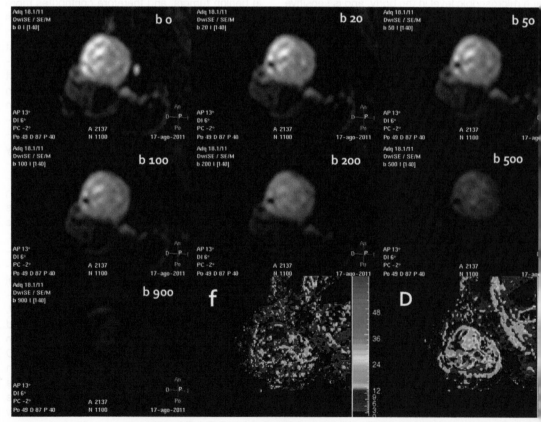

Fig. 2. Benign schwannoma. IVIM model shows a high perfusion fraction (f) (47%), without restricted diffusion (low signal), as shown on the image at b 900 s/mm², and high D value (2.29 × 10⁻³ mm²/s). This combined information on high perfusion and high diffusion favors a benign soft tissue hypervascular tumor.

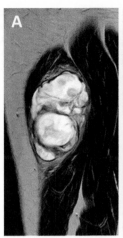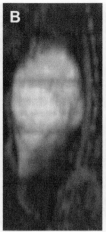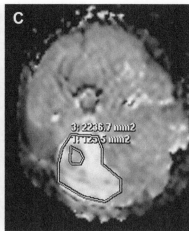

Fig. 3. Benign myxoid nerve sheath tumor. The mass shows high signal on T2-weighted imaging (*A*), DWI with b value of 1000 s/mm^2 (*B*), but lack of true restriction on ADC map (*C*) showing high value (2.2 × 10^{-3} mm^2/s). This appearance is caused by T2 shine-through effect caused by the high signal of the tumor on T2-weighted imaging sequence (*A*) related to the myxoid component of the lesion.

magnetic field. Different metabolites containing the same nucleus show characteristic chemical shifts in resonance frequency. Proton MRS peaks provide signal from water, lipid, and other metabolites, such as choline, creatine, lactate, N-acetyl-acetate, and or trimethylamine (**Fig. 5**). To date, the main diagnostic value of ^{1}H MRSI in tumors is the detection of increased levels at 3.2 ppm of choline-containing compounds or total choline, which includes contributions from choline, phosphocholine, and glycerophosphocholine.[16] MRS provides a specific curve related to the region analyzed. Multivoxel ^{1}H MRS or the single-voxel technique can be used to analyze choline peaks. The ROI to analyze should be combined with the other functional sequences in order to obtain the information within the solid areas showing early and intense contrast uptake. Detection of certain metabolites provides a noninvasive method to help distinguish malignant from nonmalignant tissue.[17,18] The lesion should be positioned in the center of the magnet and coil whenever possible, and artifacts should be avoided. The smallest ROI available (1–3.0 cm^3) should be positioned in solid and homogeneous tumor areas, to avoid hemorrhage, necrosis, and calcification. Shimming in the voxel and suppression of water are important, and are usually performed automatically by the scanner. Increased levels of choline, which is a marker of increased cell membrane turnover, has been shown to be increased in malignant tumors.[19] MRS studies on musculoskeletal tumors have produced variable results because choline level is increased in malignant as well as benign tumors.[20] Recent investigations at 3 T show that choline concentrations are notably different for benign and malignant musculoskeletal lesions, determining the absolute choline concentration at MRS by using a water-referencing method.[21]

Dynamic Contrast-enhanced Perfusion MR Imaging

DCE-MR imaging is usually performed with volumetric gradient-echo sequences (T1 or relaxivity-based methods) repeated several times after intravenous contrast agent administration.[22] The temporal resolution depends on the need for spatial resolution and filed-of-view coverage. Highly time-resolved MR angiographic sequence, named TRICKS, TRAK or TWIST depending on the vendors name's, allows the analysis of perfusion and vessels within 1 sequence (**Fig. 6**). It is advisable to perform a temporal resolution acquisition of less than 5-seconds for 4 to 5 minutes. Analysis of the DCE-MR imaging sequence can be performed using a variety of

Table 2
Signal intensity patterns to evaluate and interpret diffusion sequence and ADC maps

b = 0	b = 500–1000	ADC	Interpretation
High	High	Low	High cellularity Malignant tumor
High	High	High	Cyst/hemangioma T2 shine-through
Low	Low	Low	Fibrosis
High	Low	High	Fluid (edema) Necrosis

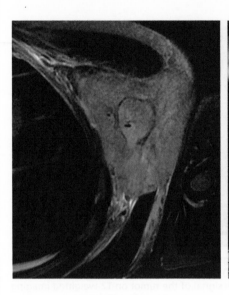 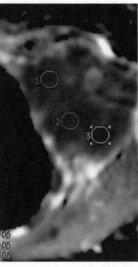

Fig. 4. Axillary lymphoma. Left axillary irregular solid mass in a 44-year-old man. The minimum ADC was 0.7 × 10^{-3} mm^2/s from the different ROIs within the tumor, as shown on the right image.

postprocessing methods and creating time-intensity curves from an ROI. Analysis can be done in a qualitative (time–signal intensity curve [TIC] profile), semiquantitative (parameters derived from changes in the signal intensity), or quantitative manner.[23] Qualitative approaches use the types of curve profile: progressive enhancement, delayed plateau, or delayed washout, corresponding with

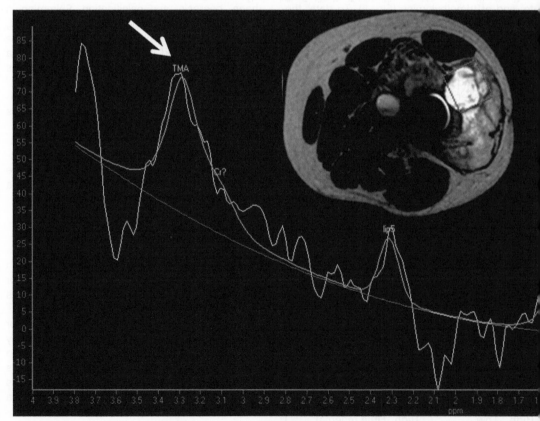

Fig. 5. Soft tissue recurrence of femoral osteosarcoma: MRS analysis shows increased level of trimethylamine (TMA) peak caused by recurrence (arrow).

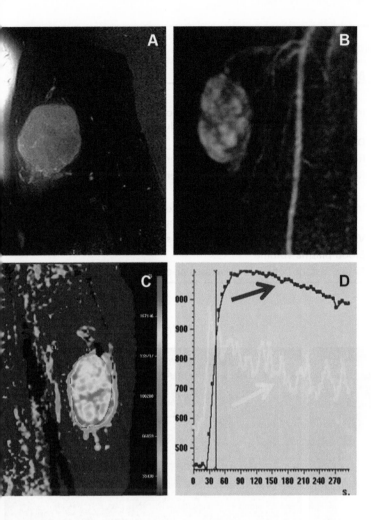

Fig. 6. Soft tissue pleomorphic sarcoma. (*A*) Coronal fat-suppressed T2-weighted image showing homogeneous high-signal-intensity tumor in the right proximal arm. (*B*) Contrast-enhanced DCE-MR imaging with high temporal resolution shows enhancement throughput of the mass on the arterial phase caused by a hypervascular malignant tumor. (*C*) The color semiquantitative vascular wash-out map and the time–signal intensity curve (*D*) shows a fast and intense wash-in and delayed washout (*yellow arrow*) compared with the enhancement curve of the artery (*blue arrow*).

curves type I, II, or III, respectively. Semiquantitative values measure and quantify, among other things, the relative signal intensity (higher postcontrast signal intensity/precontrast signal ratio), slope of the intensity-time curve (which shows speed of enhancement), or the area under the intensity-time curve (AUC). These measurements are easy to obtain in the workstations and can be represented in parametric maps, but cannot be compared among different vendors or examination times. For obtaining quantitative parameters, pharmacokinetics models defining 2 or more compartments are used, which allow quantification of various parameters: k^{trans} (transit of the contrast from the vascular compartment to the interstice through the endothelium), k_{ep} (return to the vascular compartment), and V_e (fraction of extracellular space of tumor). In addition, using these data parametric maps representing the intratumoral heterogeneity of the vascular distribution can be generated. Nonetheless, the complexity behind these parameters,

the lack of standardization, and the lack of a of universal postprocessing model or software must be taken into account. In areas in which the tumor shows high vascular permeability (such as the peripheral zone), k^{trans} values depend mainly on the flow, whereas in the center of the tumor (where permeability is the limiting factor) k^{trans} values depend on the permeability surface. Interpretation difficulties arise from the lack of standardization.[23]

The first-pass kinetics should mainly be analyzed (Table 3). Malignant lesions usually show early rapid enhancement and higher slopes, although this pattern is not specific and benign lesions might show rapid arterial enhancement (Fig. 7).[24] The entire tumor should be evaluated in order to correlate the different components of the tumor tissue before and after treatment; mainly the presence of necrosis (Fig. 8).

It is advisable to perform a delayed contrast-enhanced fat-suppressed 3D gradient-echo T1-weighted technique with isotropic voxel following

Table 3
Parameters used in clinical practice and their biological significance

Parameter Definition	Biological Significance
Semiquantitative Parameters	
Initial area under curve	Include information of blood flow, blood volume, permeability, extravascular-extracellular space volume, and microvessel density
Time to peak	Depends on tissue perfusion
Wash-in	Represents the velocity of enhancement
Washout	Represents the velocity of enhancement loss
Quantitative Parameters	
Transfer constant (k^{trans})	Influx volume transfer constant of a contrast agent from the vascular compartment to the interstitial compartment
V_e	Volume of extravascular-extracellular space per unit volume of tumor
V_p	Blood plasma volume
K_{ep}	Rate constant between extravascular-extracellular space and plasma

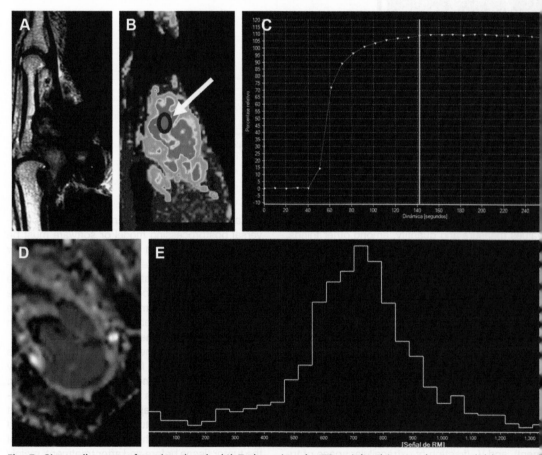

Fig. 7. Giant cell tumor of tendon sheath. (A) Turbo spin echo T2-weighted image shows a solid low-signal intensity lobulated tumor within the flexor tendon sheath of the finger. (B) Color wash-in parametric map and corresponding TIC (C) of the ROI (arrow) showing the high and rapid enhancement with a delayed plateau curve (D) ADC map on the axial image and corresponding histogram (E) shows the low ADC value of the lesion, with a mean value of 0.73×10^{-3} mm^2/s.

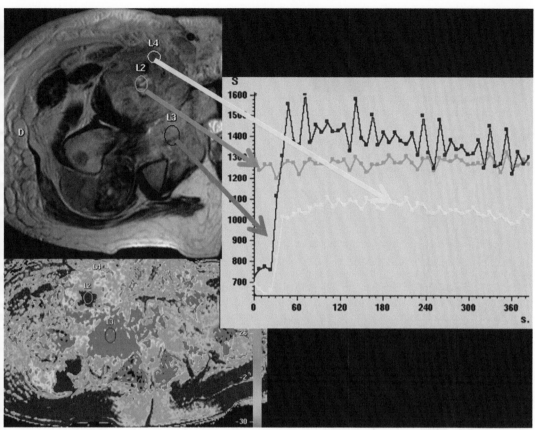

Fig. 8. Malignant soft tissue neuroendocrine tumor. Maximum relative enhancement map of DCE-MR imaging and TSE T2-weighted image shows a large, heterogeneous, solid, soft tissue lesion within the right pelvis. Different enhancement characteristics of the different components can be seen, representing the heterogeneity of this tumor. The tissue with the fastest and early contrast enhancement (*blue TIC*) is the area most representative when analyzed by biopsy, whereas the necrotic area (*green curve*), showing absence of contrast uptake, should be avoided. The anterior area of the tumor shows a moderate initial uptake of contrast and delayed plateau (*yellow curve*), indicating a less aggressive solid portion of the lesion.

the DCE-MR imaging sequence to improve the analysis of the tumor and the nearby structures. Moreover, the subtraction of the contrast-enhanced images from the unenhanced images improves the contrast between an enhancing tumor and nearby structures.[25]

DIAGNOSIS

MR imaging is not commonly a first-line technique to detect a skeletal tumor. Radiograph or ultrasonography scan are the techniques that enable detection of bone or soft tissue lesions, respectively.[3] With the advent of whole-body imaging (WB-MR imaging) including functional information from DWI (**Fig. 9**), MR imaging may become a widespread first-line tool for detection of malignancy of bone.[26] Moreover, functional techniques can provide improved tools to characterize skeletal lesions and differentiate benign from malignant lesions.

Bone Marrow Malignancy

Detection of malignancy on bone marrow using MR imaging is useful.[27] Chemical shift imaging and DWI can be used to differentiate bone marrow edema, hematopoietic marrow, or other infiltrative processes in the skeleton.[28,29] Chemical shift imaging is helpful for differentiating benign from malignant fractures in the spine or in the extremities. Using an SIR of 0.80 as a cutoff value, it has shown accuracy from 91% to 99% in differentiating malignant lesions (SIR >0.80) from benign lesions (SIR <0.80).[9]

Characterization of bone marrow malignancies on DWI is a challenge. There is some controversy in the literature regarding the role of DWI in assessing vertebral lesions. In general, ADC values in normal vertebral marrow typically range between 0.2 and 0.5 × 10^{-3} mm^2/s, whereas marrow-infiltrating lesions show values in the range of 0.7

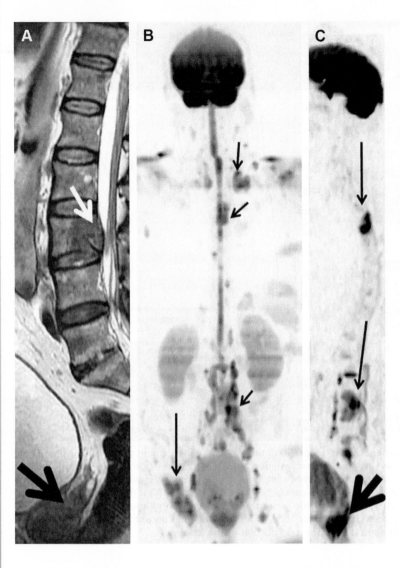

Fig. 9. Bone metastasis detection in prostate cancer. (A) Sagittal TSE T2-weighted MR imaging in a 63-year-old man to rule out lumbar herniation showing an expansive lesion at L3 (*white arrow*). (B) Coronal maximum intensity projection (MIP) of whole-body DWI (WB DWI) with high b value at inverted gray scale shows a bone lesion with diffusion restriction at the right pelvis (*long arrow*) with multiple lymph node within the mediastinum, left retroperitoneum, and pelvis (*short arrows*). (C) Sagittal MIP of WB DWI at inverted gray scale shows the multiple vertebral bone lesions (*long arrows*) and allows the unknown primary tumor in the prostate to be localized (*thick arrow*), also shown on the T2-weighted image (A). Further biopsy confirmed a prostate cancer.

to 1.0×10^{-3} mm^2/s.[30] Benign traumatic or osteoporotic fractures show even higher ADC values, generally between 1.0 and 2.0×10^{-3} mm^2/s (**Fig. 10**). Nevertheless, when interpreting the ADC of the lesion, it is essential to determine the exact age of a benign fracture, because ADC values theoretically decrease progressively until they reach the practically null values of normal bone marrow in a chronic collapse (minimal diffusion of water occurs in normal bone marrow). Therefore, evaluating the ADC in the subacute period can result in a false-positive for malignancy with ADC values within the malignant range (**Fig. 11**).

The use of DWI in the evaluation of bone marrow lesions requires knowledge of potential diagnostic pitfalls that stem from technical challenges and confounding biochemical factors that influence ADC maps[31] but are unrelated to lesion cellularity (**Table 4**). Furthermore, there are differences in the appearance of normal bone marrow in DWI and ADC according to age, anatomic location, and the dominant component of bone marrow (yellow or red bone marrow).[27] Known differences in the cellularity of normal and malignant bone marrow are reflected in the signal intensity (SI) of images with high b values and also in ADC maps.[32] The ability to use both SI and ADC values to differentiate normal and malignant bone marrow may have applications in improving skeletal tumor definitions.

Characterization

After detection of a primary musculoskeletal lesion, the next step is to determine whether the lesion is benign or malignant and whether it should be referred to biopsy to determine the histology

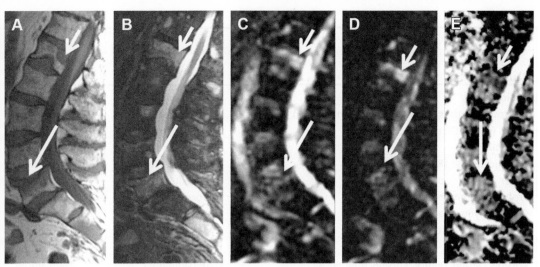

Fig. 10. Benign and malignant edema on ADC map. Lumbar spine MR imaging of a 59-year-old woman with known bone metastasis from breast cancer experiencing acute back pain. (*A*) Sagittal TSE T1-weighted image showing multiple lesions on the vertebral bodies with a nodular lesion at L1 (*short arrow*) and diffuse edema at L5 (*long arrows*). (*B*) The corresponding sagittal short tau inversion recovery (STIR) image shows a more diffuse edema at both levels, and it is difficult to differentiate whether this is infiltrative or noninfiltrative. (*C*) Sagittal DWI at b = 0 mm²/s and (*D*) at b = 800 mm²/s show the persistent high signal of the lesion at L1 level (*short arrow*) and lower signal at L5 at high b value (*long arrow*). (*E*) Sagittal ADC map confirms the low signal at L1 (*short arrow*) caused by an ADC value of 0.7 × 10⁻³ mm²/s and high signal at L5 (*long arrow*) with an ADC value of 1.6 × 10⁻³ mm²/s. The lesion at L1 is caused by a metastasis and at L5 by an insufficiency fracture, which is well depicted on the sagittal T1-weighted image (*A*) as a horizontal subcortical fracture line (*arrow*), which explains the current symptoms.

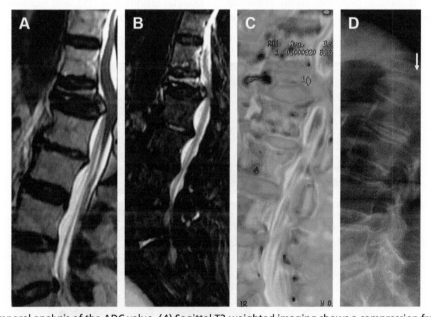

Fig. 11. Temporal analysis of the ADC value. (*A*) Sagittal T2-weighted imaging shows a compression fracture at L1 level with retropulsed posterior wall. (*B*) Sagittal DWI with high b value shows high signal of the L1 vertebral body caused by edema. (*C*) The ADC color map shows a value of 0.9 × 10⁻³ mm²/s, which is suspicious for a malignant origin of the edema, because of the low ADC value. (*D*) The plain film performed 3 months before the MR imaging showed the presence of an acute vertebral fracture (*arrow*), indicating that it was a subacute fracture, not present on a plain film performed 12 months before. The continuous process of the bone marrow edema of a benign fracture tended to normalize the ADC value close to 0 within the following weeks from the analysis performed on the current ADC map. If an ADC quantitative analysis had been performed within the acute phase of the fracture, the ADC value would probably have been greater than 2 × 10⁻³ mm²/s.

Table 4
Effects on bone marrow from different causes that affect diffusion-weighted MR imaging signal

Cause	Effect	DWI Signal
Radiotherapy	Hypocellularity	Lower signal
Marrow disorders (aplastic anemia, infections)	Hypocellularity	Lower signal
Drugs (chemotherapy, alcohol)	Hypocellularity	Lower signal
Poor nutrition	Hypocellularity	Lower signal
Chronic disease (RF, CLD, RD)	Hypocellularity	Lower signal
Older age, osteoporosis	Hypocellularity	Lower signal
Prolonged immobility	Hypocellularity	Lower signal
Children, young adults	Hypercellularity	High signal
Athlete, high altitude	Hypercellularity	High signal
Smoking	Hypercellularity	High signal
Chronic cardiac failure, chronic anemia	Hypercellularity	High signal
Pregnancy, recent pregnancy	Hypercellularity	High signal
Stimulating hematopoietic therapies	Hypercellularity	High signal

Abbreviations: CLD, chronic liver disease; RD, rheumatoid disease; RF, Renal failure.
  Adapted from Padhani AR, Koh DM, Collins DJ. Whole-body diffusion-weighted MR imaging in cancer: current statu
and research directions. Radiology 2011;261(3):708; with permission.

Morphologic imaging is not specific in differentiating benignity and malignancy. Functional imaging, mainly in clinical practice, using chemical shift imaging, DCE-MR imaging, and DWI in combination with conventional MR sequences may be useful to improve the characterization o skeletal lesions (**Fig. 12**), and moreover, to distin guish benign from malignant lesions.[33]

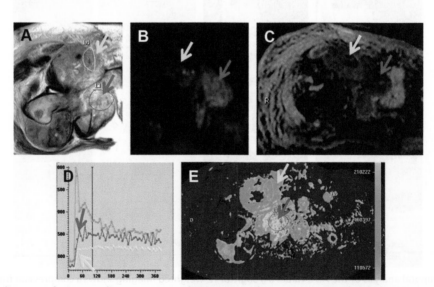

Fig. 12. Malignant soft tissue malignant neuroendocrine tumor (same case as **Fig. 8**). (*A*) TSE T2-weighted imag
showing the 2 areas to analyze (*red and yellow arrows*). (*B*) Axial DWI-weighted image at b = 1000 mm²/s show
higher signal on the posterior part (*red arrow*), corresponding with higher restriction caused by low ADC value a
analyzed on the gray-scale ADC map (*C*), ADC value of 0.7 × 10⁻³ mm²/s. The anterior part of the tumor (*yellov
arrow*) shows less restricted diffusion, shown by the lower signal on DWI (*yellow arrow*) in (*B*) and ADC value o
1.2 × 10⁻³ mm²/s. (*D*) The TIC curve shows the correspondence of the higher restriction area (*red arrow*) in (*B*
with the higher wash-in slope curve (*red arrow*). (*E*) The anterior part (*yellow area*) corresponds with the les
restricted diffusion, and also with the slower wash-in slope (*yellow arrow*).

There is overlap between enhancement characteristics of benign and malignant lesions, but certain differences can be seen. Malignant lesions usually enhance heterogeneously, show evidence of liquefaction, and do so early and rapidly in the arterial phase. Another important issue for DCE-MR imaging is the utility of direct biopsy in areas of avid contrast enhancement rather than areas of necrosis.

DWI has been used to characterize skeletal tumors, but an overlap has been identified between benign and malignant soft tissue tumors (**Fig. 13**).

Soft tissue tumors

One difficulty in characterizing soft tissue tumors is whether a tumor has a myxoid component. The discrepancies likely stem from the many factors besides lesion cellularity that influence ADC values, such as the composition of the tumor matrix, the presence of spontaneous necrosis, and different imaging protocols performed for DWI.[12,34] An understanding of the morphologic MR imaging appearance, as well as the perfusion and DWI characteristics of myxoid tumors, may permit a more accurate diagnosis in cases of indeterminate soft tissue masses. In general, the lower the ADC, the higher the likelihood of malignancy.

The combination of findings using DWI, perfusion, and morphologic sequences helps to differentiate abscesses from necrotic neoplasms. The abscess cavity shows markedly reduced ADC in the necrotic center, whereas the necrotic center of a neoplasm tends to have more facilitated diffusion. Moreover malignant tumors tend to have more restricted diffusion on the ADC map in the solid part of the tumor.[8]

DWI can help to differentiate chronic expanding hematomas (CEHs) from hemorrhagic malignant tumors. The ADC value of CEHs has been shown to be higher than that of malignant soft tissue tumor.[35]

Fibrous tumors are common soft tissue tumors seen on MR imaging, showing typical findings as bands of low signal intensity and contrast enhancement. Although these findings are seen in benign and malignant fibrous tumors, benign and intermediate fibrous tumors usually have facilitated diffusion, whereas malignant tumors have restricted diffusion on the ADC map. DWI can help to differentiate myositis ossificans from a malignant tumor, because it presents high ADC, whereas the perfusion study may show neovascularity and may mimic a malignant neoplasm.[8]

Certain tumors with high cellularity, such as lymphoma or Ewing sarcoma, have shown characteristically low ADC values.[36]

Bone tumors

Differentiation between enchondroma and chondrosarcoma grade I (in the World Health Organization 2013 classification this group is now classified as intermediate and is named atypical cartilaginous

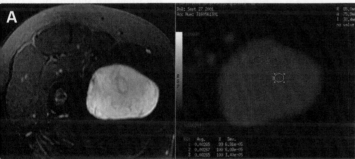
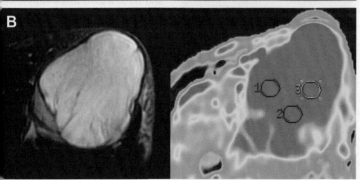

Fig. 13. Overlap ADC values on benign and malignant myxoid tumors. (A) An 11-year-old boy with a cystic-appearing soft tissue tumor on the medial compartment of the right thigh on axial T2-weighted fat-suppressed image. The corresponding ADC map on the gray scale showed a value of 2.65×10^{-3} mm^2/s. Final histologic diagnosis was intramuscular myxoma. (B) A 65-year-old man with a cystic-appearing soft tissue mass on the medial compartment of the right thigh, on axial T2-weighted fat-suppressed imaging. The lowest ADC value on the corresponding color map (from the 3 different ROIs shown) was 2.60×10^{-3} mm^2/s. Final histologic diagnosis was myxofibrosarcoma.

tumor/chondrosarcoma grade I) is difficult clinically, on imaging studies and also on histology.[37] Not only diagnostic parameters to differentiate these entities are controversial; strategies for treatment are also controversial. Functional imaging, in particular DCE-MR imaging, has a role in differentiating benign from malignant cartilaginous tumors. Chondrosarcoma grade I or atypical cartilaginous tumor typically enhances within 10 seconds of arterial enhancement. However, enchondroma enhances after 10 seconds or not at all. In contrast, DWI cannot be used in the differentiation of enchondroma from low-grade chondrosarcoma because high ADC values and facilitated diffusion on ADC maps are shown by both benign and malignant cartilaginous tumors (Fig. 14) because of their high chondroid matrix content, as Hayashida and colleagues[32] have described.

It is mandatory to apply multiple areas of interest within a heterogeneous mass to search the regions with the lowest ADC and also with earlier and rapid enhancement on DCE-MR imaging as general biomarkers of malignancy. This procedure should apply for bone tumors and for soft tissue as well.

STAGING

MR imaging has an important role in evaluating the extension of malignant skeletal tumors before treatment.[38] The most important considerations in staging the local extent of a tumor include tumor margins and size; tumor extension beyond the anatomic compartment; tumor invasion of bone, joint, muscle, and neurovascular bundle; and tumor location relative to deep fascia. The initial slopes of tumor and nontumor tissues differ significantly (Fig. 15). Therefore, DCE-MR imaging may improve the delineation of tumor margins because enhancement of tumor tissue is earlier and faster than that of peritumoral edema.[25] MR imaging has been proved to be an accurate and reliable imaging modality in local tumor staging in patients with soft tissue sarcoma; in helping predict osseous invasion; and in assessing encasement of arteries, veins, and nerves if the contact between tumor and vascular or neural circumference exceeds 180°, as assessed on axial T2-weighted images.[39] MR angiography may help to evaluate vascular invasion of bone sarcomas. It is useful for the mapping of major arteries, but

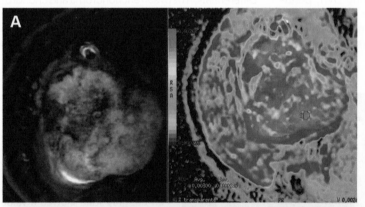
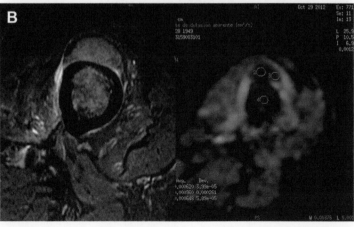

Fig. 14. Different ADC values on chondrosarcoma. (A) Axial T2-weighted fat-suppressed image shows a mass in the right humerus and color ADC map shows an ADC value of 2.90×10^{-3} mm²/s (from the small ROI shown) on a chondrosarcoma grade II. (B) Axial T2-weighted fat-suppressed image shows a mass in the left femur and gray-scale ADC map shows an ADC value of 0.9×10^{-3} mm²/s on a chondrosarcoma grade I. Different ADC values for the same diagnosis are related to different tissue analyzed within the different ROI performed. ROI of (A) is within a myxoid tissue and (B) in a solid tissue with lower ADC value.

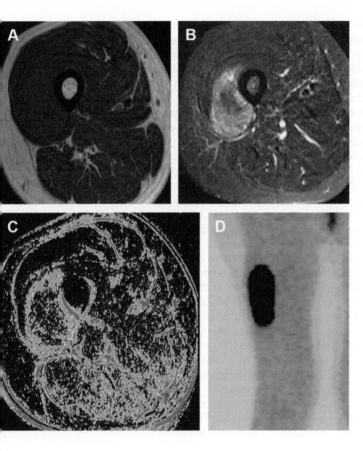

Fig. 15. Soft tissue Ewing sarcoma. (A) Axial T1-weighted image of the right thigh does not show signal intensity changes within the bone marrow of the femur. (B) Axial post-contrast fat-suppressed T1-weighted image shows an enhancing mass with central necrosis and absence of peritumoral enhancement changes. (C) Axial wash-in color map from DCE-MR imaging shows the early peripheral-rim enhancement of the tumor without any early uptake within nearby structures. (D) PET-fluorodeoxyglucose coronal view confirms the absence of tumor extension beyond the lesion.

for assessing vascular invasion, axial images are important to assess the relationship between the tumor and the blood vessels.[40]

POSTTREATMENT EVALUATION

After detection, local staging, biopsy, and initial treatment of skeletal tumor, the radiologist may have to assess response to therapy. It might be necessary to evaluate changes before surgery, and after chemotherapy and/or radiation therapy to define the extent of the lesion after treatment and to help determine treatment response.[41] Another important task of radiologists is to perform MR imaging follow-up after surgery or radiotherapy to distinguish postoperative fibrosis and inflammation from residual or recurrent tumor.[42]

The potential use of ^{18}F-fluorodeoxyglucose (FDG)-PET in the evaluation of posttreatment changes in skeletal sarcomas is still questionable because inflammatory tissue overlaps that of residual or recurrent tumor. However, ^{18}F-FDG-PET in conjunction with MR imaging seems particularly useful in patients with extensive histories of surgery.[43]

Preoperative Treatment Response

The most reliable factor in predicting treatment response, assessing the effectiveness of therapy, planning further treatment, and for predicting survival and risk of local recurrence is the percentage of tumor necrosis seen at histologic examination after surgery. Histologic necrosis of 90% to 95% has been established as a criterion for responder on bone sarcoma; although not well established for soft tissue sarcomas, it has shown good outcomes in patients with 95% necrosis.[44]

Tumor size criteria have been shown to be insufficient to render tumor response.[45] MR imaging using functional acquisitions could be beneficial as a presurgical measure of response. Predicting treatment response before surgery could result in an alteration of the chemotherapy regimen for the patient, a change in the timing of surgery, and possibly a change in the extent of surgery. The most powerful functional MR imaging technique used to differentiate responders from nonresponders is DCE-MR imaging, as described earlier. An increase, no change, or even a slight decrease in the amplitude of the TIC and in the slope of the curve (percentage of increase of signal intensity per minute) during follow-up indicates poor response to treatment.[8,25] Changes in the TIC with a decrease of at least 60% in slope indicate greater than 90% necrosis, which is considered a good response.[22] The qualitative analysis of the first-pass images allows clinicians to detect perfused viable tumor that suggest that more than 10% of viable tumor is present. Moreover, DCE-MR imaging allows clinicians to differentiate the rapid enhancement pattern of viable tumor from slowly enhancing inflammation and fibrosis.

ADC values may also be used to differentiate viable tumor tissue and necrotic areas with DWI (Fig. 16). A direct relationship has been observed in patients with osteosarcoma between increase of ADC and extent of tumor necrosis.[46] The pretherapeutic and posttherapeutic diffusivities of tumor tissue have shown significant differences in ADC values for osteosarcoma.[47] There is no specific threshold to determine responder from nonresponder, but it is likely that a change in ADC value in posttreatment from pretreatment signifies some measure of response (Fig. 17, Table 5).

Posttherapy Follow-up

MR imaging is the primary imaging modality to evaluate posttherapy follow-up. Although posttreatment changes could mimic or obscure local recurrence on MR imaging, a systematic approach to, and knowledge of, the features of recurrence versus therapeutic change allows their differentiation in almost all cases.

Conventional MR imaging sequences, such as T2-weighted images, have shown utility in ruling out recurrent tumor in the absence of abnormal signal intensity.[48] When a recurrent tumor is present, it can be obvious on nonenhanced images. However, postoperative inflammation or fibrosis can appear as a masslike lesion. Thus, DCE-MR imaging sequences should be routinely performed to detect recurrence when T2-weighted images show signal intensity abnormalities (Fig. 18). Tumor tissue, either residual or recurrent, enhances early and more rapidly during the first pass of contrast, whereas reactive tissue or a pseudomass resulting from posttherapeutic changes enhances later and more slowly (Fig. 19).

DWI can help to assess activity of residual disease after treatment and to detect early recurrence at a time when a salvage therapy may still be effective.[49] DWI has shown significantly higher diffusion in hygromas (Fig. 20) than in viable recurrent tumor.[50]

Radiation changes are readily identified in both bone and soft tissue. Following radiation therapy, patients may develop inflammatory tissue caused

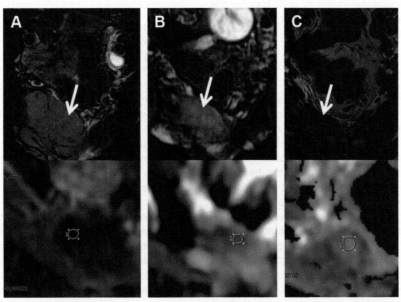

Fig. 16. Evaluation response to Ewing sarcoma with DWI and ADC evaluation in a 14-year-old girl with a sacral mass (arrows). (A–C) Axial fat-suppressed T2-weighted images with corresponding ADC maps (bottom) before (A) 2 months (B), and 4 months (C) after treatment. The initial ADC of 0.69×10^{-3} mm²/s (A, bottom) is gradually increasing after chemotherapy up to 1.7×10^{-3} mm²/s (C, bottom), indicating the presence of tumor necrosis and good response. ADC values are obtained from the ROIs shown in the ADC maps (bottom).

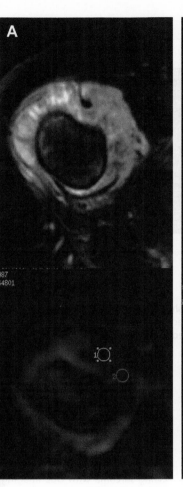
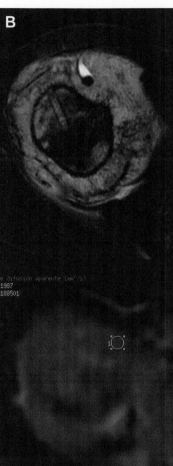

Fig. 17. Poor response of osteosarcoma of the humerus in a 21-year-old man. (A, B) Axial fat-suppressed T1-weighted images with corresponding ADC maps (*bottom*) before treatment (A) and 2 months after treatment (B). The initial ADC of 1.69×10^{-3} mm^2/s (A, *bottom*) increased after chemotherapy to 2.07×10^{-3} mm^2/s (B, *bottom*). In spite of an increase of 0.4×10^{-3} mm^2/s, the final histology report showed tumoral necrosis less than 90%. ADC values are obtained on the ROIs shown at the bottom images.

by granulation tissue or induced neovascularization. Differentiation of a reactive mass with recurrent tissue may be difficult in the first 3 to 6 months after irradiation. DCE-MR imaging is the technique of choice to differentiate recurrence from fibrotic tissue. Tumor recurrence enhances fast during the first pass, whereas reactive tissue enhances later and more slowly.[25]

Table 5
Multiparametric MR imaging parameters: correlation with response to neoadjuvant chemotherapy/radiotherapy

Sequence	Response to Therapy	
	Good	**Poor**
T2-weighted imaging	No tumor High signal in bone marrow (radiotherapy)	Residual/increased soft tissue mass Increased extent of bone marrow invasion
Spectroscopy	Increased choline peak	No choline peak
Diffusion	Increased ADC values	Low ADC values
Perfusion	Change to slow/absent enhancement	Persistent fast/intense enhancement

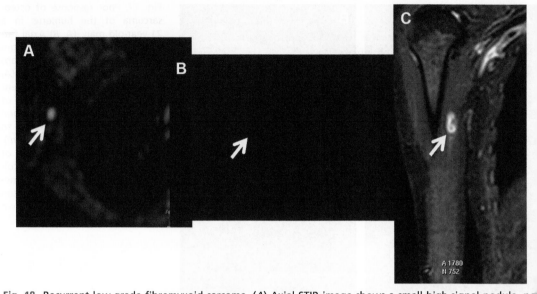

Fig. 18. Recurrent low-grade fibromyxoid sarcoma. (*A*) Axial STIR image shows a small high-signal nodule, no depicted on the DWI image (*B*) and well shown on the coronal T1-weighted fat-suppressed image after contras enhancement (*C*). DWI fails to detect the recurrence as an area of restricted diffusion, because of its myxoid na ture. ADC value was 2.1×10^{-3} mm^2/s.

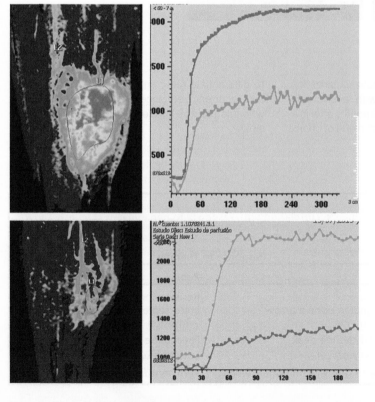

Fig. 19. Evaluation of response o Ewing sarcoma with DCE imaging Upper images show pretreatmen DCE color parametric MR imagin of the heterogeneous soft tissu mass with a fast wash-in curv (*red curve*). Bottom images show MR imaging performed 3 month after chemotherapy, showing pa tial response caused by a signifi cantly slower wash-in of the curv within the tumor (*red curve*). Gree curves correspond to the enhance ment of the artery.

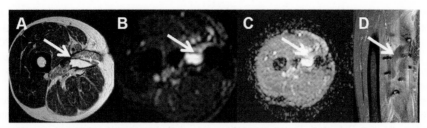

Fig. 20. Follow-up posttreatment imaging of a myxoid liposarcoma in a 53-year-old man. (*A*) Axial T2-weighted image 6 months after surgery and radiotherapy, showing a high-signal-intensity lesion on the surgical bed (*arrow*). (*B*) The corresponding axial DWI at high b value and the ADC map (*C*) show high signal caused by high ADC values related to a hygroma, caused by a T2 shine-through effect corresponding with a cystic fluid-filled lesion. (*D*) Postcontrast fat-suppressed T1-weighted image confirms the absence of enhancement of the fluid in the postsurgical lesion, without evidence of recurrence.

SUMMARY

Functional, multiparametric MR imaging techniques allow the management of malignant skeletal tumors combining anatomy, diffusion, metabolic, and vascular information within a single examination. Advanced MR imaging has a prime role in the evaluation of musculoskeletal tumors using morphologic sequences, DWI, perfusion, and spectroscopy to provide additional data on the detection, characterization, staging, and follow-up after treatment.

REFERENCES

1. Alyas F, James SL, Davies AM, et al. The role of MR imaging in the diagnostic characterisation of appendicular bone tumours and tumour-like conditions. Eur Radiol 2007;17(10):2675–86.

2. Sherman CE, O'Connor MI. Musculoskeletal tumor imaging: an orthopedic oncologist perspective. Semin Musculoskelet Radiol 2013;17(2):221–6.

3. Wu JS, Hochman MG. Soft-tissue tumors and tumor-like lesions: a systematic imaging approach. Radiology 2009;253(2):297–316.

4. Nascimento D, Suchard G, Hatem M, et al. The role of magnetic resonance imaging in the evaluation of bone tumours and tumour-like lesions. Insights Imaging 2014;5(4):419–40.

5. Kransdorf MJ, Bridges MD. Current developments and recent advances in musculoskeletal tumor imaging. Semin Musculoskelet Radiol 2013;17(2):145–55.

6. Fayad LM, Jacobs MA, Wang X, et al. Musculoskeletal tumors: how to use anatomic, functional, and metabolic MR techniques. Radiology 2012;265(2):340–56.

7. Jackson A, O'Connor JP. Imaging angiogenesis. In: Luna A, Vilanova JC Jr, de Cruz LC, et al, editors. Functional imaging in oncology: clinical applications. Berlin: Springer; 2014. p. 127–46.

8. Costa FM, Canella C, Gasparetto E. Advanced magnetic resonance imaging techniques in the evaluation of musculoskeletal tumors. Radiol Clin North Am 2011;49(6):1325–58, vii–viii.

9. Martel Villagrán J, Bueno Horcajadas Á, Pérez Fernández E, et al. Accuracy of magnetic resonance imaging in differentiating between benign and malignant vertebral lesions: role of diffusion-weighted imaging, in-phase/opposed-phase imaging and apparent diffusion coefficient. Radiologia 2015;57(2):142–9.

10. Berglund J, Johansson L, Ahlström H, et al. Three-point Dixon method enables whole-body water and fat imaging of obese subjects. Magn Reson Med 2010;63(6):1659–68.

11. Koh DM, Lee JM, Bittencourt LK, et al. Body diffusion-weighted MR imaging in oncology: imaging at 3T, in press.

12. Subhawong TK, Jacobs MA, Fayad LM. Diffusion-weighted MR imaging for characterizing musculoskeletal lesions. Radiographics 2014;34(5):1163–77.

13. Mannelli L, Nougaret S, Vargas HA, et al. Advances in diffusion-weighted imaging. Radiol Clin North Am 2015;53(3):569–81.

14. Subhawong TK, Jacobs MA, Fayad LM. Insights into quantitative diffusion-weighted MRI for musculoskeletal tumor imaging. AJR Am J Roentgenol 2014;203(3):560–72.

15. Oka K, Yakushiji T, Sato H, et al. The value of diffusion-weighted imaging for monitoring the chemotherapeutic response of osteosarcoma: a comparison between average apparent diffusion coefficient and minimum apparent diffusion coefficient. Skeletal Radiol 2010;39(2):141–6.

16. Deshmukh S, Subhawong T, Carrino JA, et al. Role of MR spectroscopy in musculoskeletal imaging. Indian J Radiol Imaging 2014;24(3):210–6.

17. Fayad LM, Bluemke DA, McCarthy EF, et al. Musculoskeletal tumors: use of proton MR spectroscopic imaging for characterization. J Magn Reson Imaging 2006;23(1):23–8.

18. Wang CK, Li CW, Hsieh TJ, et al. Characterization of bone and soft-tissue tumors with in vivo 1H MR spectroscopy: initial results. Radiology 2004; 232(2):599–605.

19. Fayad LM, Wang X, Salibi N, et al. A feasibility study of quantitative molecular characterization of musculoskeletal lesions by proton MR spectroscopy at 3 T. AJR Am J Roentgenol 2010;195(1):W69–75.

20. Fayad LM, Wang X, Blakeley JO, et al. Characterization of peripheral nerve sheath tumors with 3T proton MR spectroscopy. AJNR Am J Neuroradiol 2014; 35(5):1035–41.

21. Lee CW, Lee JH, Kim DH, et al. Proton magnetic resonance spectroscopy of musculoskeletal lesions at 3 T with metabolite quantification. Clin Imaging 2010;34(1):47–52.

22. Erlemann R, Vassallo P, Bongartz G, et al. Musculoskeletal neoplasms: fast low-angle shot MR imaging with and without Gd-DTPA. Radiology 1990;176(2): 489–95.

23. García-Figueiras R, Padhani AR, Beer AJ, et al. Imaging of tumor angiogenesis for radiologists-part 1: biological and technical basis. Curr Probl Diagn Radiol 2015;44(5):407–24.

24. van Rijswijk CS, Geirnaerdt MJ, Hogendoorn PC, et al. Soft-tissue tumors: value of static and dynamic gadopentetate dimeglumine-enhanced MR imaging in prediction of malignancy. Radiology 2004;233(2): 493–502.

25. Verstraete KL, Lang P. Bone and soft tissue tumors: the role of contrast agents for MR imaging. Eur J Radiol 2000;34(3):229–46.

26. Vilanova JC, Barcelo J. Diffusion-weighted whole-body MR screening. Eur J Radiol 2008;67(3):440–7.

27. Dietrich O, Biffar A, Reiser MF, et al. Diffusion-weighted imaging of bone marrow. Semin Musculoskelet Radiol 2009;13(2):134–44.

28. Padhani AR, van Ree K, Collins DJ, et al. Assessing the relation between bone marrow signal intensity and apparent diffusion coefficient in diffusion-weighted MRI. AJR Am J Roentgenol 2013;200(1): 163–70.

29. Fayad LM, Kamel IR, Kawamoto S, et al. Distinguishing stress fractures from pathologic fractures: a multimodality approach. Skeletal Radiol 2005;34(5): 245–59.

30. Balliu E, Vilanova JC, Peláez I, et al. Diagnostic value of apparent diffusion coefficients to differentiate benign from malignant vertebral bone marrow lesions. Eur J Radiol 2009;69(3):560–6.

31. Padhani AR, Koh DM, Collins DJ. Whole-body diffusion-weighted MR imaging in cancer: current status and research directions. Radiology 2011; 261(3):700–18.

32. Hayashida Y, Hirai T, Yakushiji T, et al. Evaluation of diffusion-weighted imaging for the differential diagnosis of poorly contrast-enhanced and T2-prolonged bone masses: initial experience. J Magn Reson Imaging 2006;23(3):377–82.

33. Costa FM, Ferreira EC, Vianna EM. Diffusion-weighted magnetic resonance imaging for the evaluation of musculoskeletal tumors. Magn Reson Imaging Clin North Am 2011;19(1):159–80.

34. van Rijswijk CS, Kunz P, Hogendoorn PC, et al. Diffusion-weighted MRI in the characterization of soft tissue tumors. J Magn Reson Imaging 2002;15(3): 302–7.

35. Oka K, Yakushiji T, Sato H, et al. Ability of diffusion-weighted imaging for the differential diagnosis between chronic expanding hematomas and malignant soft tissue tumors. J Magn Reson Imaging 2008;28(5):1195–200.

36. Nagata S, Nishimura H, Uchida M, et al. Usefulness of diffusion-weighted MRI in differentiating benign from malignant musculoskeletal tumors. Nihon Igaku Hōshasen Gakkai Zasshi 2005;65(1):30–6 [in Japanese].

37. Geirnaerdt MJ, Hogendoorn PC, Bloem JL, et al. Cartilaginous tumors: fast contrast-enhanced MR imaging. Radiology 2000;214(2):539–46.

38. Beaman FD, Kransdorf MJ, Andrews TR, et al. Superficial soft-tissue masses: analysis, diagnosis, and differential considerations. Radiographics 2007;27(2):509–23.

39. Holzapfel K, Regler J, Baum T, et al. Local staging of soft-tissue sarcoma: emphasis on assessment of neurovascular encasement–value of MR imaging in 174 confirmed cases. Radiology 2015;275:501–9.

40. Ehara S. MR imaging in staging of bone tumors. Cancer Imaging 2006;6:158–62.

41. Beaman FD, Jelinek JS, Priebat DA. Current imaging and therapy of malignant soft tissue tumors and tumor-like lesions. Semin Musculoskelet Radiol 2013;17(2):168–76.

42. Del Grande F, Subhawong T, Weber K, et al. Detection of soft-tissue sarcoma recurrence: added value of functional MR imaging techniques at 3.0 T. Radiology 2014;271(2):499–511.

43. Gaston LL, Di Bella C, Slavin J, et al. 18F-FDG PET response to neoadjuvant chemotherapy for Ewing sarcoma and osteosarcoma are different. Skeletal Radiol 2011;40(8):1007–15.

44. Donahue TR, Kattan MW, Nelson SD, et al. Evaluation of neoadjuvant therapy and histopathologic response in primary, high-grade retroperitoneal sarcomas using the sarcoma nomogram. Cancer 2010; 116(16):3883–91.

45. Stacchiotti S, Collini P, Messina A, et al. High-grade soft-tissue sarcomas: tumor response assessment-pilot study to assess the correlation between radiologic and pathologic response by using RECIST and Choi criteria. Radiology 2009;251(2): 447–56.

46. Dudeck O, Zeile M, Pink D, et al. Diffusion-weighted magnetic resonance imaging allows monitoring of anticancer treatment effects in patients with soft tissue sarcomas. J Magn Reson Imaging 2008; 27(5):1109–13.

7. Uhl M, Saueressig U, Koehler G, et al. Evaluation of tumour necrosis during chemotherapy with diffusion-weighted MR imaging: preliminary results in osteosarcomas. Pediatr Radiol 2006;36(12):1306–11.

8. Davies AM, Vanel D. Follow-up of musculoskeletal tumors. I. Local recurrence. Eur Radiol 1998;8(5): 791–9.

49. Padhani AR, Koh DM. Diffusion MR imaging for monitoring of treatment response. Magn Reson Clin North Am 2011;19(1):181–209.

50. Baur A, Huber A, Arbogast S, et al. Diffusion-weighted imaging of tumor recurrencies and post-therapeutical soft-tissue changes in humans. Eur Radiol 2001;11(5):828–33.

Therapy Monitoring with Functional and Molecular MR Imaging

Roberto García-Figueiras, MD, PhD[a],*, Anwar R. Padhani, MBBS, FRCP, FRCR[b],
Sandra Baleato-González, MD, PhD[a]

KEYWORDS

- Oncology • Anticancer treatments • Tumor response • Functional imaging • MR imaging
- Diffusion MR imaging • Perfusion imaging/methods • Multiparametric imaging

KEY POINTS

- MR imaging offers an attractive combination of anatomic, physiologic, and molecular information of tumor phenotype.
- MR imaging findings of tumor response depend on tumor type, on anatomic locations, on the mechanism of action of therapy given, and on the imaging techniques.
- Multiparametric MR imaging has demonstrated to be a useful tool for tumor response evaluation in multiple tumor types.

INTRODUCTION

Historically, cancer therapy has been based on different combinations of surgery, radiotherapy (RTP), and chemotherapy (CTP). These therapies have proven value but have also shown obvious limitations (eg, RTP and CTP do not kill cancer cells specifically) with treatment-related side effects commonly encountered. Recently, there has been a continuous effort in order to develop oncologic therapies (OTs) designed to target and disrupt specific tumor hallmarks (angiogenesis, metabolism, proliferation, and invasiveness) and genetic-related tumor changes (eg, epidermal growth factor receptor [EGFR] or anaplastic lymphoma kinase [ALK] mutations).[1,2] Many advances in our understanding of key biological processes that are altered in tumors have been translated into the development of these OTs, including antiangiogenic/antivascular drugs, drugs interfering with tumor growth signaling (EGFR, ALK, tyrosine-protein kinase Kit [c-KIT], and pathways mediating their downstream effects), hormonal therapy (HT), immunotherapy (IT), and interventional techniques (eg, embolization or ablation).[1–4] In this scenario, the effectiveness of these approaches needs to be evaluated, in particular the onset, duration, and heterogeneity of benefits requires assessment.

Intrinsically magnetic resonance (MR) offers a combination of anatomic, physiologic, and molecular information, which makes MR an ideal tool for evaluating different aspects of the cancer phenotype in vivo.[5] Many functional and molecular imaging (FMI) techniques that are available on MR imaging systems include dynamic contrast-enhanced MR imaging (DCE-MR imaging),

Disclosure statement: Dr A.R. Padhani serves on the advisory board for Siemens Healthcare Speakers Bureau, Siemens Healthcare, Johnson & Johnson. He is also a researcher for Siemens Healthcare. Drs R. García-Figueiras and S. Baleato-González have nothing to disclose.
[a] Department of Radiology, Complexo Hospitalario de Santiago de Compostela (CHUS), Choupana s/n, Santiago de Compostela 15706, Spain; [b] Paul Strickland Scanner Centre, Mount Vernon Cancer Centre, Northwood, Middlesex HA6 2RN, UK
* Corresponding author.
E-mail address: roberto.garcia.figueiras@sergas.es

dynamic susceptibility contrast-enhanced MR imaging (DSC-MR imaging), diffusion-weighted MR imaging (DW-MR imaging), and Magnetic resonance spectroscopy and spectroscopic imaging (MRS/I).[5–13] These noninvasive FMI techniques can demonstrate the spatial and temporal distribution of important tumor characteristics. They also provide quantitative biomarkers for the objective assessment of physiologic and molecular processes and, thus, enable assessment of changes in response to therapy. Understanding the relationship between tumor hallmarks, therapy effects, and MR imaging findings is essential for an adequate evaluation of OTs. In this article, the authors describe the role of functional MR imaging in oncology for therapy monitoring.

MR IMAGING TECHNIQUES FOR THE EVALUATION OF TUMOR PHENOTYPE

When considering therapy effects on tumors, imaging observations are sometimes difficult to interpret. Imaging findings seem to depend on anatomic locations, on interactions between specific tissue characteristics and the mechanism of action of therapy given, and on the imaging techniques making the observations. Different FM–MR imaging techniques are available in modern scanners (Table 1).[5–13] MR-based FMI techniques are increasingly being used to monitor the tumor response to therapies in daily clinical practice. MR imaging is able to predict the success of therapy before size changes become evident, and FM–MR imaging methods are increasingly being used as biomarkers of response in early phase drug development.

TUMOR RESPONSE ASSESSMENT USING MR IMAGING

Tumor and normal tissue response evaluations are critical roles of imaging in oncology. In this setting, imaging findings depend highly on the type and method of therapy delivery, the timing of treatment, and the imaging technique being used to observe the effects (Table 2). Additionally, combined therapies are increasingly being used in many tumor types, which may sometimes make it difficult to separate the net effect on imaging findings of every type of therapy.

Conventional Oncologic Therapies: Chemotherapy and Radiotherapy

CTP causes cellular lysis often via dominant necrosis or apoptotic mechanisms. On DW-MR imaging, cellular lysis results in increased water diffusion, which increases the apparent diffusion

coefficient (ADC) values.[8–10] Elevations of ADC depend on the degree of cell kill and reactive inflammatory changes if any. Early increases in ADC often precede any change in the tumor size and may be used in the early assessment of response. The use of histogram analysis of ADC values has been shown to be more sensitive to detect effective treatment response than average tumor ADC change or shrinkage of tumor. In patients with successful treatment, the ADC histogram shifts to higher values, in contrast to nonresponders whereby no shift or shift to lower values is observed[14] (Fig. 1). In the case of bone metastatic involvement, whole-body MR imaging (WB-MR imaging) is increasingly being used to evaluate metastatic bone disease and to monitor its therapeutic response.[11,15,16] Effective tumor response results in greater water diffusivity manifested as lower signal intensity on high b-value images, reductions in the extent of bone disease usually accompanied by higher ADC values.[8–1] However, the extent of ADC increases with therapy (including CTP) is very variable and depends on the mechanism of cell kill and the complexity of bone marrow (BM) composition (hematologic cells, bone cells, fat, tumor involvement, and so forth), which can be independently altered by accompanying therapies and their effects. So granulocyte colony-stimulating factor (G-CSF when used to support CTP can increase background high b-value image intensity due to normal BM hyperplasia, and HT can cause increased BM fat so lowering high b-value signal intensity. In the latter setting, a particular difficulty is the presence of fat intermixed with tumor infiltration as seen in myeloma or return of marrow fat infiltration that usually accompanies response and can counteract expected increases in ADC. This feature may explain the smaller ADC increases associated with bone disease responding to therapy.[15,1] Conventional mono-exponential diffusion MR imaging evaluation assumes a Gaussian behavior of diffusion process (ie, free and unrestricted diffusion of water). However, in many biological tissues, the water diffusion process is no longer Gaussian, a feature noticeable on ultrahigh b value images (>1500 s/mm^2). Diffusional kurtosis imaging (DKI) quantifies the deviation of tissue diffusion from a Gaussian pattern.[12] Recently the clinical value of DKI for tumor response evaluation has been undertaken. Chen and colleagues[17] report that DKI might be superior to mono-exponentially derived ADC values for predicting early response to neoadjuvant CTP in patients with nasopharyngeal carcinoma; the latter is probably related to changes in intracellular complexity. Tumor cell kill also causes a

An overview of main MR-based imaging techniques for the evaluation of cancers

MR Imaging Technique	Biological Bases of Imaging Technique	Evaluation Parameters Obtained	Pathophysiologic Correlation	Advantages	Disadvantages
DCE-MR imaging	Contrast medium uptake rates Transfer rates Extracellular volume Plasma volume fraction	• Qualitative: evaluation of the type of time/signal intensity curve • Semiquantitative evaluation: wash-in, washout, time to peak enhancement, and so forth • Quantitative analysis (based on mathematical models): initial area under gadolinium curve, K^{trans} and rate constant (kep), leakage space fraction (ve), fractional plasma volume (vp)	Vessel density Vascular permeability Perfusion Extravascular space Plasma volume	Low toxicity of contrast agents No ionizing radiation Versatility in pulse sequences	Complex biological explanation of many parameters Complex analysis in quantitative models
DSC-MR imaging	Contrast medium uptake rate in tissues, which is influenced by: • Perfusion rates • Blood volume and blood flow	• Qualitative: evaluation of the type of time/signal intensity curve • Semiquantitative evaluation: relative blood flow, relative blood volume, transit time	Vessel density Perfusion Vessel size	Availability Low cost	Semiquantitative models Technical complexity in extracranial lesions
Imaging techniques based on water diffusion	Diffusivity of water - monoexponential analysis (DWI) Perfusion component: IVIM Structural complexity: Diffusion Kurtosis Imaging (DKI)	• ADC • f • Diffusion (D) ○ Non-Gaussian diffusion coefficient (D) and deviations from normal distribution (K)	Tissue architecture: cell density & size, extracellular space tortuosity, gland formation, cell membrane integrity, necrosis Microvessel perfusion Quantifying the nongaussianity of any distribution and may evaluate membrane integrity	Availability No contrast agents No ionizing radiation	Technical complexity of advanced techniques (IVIM and DKI)
Magnetic resonance spectroscopy and spectroscopic imaging (MRS/I)	Chemical environment of the nuclear spin, such as number of chemical bonds, neighboring nuclei, and overall chemical structure	Ratios between metabolites Abnormal peaks of metabolites Absence of normal metabolites	Analysis of metabolic pathways	Specificity No contrast media	Technical complexity Difficult analysis

Abbreviations: ADC, apparent diffusion coefficient; D, non-Gaussian diffusion coefficient; DKI, diffusional kurtosis imaging; DWI, diffusion-weighted imaging; f, perfusion fraction; IVIM, intravoxel incoherent motion; K, kurtosis; kep, rate constant; K^{trans}, transfer constant; ve, leakage space fraction; vp, plasma volume.

Table 2
General rules for functional imaging evaluation of the effects of main oncologic therapies (Note: based on the limited literature available in many of these therapies)

Type of Therapy	Perfusion/Permeability-Related Parameters	Diffusion-Related Parameters (ADC)
Antiangiogenic therapy		
Early effect (normalization)	Variable effects on perfusion with a decreased permeability	Decrease • Reductions in blood flow and in extravascular extracellular space lead to impeded water movement in the extracellular space. • Decreases in ADC are seen within 1–2 wk for antiangiogenic agents.
Late effect	Decrease	Increase • Increases are secondary to late tumor necrosis.
Vascular disrupting agents		
Early effect	Decrease	Decrease • Decreases in ADC are seen within 2–4 h for VDAs agents.
Late effect	Increase in tumor periphery due to tumor repopulation	Variable • ADC can decrease mainly in tumor periphery because of tumor repopulation.
RTP		
Early effect (hyperemia)	Increase	Variable • Early RTP causes increases in ADC due to immediate vasodilation-perfusion effects, which effectively counteract the effects of cell swelling.
Late effect	Decrease	Increase • There is marked increase secondary to T2-shine through due to massive liquefactive necrosis.
CTP (mainly a late effect)	Decrease • Loss of cytokine support following cell death	Variable • Increases in ADC are within a few days, but duration of effects can be variable and transient. • Massive necrosis may cause a marked ADC increase secondary to T2-shine through. • At bone marrow, bony sclerosis and secondary CTP may induce marrow fibrosis and also lower ADC values.
Other target therapies		
EGFR/HER2	No definitive data	No definitive data
KIT receptors	Decrease	Increase
PI3K/AKT/mTOR and RAS-RAF-MAPK pathways	No definitive data	No definitive data
MET pathway	No definitive data	No definitive data
Locoregional therapies		
RFA	Decrease or absent • Excepting peripheral ring area • Time courses of changes not well defined	Early decreases in ADC values • Time course of changes in ADC within different organs are not yet fully established.

(continued on next page)

Table 2
(continued)

Type of Therapy	Perfusion/Permeability-Related Parameters	Diffusion-Related Parameters (ADC)
TACE	Decrease or absent	Increase • Tumor cell death is from ischemia and treatment-induced liquefactive necrosis.
Immunotherapy	No definitive data • Variable changes depending on tumor type	Increase
Hormonotherapy	Decrease	Variable • Androgen deprivation in bone metastases can lead to initial ADC increases with cell killing with reductions later due to healing. • Androgen deprivation therapy causes diverse morphologic and metabolic changes in the prostate gland depending on the type (single therapy or combined agents) and duration of therapy.

Abbreviations: ADC, apparent diffusion coefficient; mTOR, mammalian target of rapamycin; PI3K, phosphoinositide-3-kinase; TACE, transarterial chemoembolization; VDAs, vascular disruptive agents.

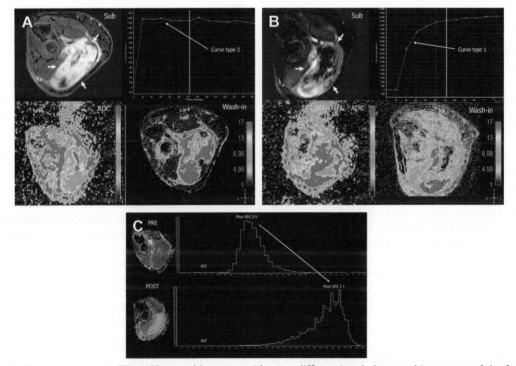

Fig. 1. Tumor response to CTP. A 67-year-old woman with an undifferentiated pleomorphic sarcoma of the forearm (*short arrows* in *A* and *B*) treated with 3 cycles of CTP (gemcitabine + docetaxel). Multiparametric MR examination including a DCE-MR imaging–derived subtraction image (maximum enhancement phase minus unenhanced phase) (sub), a signal intensity/time curve, and DCE-MR imaging–derived wash-in and ADC parametric maps pretherapy (*A*) and 3 months (*B*) following therapy. MR examinations demonstrated a change in the signal intensity/time curve from type 2 to type 1 and increased ADC values represented on histograms (*C*) following CTP (mean ADC pretherapy 0.9×10^{-3} mm^2/s vs 2.1×10^{-3} mm^2/s after therapy). Notice changes in functional MR imaging, without significant modification of tumor volume with therapy.

subsequent withdrawal of angiogenic cytokines, which explains the indirect antivascular effect of CTP. On DCE imaging, a favorable tumor response to CTP results in decreases in the rate and magnitude of enhancement in several tumor types. The magnitude of antiangiogenic response to neoadjuvant CTP demonstrated by DCE-MR imaging can be predictive of overall and disease-free survival in some solid cancers but also in hematologic malignancies.[7,8] In this setting, a change in signal intensity-time curves shape of 1 or more points was significant for overall 5-year survival in patients with breast cancer (BC) scored using a 5-curve–type classification schema encompassing wash-in and wash-out phases.[18]

Response to CTP or radiation is usually associated on MRS/I with a decline in the levels of choline-containing metabolites and other tumor-associated metabolites. For example, in breast cancer, a reduction of total choline between pre-treatment and within 24 hours of the first CTP dose was significantly correlated with subsequent changes in tumor size.[19]

In the case of RTP, accurate disease localization is critical in order to prevent marginal misses and to maximally spare important normal organs at risk with dose escalation treatment strategies. In this setting, biological target volume definitions determined on physiologic, metabolic, and molecular MR imaging is actively being explored as a tool for RTP planning in different tumors.[20–22] As a general rule, RTP induces similar changes than CTP on DW imaging (DWI) with added bystander effects on exposed adjacent tissues (Figs. 2 and 3). DWI has demonstrated significant value in tumor response evaluation after RTP in brain, rectal, prostate, head and neck, and gynecological tumors.[8,23] ADC increases occur as early as 24 to 72 hours after a single large fraction of radiation in radiosensitive tumors. Conversely, a failure to increase ADC values can be an indicator of radioresistance. Furthermore, increases in ADC values seem to occur incrementally in fractionated regimens, with the greatest increases visible toward the end of therapy. These ADC increases are mainly related to tumor cell death and the development of edema and inflammation. The clinical value of DKI for the evaluation of tumor response to RTP has not been established (Fig. 4). Concerning DCE-MR imaging findings, initial increases of enhancement corresponding to the recognized acute hyperemic response can be depicted[7] (Fig. 5). In addition DCE-MR imaging may identify the sub-volume of the tumor resistant to RTP during the course of treatment, which can have substantial implications in RTP. Best local control and overall survival (OS) rates are achieved in

those patients who have no or small subvolumes of tumors with poor enhancement pretreatment. Interestingly, RTP-induced hyperemia occurring early in tumors that initially show poor enhancement results in improved tumor local control and OS, compared with patients having persistent poor enhancement along the course of treatment.[24] The latter suggests that improved tumor oxygenation resulting from initial RTP fractions are reversing tumor hypoxia and so improving the effectiveness of RTP. Therefore, radiation induced changes in lesions can mimic tumor recurrence with an increase in the degree of enhancement and perilesional edema, a pitfall to be aware of. FMI may, thus, overcome the limitations of morphology-based conventional MR imaging after RTP. For example, a decrease of relative cerebral blood volume values in brain radiated tumors indicates a tumor response to therapy regardless of increases in tumor volume.[2] Finally, alterations more than the response patterns of tumors treated by combining therapies included with RTP, such as chemoradiotherapy need to be considered. Increased contrast enhancement or edema that occurs following RTP associated with temozolomide can mimic tumor recurrence, which is named pseudoprogression; in these circumstances, lower blood volume can help to distinguish between active disease and CRT-induced necrosis.[26]

In the case of MRS/I, this technique may show a potential in monitoring metabolic response after RTP and in predicting patients' outcomes (see Fig. 3). For example, patients with prostate cancer (PC) demonstrating a choline (Cho) +creatine/citrate ratio less than 0.2 following RTP did not show biochemical relapse at 24 months.[27]

Targeted Therapies

Tumors are often physiologically dependent on the continued activity of specific activated or overexpressed oncogenes and pathways for the maintenance of their malignant phenotype. Targeted therapy refers to a new generation of cancer drugs designed to interfere with specific molecules that is thought to have a critical role in in cancer cell growth, survival, or progression.

Tumor angiogenesis: antiangiogenic and antivascular therapies

Tumor angiogenesis results in the development of a heterogeneous and disorganized network of tortuous and dilated vessels, which show increased microvessel permeability. Solid tumor vasculature is highly heterogeneous, which presents challenges to antiangiogenic therapy (AAT) as well as the evaluation of its therapeutic

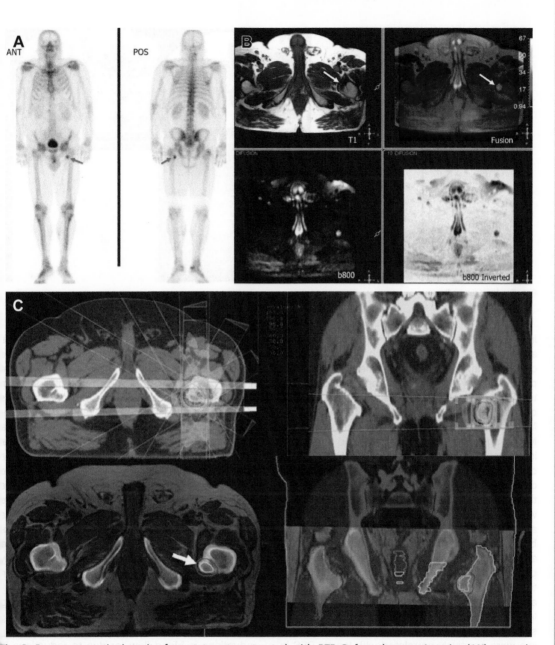

Fig. 2. Bone metastatic deposit of prostate cancer treated with RTP. Before therapy, Anterior (AN), posterior (POS), bone scan projections (A) and a series of MR images (B), including T1-weighted image, fused image super-imposing axial T1-weighted MR image, and color-coded map derived from the b800 s/mm² DWI, DW b800 s/mm² image, and inverted gray scale from the same diffusion image. Baseline images (prostate-specific antigen [PSA] value: 18 ng/mL) depicted oligometastatic disease with a deposit in proximal left femur (white arrow), which showed increased tracer uptake on the bone scan (red arrows) and a restricted motion of free water on DWI. RTP (C) was performed using for planning both CT (upper row) and MR (bottom row) scans were used for radi-ation therapy guide (C). Following therapy, bone scan (D) and MR images (E) demonstrated a complete response of the bone lesion (PSA value: 5.3 ng/mL). Treatment of oligometastatic disease is designed to postpone onset of androgen deprivation therapy and its anticipated side effects until a larger burden of disease emerges.

efficacy.[6] Tumor angiogenesis is an attractive target for anticancer therapy, mainly based on the inhibition of growth factors/signaling pathways necessary for the angiogenic process or targeting

the established tumor vasculature (vascular disruptive agents [VDAs]). Antiangiogenic agents have been approved for using as a single agent or in combination in several indications,

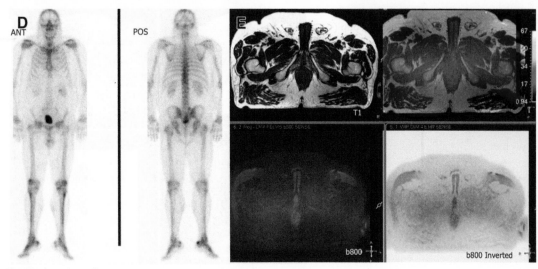

Fig. 2. (*continued*)

including colorectal, lung, ovarian, and renal metastatic cancer; hepatocellular carcinoma (HCC); glioblastoma; and neuroendocrine tumors. On its part, VDAs have not yet been approved for clinical use.[6,7,28] Indirect measurements of angiogenesis can be performed noninvasively using different MR-based imaging techniques, including DCE-MR imaging, DSC-MR imaging, and intravoxel incoherent motion (IVIM).[6] DCE-MR imaging–derived parameters allow the monitoring of changes in tumor vascularization secondary to therapy. Unfortunately, our understanding of what determines response and resistance to these agents is limited. Up to date, no definitive imaging biomarker has been validated[29]; although the administration of AAT has been shown to extend progression-free survival (PFS) and OS in different tumors, the correlation between imaging changes and patient outcomes has not been clearly established yet. However, 2 studies in renal cancer showed that high transfer constant (K^{trans}) at baseline were positively correlated with longer PFS in patients treated with sorafenib.[30,31] The main effects of successful therapy using antiangiogenic drugs and VDAs consist of reductions in perfusion and permeability-related parameters, improved blood flow in mature vessels, and areas of devascularization, all consistent with vascular pruning (Fig. 6). Vascular endothelial growth factor (VEGF)-specific inhibition induces rapid structural and functional effects with downstream significant antitumor activity within one cycle of therapy.[32] The effects of AAT are not immediate, arising at least 1 to 2 days after drug administration and being usually maximal at 10 to 14 days, whereas VDAs cause rapid shutdown of the vasculature

within minutes to hours of drug administration However, reversibility of VDAs effects can be visible with tumor regrowth from a residual viable rim after treatment.[7,8,33,34] As a potential solution for this last phenomenon, combined treatment of a VDA and AAT have been evaluated.[35] In clinical practice, there is a great heterogeneity in tumor response to AAT with a variable degree of change in size, in enhancement, and in the degree of response between lesions.[36] Finally, specific clinical scenarios need to be considered. In the case of antiangiogenic therapies in high-grade gliomas, these drugs induce an early change in vascular permeability with a normalization of the blood-brain barrier, which produce a rapid decrease in contrast enhancement independently of the degree of tumor response, a phenomenon termed pseudoresponse[26] (Fig. 7).

DW-MR imaging may also evaluate AAT and VDAs. These agents cause early slight reductions in tumor ADC values, related to cellular swelling reductions in blood flow, or due to reductions in extracellular-extravascular space.[37,38] After this transient decrease in ADC values, the collapsed cell membranes and decreased cellularity secondary to tumor necrosis usually causes increased ADC values[8,10] (Fig. 8). Microvessel perfusion also alters water diffusion and ADC measurements. Perfusion components are readily visualized on DW images obtained at low b-values (<200 s/mm^2) and can be assessed quantitatively using IVIM analysis, which permits the separation and quantification of diffusion and perfusion effects.[6] Different studies found an early reduction in IVIM-related parameters at 4 hours after VDA administration. An early recovery of these

A

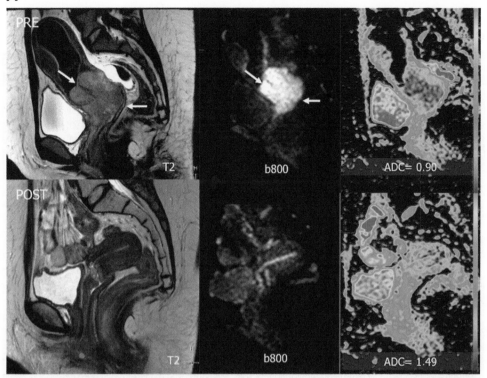

B

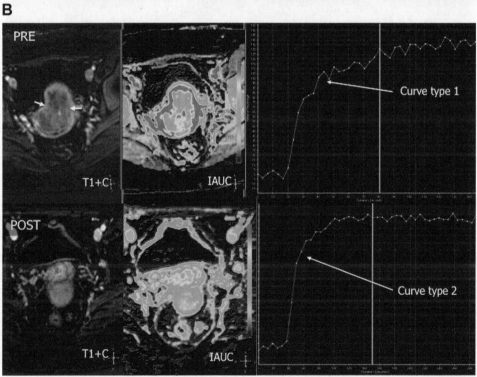

Fig. 3. Combined radiochemotherapy. A 35-year-old woman with cervical cancer (*arrows*). Multiparametric evaluation before (PRE) and after chemoradiotherapy (POST), including sagittal T2-weighted and DW (b800 s/mm²) images and ADC color-coded parametric maps (*A*), axial contrast-enhanced fat-saturation T1-weighted, initial area under the curve (IAUC) parametric maps, and signal intensity/time curve (*B*), and single-voxel MR spectroscopy (MRS/I) and single-voxel MR spectroscopy (MRS) (*C*). Imaging evaluation evidenced a large cervical mass with diffusion restriction (ADC before therapy 0.9×10^{-3} mm²/s), hypovascular behavior, and an increased choline peak (Cho). Following therapy there is a complete tumor response with increased ADC values (ADC after therapy 1.49×10^{-3} mm²/s), improvement of the vascularization in the cervical area, and disappearance of the abnormal Cho peak on MRS.

C

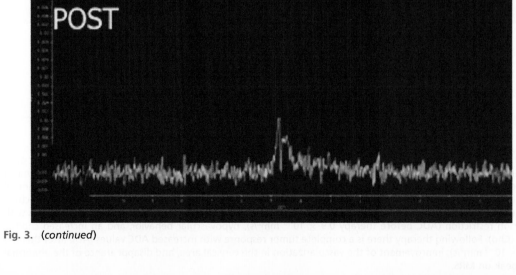

Fig. 3. (continued)

parameters (at 24 hours) was associated to tumor revascularization.[39,40] However, a poor measurement reproducibility of the perfusion fraction and pseudodiffusion coefficient, especially in apparently hypovascular lesions, may limit its value.[41,42]

Targeted therapies blocking tumor proliferation and metabolism

Different intracellular pathways are involved in tumor proliferation and metabolic activity regulation: (1) the EGFR family (EGFR and HER2 [human epidermal growth factor receptor 2]), (2) KIT receptor, (3) ALK, and (4) pathways mediate their downstream effects, which include phosphoinositide-3-kinase/AKT/mammalian target of rapamycin (mTOR) (PI3K/AKT/mTOR) pathway, and the RAS-RAF-MAPK pathway.

Anti–epidermal growth factor receptor/HER2 drugs There is a very limited evaluation of EGFR inhibitors with FM–MR imaging techniques.[43] DCE-MR imaging did not show a significant change in quantitative parameters in patients treated with EGFR inhibitors alone or with combined therapy including these agents[44–46] (Fig. 9).

Anti–anaplastic lymphoma kinase drugs There are no clinical reports in the literature of the use of FM–MR imaging for the evaluation of the response to therapy in ALK-positive tumors. Preclinical data have suggested that ALK-mutated neuroblastomas showed a apparent transverse relaxation rate, a feature that may be useful in the future for response assessment.[47]

Drugs inhibiting c-KIT pathway Drugs targeting the c-KIT pathway have been mainly focused in gastrointestinal stromal tumors treated with imatinib. Different studies have explored the role of DW-MR imaging compared with PET for evaluating tumor response.[48–51] Responders showed an increase in ADC values between 44.8% and 75.0% after 7 to 12 days of imatinib treatment.[48,49] Different multi-targeted tyrosine kinase inhibitors have shown activity against the c-KIT pathway in different tumor types, including sunitinib, pazopanib, and axitinib (renal cancer), cediranib or vandetinib (glioblastomas), telatinib, and so forth. However, many of them showed a predominant activity against the VEGF pathway, which explains DCE-MR imaging preclinical findings with a decrease in vascular permeability estimated by K^{trans}.[52]

Pathways mediating downstream effects of epidermal growth factor receptor, anaplastic lymphoma kinase, and c-KIT The PI3K/AKT/mTOR pathway stimulates protein synthesis,

glucose metabolism, cellular migration, cell survival, and angiogenesis in tumors (Fig. 10).[28] One experimental study has suggested that DW-MR imaging could discriminate between a strong and weak tumor response to PI3K/AKT/mTOR inhibition in ovarian cancer xenografts.[53] Beside this, a consistent decrease in total Cho levels measured by MRS/I was observed after inhibition of PI3K and RAS-RAF-MEK signaling.[52] However, DCE-MR imaging did not show any net change in K^{trans} in patients with advanced cancer treated with everolimus in combination with cetuximab.[46]

The BRAF proto-oncogene activates RAF/MEK/ERK signaling, a major driver of carcinogenesis in various malignancies, most notably in melanoma[54] (Fig. 11). DWI has demonstrated ADC increases following treatment with the MEK-inhibitor selumetinib in human melanoma and colon cancer xenografts, which were correlated to a significant increase in tumor necrosis.[55] Furthermore, inhibition of the MEK pathway decreases lactate production in human cancer cells allowing monitoring of drug effects by MRS/I.[56]

Tumor invasiveness
The MET pathway promotes tumor growth, invasion, and dissemination in cancer. Abnormal MET activation is associated with poor clinical outcomes in patients with cancer. Several MET inhibitors have been introduced into the clinic, including cabozantinib, which is currently being evaluated in metastatic PC (see Fig. 8), and tivantinib. There is limited experience evaluating the MET pathway using MR imaging. Preclinical studies in patients with metastatic PC treated with cabozantinib showed statistically significantly increases in ADC values that were associated with extensive necrosis of the lesions.[57] On its part, no significant change in DCE-MR imaging parameters was observed after tivantinib treatment.[58,59]

Hormonal Therapy

HT blocks the effects of hormones in tumors, mainly in BC and PC. Androgen deprivation therapy causes diverse morphologic and metabolic changes in the prostate gland depending on the type (single therapy or combined agents) and duration of therapy.[60] To date, HT is also an established therapy for metastatic BC and PC. WB-MR imaging is increasingly being used to monitor the therapeutic response in this setting.[15,16,61] Tumor response is also associated with increases in ADC values.[8–11] However, the extent of ADC increases with HT seems to be less marked than with other therapies (CTP, RTP, and so forth) possibly because cell death is less likely to be

A

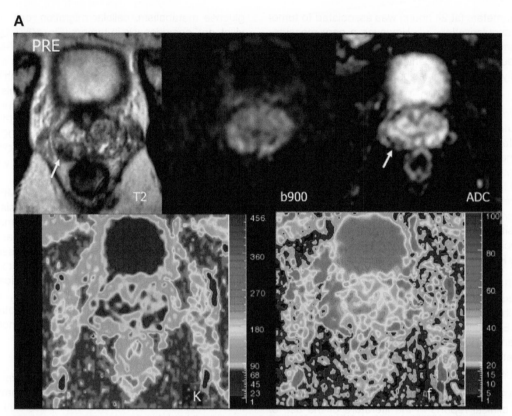

B

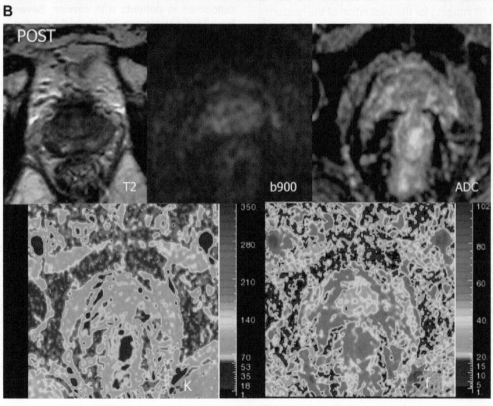

A   **B**

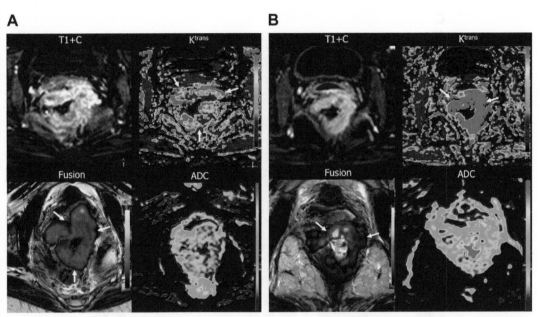

Fig. 5. Hyperemic response in RTP. A 64-year-old woman with rectal cancer stage cT4b cN2 cM0 (*white arrows*) under radiochemotherapy. Fat-saturated contrast-enhanced T1-weighted (T1+C) images, transfer constant (K^{trans}) parametric maps, fused images superimposing axial T2-weighted MR image and color-coded map derived from the b1000 s/mm² DWI, and ADC color-coded parametric maps obtained before therapy (*A*), 2 weeks from the beginning of the treatment (*B*), and 1 month later after therapy. DCE-MR imaging demonstrated an increased tumor enhancement and higher K^{trans} values in the rectal mass indicating hyperemia secondary to RTP in the middle of the treatment, which should not be considered as tumor progression (*B*). However, tumor response was clearly depicted when fused images including DWI information are compared at this point with increase in ADC values (ADC before therapy 0.79×10^{-3} mm²/s; ADC first evaluation 1.08×10^{-3} mm²/s). ADC increases are due to a combination of increased perfusion and cell kill. At the end of the therapy (*C*), tumor shrinkage has occurred morphologically and is evident on DCE-MR imaging. Note how ADC decreases slightly compared with the middle examination due to tumor sloughing. Final pathology staging was ypT2 ypN1.

associated with inflammation.[62] Novel hormone therapy (eg, abiraterone acetate and enzalutamide), IT (sipuleucel-T), and novel CTP agents, such as cabazitaxel, active against docetaxel-resistant cells could be used in PC (**Fig. 12**). Abiraterone inhibits the action of 17 α-hydroxylase/C17,20 lyase, which blocks the formation of dehydroepiandrosterone and androstenedione, androgen precursors of testosterone.

Enzalutamide is an androgen receptor antagonist drug. Different reviews have reinforced the emerging role of MR imaging (including DWI) for the detection of metastases in PC and its ability to measure tumor responses with important implications in treatment decision making. However, current opinion is that MR imaging availability is too low for its widespread adoption as a first-line imaging tool in this setting.[63,64]

Fig. 4. DKI. A 67-year-old man with a prostate carcinoma in the right peripheral zone of midgland (*white arrow*). T2-weighted and DWI (b900 s/mm²) and ADC parametric maps (based on a mono-exponential analysis of diffusion), kurtosis (K) (derived from diffusion at ultrahigh b values analyzed with a diffusion kurtosis imaging non-Gaussian model) and perfusion fraction (f) parametric maps (derived from an intravoxel incoherent motion model [IVIM]) of the prostate gland before (*A*) and after therapy (*B*). Before therapy, tumor showed a restricted diffusion (ADC = 0.65×10^{-3} mm²/s) and apparent diffusional kurtosis value (K = 1.5) and also demonstrated decreased values of the perfusion fraction (f = 23%). Diffusion coefficient and diffusivity parametric maps (not shown) also demonstrated reduced values in tumor comparing with contralateral peripheral gland. Following RTP, tumor area showed increased ADC (0.97×10^{-3} mm²/s) and a decreased kurtosis (K = 0.7). The last one suggested a decreased cellular complexity with treatment response. Perfusion fraction values showed minimal changes (f = 25%). (*Courtesy of* Antonio Luna, MD, Department of Radiology, Clínica Las Nieves SERCOSA, Health Time, Jaén, Spain.)

C

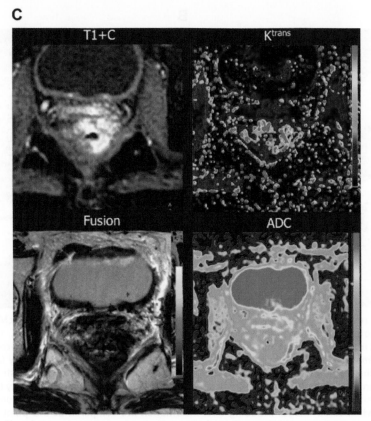

Fig. 5. (*continued*)

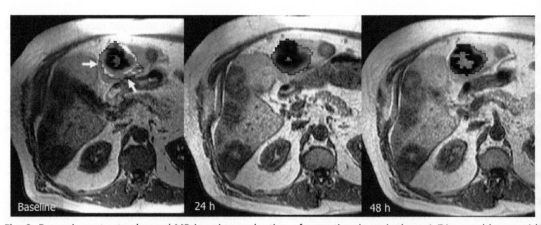

Fig. 6. Dynamic contrast-enhanced MR imaging evaluation of an antiangiogenic drug. A 74-year-old man with multiple colorectal cancer liver metastases treated with bevacizumab, a recombinant humanized monoclonal antibody that blocks angiogenesis by inhibiting vascular endothelial growth factor A. DCE–MR imaging evaluation (extended Tofts model with individually measured arterial input function) corresponding to one of the metastases (*arrows*) at baseline and 24 hours and 48 hours following the administration of the antiangiogenic agent showed early changes of the transfer constant. (*Courtesy of* James O'Connor, MA, PhD, FRCR, Cancer Imaging Centre in Cambridge and Manchester, University of Manchester; and *Data from* O'Connor JP, Carano RA, Clamp AR, et al. Quantifying antivascular effects of monoclonal antibodies to vascular endothelial growth factor: insights from imaging. Clin Cancer Res 2009;15(21):6674–82.)

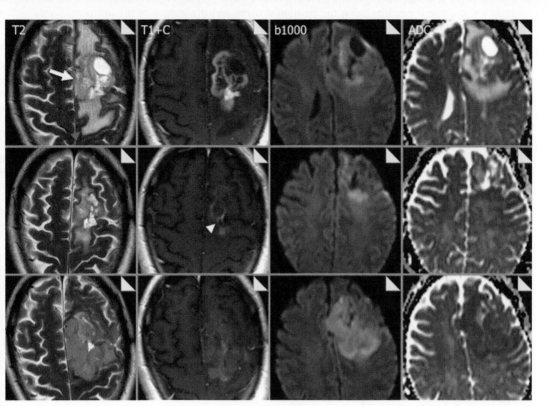

Fig. 7. Pseudoresponse. Glioblastoma under bevacizumab therapy. (*Left to right columns*) T2-weighted, contrast-enhanced T1-weighted, and DW (b1000 s/mm^2) images and ADC parametric maps baseline and following therapy (*middle and bottom rows*). Baseline images (*top row*) depicted a brain mass in the left frontal lobe (*arrows*), which showed an extensive area of associated vasogenic edema (*red arrowheads*). Following therapy, note how the ADC values progressively went down because of tumor progression. However, there was a decrease in both enhancement (*white arrowhead*) and edema due to the presence of less fluid in the extracellular/extra-vascular space (secondary to the effect of the AAT on vascular permeability), which could suggest tumor response.

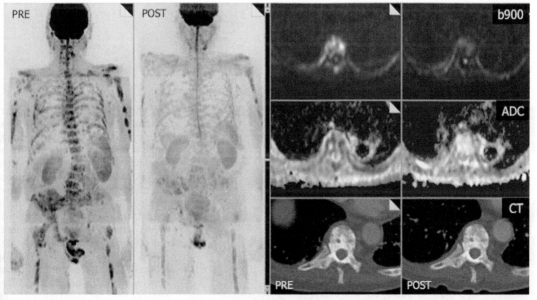

Fig. 8. DWI evaluation of an anti-VEGFR agent. A 72-year-old man with a metastatic castration-resistant PC. Baseline and after therapy. WB-DW MR imaging (inverted scale, b900 s/mm^2 images) (*left images*) and DWI (b900 s/mm^2), ADC parametric maps, and computed tomography (CT) image acquired before (*right rows*) (PRE) and 3 weeks after therapy with cabozantinib (an anti-VEGF & c-MET inhibitor) (POST). Baseline WB examination demonstrated a diffuse pattern of metastatic bone disease (low-signal intensity foci, *left image*), which showed restriction of the diffusion on b900 images and ADC parametric maps. Following therapy, tumor response was clearly seen on diffusion-related images. However, conventional CT did not depict significant changes.

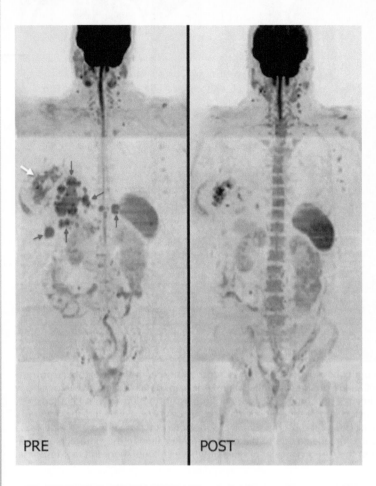

PRE

POST

Fig. 9. Anti-HER2 therapy. Inflamma tory BC (*white arrow*) with liver metas tases (*red arrows*). Two examination performed 5 months apart are shown WB-DW MR imaging (inverted scale b800 s/mm² images) before (*PRE*) and 5 months later after therapy with gemcitabine1carboplatin1trastuzumab (an anti-HER2 agent) (*POST*). Image evidenced partial response with reduction of the size of the breas tumor and almost complete disap pearance of liver metastatic deposit after therapy.

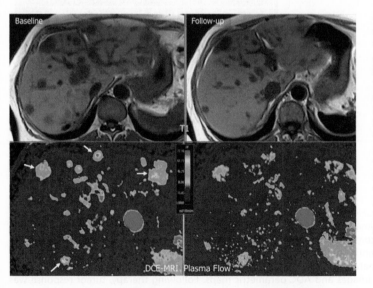

Baseline

Follow-up

DCE-MRI Plasma Flow

Fig. 10. mTOR inhibitors. A 57-year old patient with metastasized rena cell carcinoma. T1-weighted image and plasma-flow parametric map baseline (*left column*) and afte treatment with the mTOR-inhibito everolimus (*right*). Baseline show multiple hypervascular intrahepati metastases (*arrows* in some o them). After 56 days of treatment reduction of tumor size was de tected. Tumor perfusion wa reduced but still evident. The pa tient went on to progression afte another 56 days. (*Courtesy of* Mik Notohamiprodjo, MD, Diagnosti sche und interventionelle Radiolo gie Universitätsklinikum Tübingen Tübingen, Germany.)

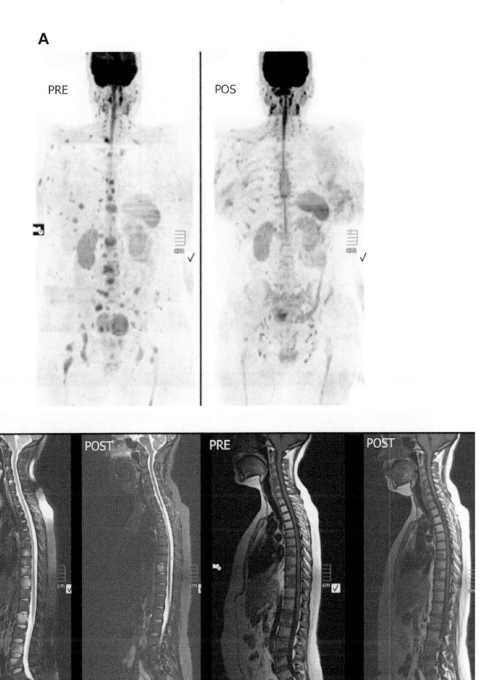

Fig. 11. BRAF and MEK pathways. A patient with a BRAF (V600)-mutated metastatic melanoma. Baseline images (PRE) and images obtained after treatment with a combination of dabrafenib (BRAF inhibitor) and trametinib (MEK inhibitor) (POST). Baseline images depicted a diffuse pattern of metastatic disease. Note the changes on WB-DW MR imaging (inverted scale, b900 s/mm² images) (A) and on whole-spine sagittal T2-weighted and T1-weighted images (B) related to partial tumor response with almost complete resolution of many of the tumor metastatic deposits.

A

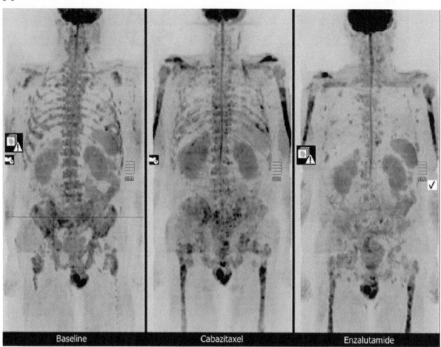

Baseline   Cabazitaxel   Enzalutamide

B

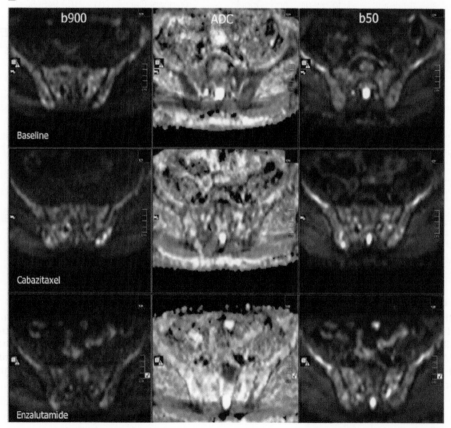

b900   ADC   b50

Baseline

Cabazitaxel

Enzalutamide

Immunotherapy

Cancer IT is an emerging antitumor strategy that is being increasingly used in the clinic for treatment of PC, BC, renal cancer, lung tumors, lymphoma, glioblastoma, and melanoma[65,66] (Fig. 13). IT is based on 2 main mechanisms of action: antibody therapies against known immunogenic cancer cell-related antigens (passive IT) and response modulation of the immune system by activating both cell-mediated and humoral immunity (active IT).[65] It is important to consider that current response and follow-up criteria must be made sufficiently flexible for an adequate evaluation of these new therapeutic agents with unique mechanisms of action, because they may be associated with features during treatment suggestive of progressive disease despite clinical benefit. To date, the clinical role of FMI techniques to monitor IT effects is limited to the experimental field. However, in the case of patients with lymphoma (including a group treated with IT), WB-DW-MR imaging may be a useful alternative to PET/computed tomography (CT) for treatment response assessment. Mayerhoefer and colleagues[67] used the International Harmonization Project criteria of the International Working Group for evaluating both the PET and the diffusion images. In the experimental field, Lazovic and colleagues[68] reported that ADC was significantly increased at 2 and 3 days after treatment of glioblastoma with IT. On its part, DCE-MR imaging parameters, except the extracellular-extravascular volume fraction (ve), did not show significant changes in a similar study.[69,70]

Interventional Techniques

Response to transarterial chemoembolization (TACE) causes cystic and necrotic changes in lesions. FMI evaluation demonstrates an early reduction of ADC values a few hours following therapy, after which consistent increases in ADC values occur, coinciding with the development of cystic and necrotic changes.[10,71] Kamel and colleagues[71] reported that these increases in ADC values became most apparent after 1 to 2 weeks and returned to the baseline values by 4 weeks. On its part, reductions in the degree of enhancement were seen immediately on DCE-MR imaging images after TACE and were sustained over the observation period. Contrast-enhanced and diffusion-based 3-dimensional quantitative imaging were demonstrated as feasible in the analysis of tumor response after intra-arterial therapy and are preferable to size-based criteria (modified response evaluation criteria in solid tumors [mRECIST] and quantitative European Association for the Study of the Liver [qEASL]) in different tumor types. Both volumetric techniques showed similar accuracy in determining the extent of pathologic tumor necrosis after TACE.[72,73] DKI may be a useful tool for the assessment of post-therapeutic response in HCC. Goshima and colleagues[74] reported that the mean kurtosis value was significantly higher for viable areas in HCCs with a significant decrease of this parameter in the HCCs that were completely necrotic after TACE or radiofrequency ablation (RFA). Besides, the diagnostic performance for the detection of HCC viability was greater with DKI than with conventional mono-exponential analysis (ADC) of diffusion.

Concerning radioembolization, DWI seems superior to PET/CT for early response assessment (within 6 weeks before) in patients who undergo Yttrium-90 microspheres radioembolization for hepatic metastases.[75] On its part, mRECIST and volumetric ADC performed better than traditional size RECIST or volumetric parameters in detecting imaging response to Y90; however, a complete pathologic necrosis cannot be predicted by any criteria.[76] Schelhorn and colleagues[77] reported that additional DWI does not substantially improve

Fig. 12. Hormonotherapy. Serial changes in advanced metastatic castration-resistant PC (mCRPC) responding to enzalutamide (an androgen receptor antagonist drug). A 74-year-old man with metastatic castration-resistant PC to bone after docetaxel CTP. Serial changes on WB-DWI (inverted scale, b900 s/mm²) before treatment (prostate-specific antigen [PSA] value: 1080 ng/mL), after cabazitaxel (an inhibitor of 17a-hydroxylase that reduces testosterone production by both the testes and adrenal glands) (PSA value: 1800 ng/mL), and after enzalutamide (an androgen receptor antagonist drug) (PSA value: 180 ng/mL) (A). Disease progression (increasing signal in humeri and femora) was seen on cabazitaxel. Note reductions in signal in the axial skeleton on enzalutamide, although persistent disease continued to be seen in the humeri and femora. Such spatial heterogeneity of response is commonly encountered in mCRPC. DW b900 s/mm² images, ADC parametric maps, and b50 s/mm² images at the 3 corresponding time points (top to bottom) obtained at the level of the sacrum (B). Although small focal areas of high ADC values were seen after cabazitaxel (middle row), areas of nonresponse were visible indicating poor overall response. There were uniform increases in ADC values after enzalutamide consistent with marked cell kill.

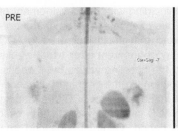
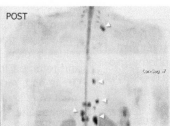

Fig. 13. Immunotherapy. Maximum intensity projection images of diffusion examination (inverted gray scale, b900 s/mm² images) of the thorax before (*left*) and after (*right*) the administration of ipilimumab in a patient with melanoma evidenced disease progression at the level of multiple lymph nodes in the mediastinum (*arrowheads*).

therapy response evaluation in HCC after radioembolization in comparison with MR imaging using hepatocyte-specific contrast agents.

RFA causes heterogeneous appearances on ADC maps in the ablated areas, reflecting different treatment effects, such as interstitial edema, hemorrhage, carbonization, necrosis, and fibrosis.[8–10,78] A common early postablative DWI finding is a hyperintense rim with decreased ADC surrounding the hypointense zone of coagulative necrosis.[79] Posteriorly, significantly higher ADC values at 1 and 6 months after RFA were depicted.[80] Finally, early diagnosis of small-volume recurrences following local hepatic tumor ablation may be improved with the use of PET/MR imaging.[81,82] In the case of cryoablation, imaging findings seem to be different. Treated lesions often demonstrate MR imaging contrast enhancement following successful percutaneous cryoablation, which does not suggests residual tumor.[83] The effects of high-intensity focused ultrasound have been investigated using MR imaging. Initial reductions in ADC values within ablated tissues were observed in combination with decreasing contrast enhancement. Increasing ADC values were presumed to reflect cell loss and liquefactive necrosis.[8–10,84]

A recent technique called irreversible electroporation has proven successful in treating tumors. This procedure is done using small electrodes to apply short repetitive bursts of electricity, which produce the formation of nanoscale pores within the cell membrane changing transmembrane potential and causing cell dead. Experimental models showed that ADC and kurtosis values could be used to detect therapy effects.[85,86] However, in clinical practice, ADC values did not show statistically significant differences between the baseline examination and the reassessment after 1 month in the case of patients with HCC.[87]

Other Therapeutic Agents in Cancer

Currently, many tumor pathways and anticancer therapies are under investigation. The ubiquitin-proteasome pathway regulates intracellular protein degradation and plays a significant role in multiple myeloma (MM). Bortezomib has been a major breakthrough in the treatment of MM. WB-MR imaging is increasingly used to evaluate MM and to monitor therapeutic response (**Fig. 14**). Evaluation of MM response with conventional MR imaging sequences often provides false-positive results because of persistent nonviable lesions. DW-MR imaging improves the results of MR imaging for a most accurate detection of response.[88] Giles and colleagues[89] reported that WB-DWI could demonstrate changes in mean ADC values of the BM (assessing the entire skeleton) in patients receiving different combinations of treatment regimes. The mean ADC increased in 95% of responding patients (related to tumor cell lysis) and decreased in all nonresponders. Beside this, an increase of ADC by 3.3% was associated with response (sensitivity 90%, specificity 100%).

Heat shock protein 90 [HSP90] is a chaperone (protein that plays a role in the conformational stability, maturation, and function of other proteins that it is essential for oncogenic transformation.[90] A study has shown that the inhibition of HSP90 was associated with an elevation in Cho levels on MRS/I.[91]

ONCOLOGIC-RELATED IMAGING FINDINGS
Bone-Targeted Therapies

Tumor invasion into bone is associated with osteoclast and osteoblast activation and liberation of growth factors from the bone matrix, which enhance tumor growth. In this context, there is an emerging role for bone-related oncologic therapies, which decrease the incidence of skeletal complications and can also have direct antitumor activity. Bone microenvironment could be targeted using different agents, including bisphosphonates, therapies directed against the receptor activator of nuclear factor kappa B ligand (ie, denosumab) and the transforming growth factor-β, and WNT signaling pathway inhibitors (Dickkopf-related protein 1 [DKK1]).[92] Changes in bone

A

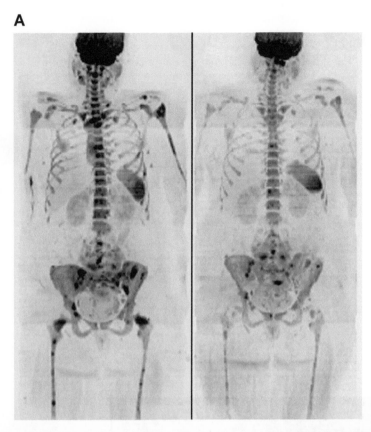

B

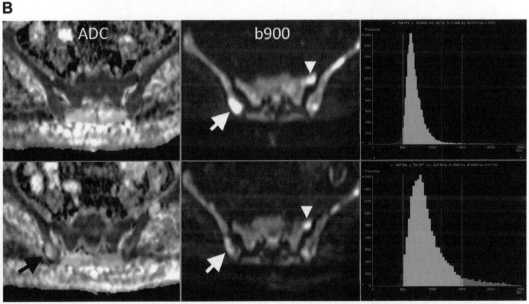

Fig. 14. Proteosome inhibitors. A 42-year-old woman with multiple myeloma being treated with bortezomib (a proteosome inhibitor). Two examinations performed before and after therapy are shown. WB-DW MR imaging (inverted gray scale, b900 s/mm² images) (A) showed tumor response with decreasing signal intensity and extent of the bony marrow disease. Detailed evaluation regarding the degree of signal intensity on high b-value (b900 s/mm²) images and ADC values (B) in the pelvis showed reductions in the signal intensity of lesions in sacrum (white arrows) and iliac bones (white arrowheads) and increased ADC values (black arrow).

A

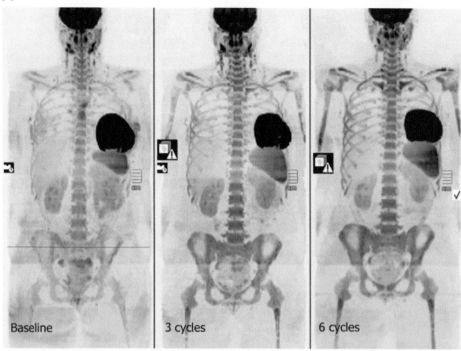

Baseline   3 cycles   6 cycles

B

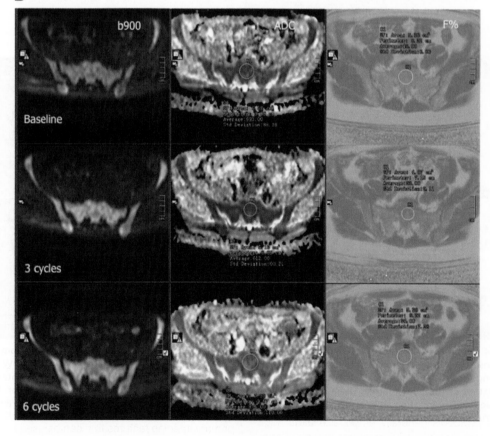